Quick Reference Dictionary
of Eyecare Terminology

Fifth Edition

Quick Reference Dictionary of Eyecare Terminology

Fifth Edition

EDITED BY

Janice K. Ledford, COMT

Joseph Hoffman

PRONUNCIATIONS BY

Al Lens, COMT

SLACK
INCORPORATED

Delivering the best in health care information
and education worldwide

www.slackbooks.com

ISBN: 978-1-55642-805-0

Contact SLACK Incorporated for more information about other books in this field or about the availability of our books from distributors outside the United States.

Published by: SLACK Incorporated
                   6900 Grove Road
                   Thorofare, NJ 08086 USA
                   Telephone: 856-848-1000
                   Fax: 856-853-5991
                   www.slackbooks.com

Library of Congress Cataloging-in-Publication Data

Quick reference dictionary of eyecare terminology / edited by Janice K. Ledford, Joseph Hoffman ; pronunciations by Al Lens. -- 5th ed.
      p. ; cm.
   Includes bibliographical references and index.
   ISBN 978-1-55642-805-0 (alk. paper)
   1. Ophthalmology--Dictionaries. I. Ledford, Janice K. II. Hoffman, Joseph, 1961- III. Lens, Al.
   [DNLM: 1. Eye Diseases--therapy--Terminology--English. 2. Ophthalmology--Terminology--English. WW 15 Q65 2008]

   RE21.H64 2008
   617.7003--dc22
                              2007028047

Printed in the United States of America.

Last digit is print number: 10 9 8 7 6 5 4 3 2

Dedication, Fifth Edition

For Paula Calaway, of blessed memory.
Now we can both remember.
Jan Ledford

Dedication, Fourth Edition

For Bernie Calaway, who thinks like me
and loves words just as much.
Jan Ledford

Dedication, Third Edition

Dedicated, for my part, to the Mighty Girl Writers:
Londa, Pam, Eva, and Dee.
Jan Ledford

CONTENTS

ACKNOWLEDGMENTS, FIFTH EDITION

Crunch-time is here, as it always is at the deadline of a project, but writing the acknowledgments is a pleasure. Some of my supporters are still hanging about and others have moved on. For this fifth edition, I am indebted to Al Lens, COMT, who makes his debut on this particular project with the pronunciations. Other professional associates who contributed are Charles G. Kirby, MD (who also helps keep me going … AND employed!); Barbara Brown, CO, Med; Brian Duvall, OD; Robert Kershner, MD; John Berdahl, MD; and Johnny Gayton, MD. In the private sector, my appreciation goes to Bernie Calaway (for editing duties), Pam Keyser (who helped wade through the drug tables), Tammy Langley (who gave the manuscript the once-over), and my son, Collin (who, as always, helped with my computer troubles). The English-to-Spanish ophthalmic history translation was a special challenge, and I was assisted by Holly and Brandon Smith (and their friend, who wishes to remain anonymous), Ben Unger, Sara Kennedy, and Victor Moraloza. My colleagues at SLACK Incorporated are stalwart as ever, and I especially thank Jennifer Briggs and John Bond.

Jan Ledford, COMT

ACKNOWLEDGMENTS, FOURTH EDITION

It hardly seems that 2 years have gone by since I took on the QRD and debuted with the third edition. Once again, Joe Hoffman has been of particular help, especially regarding the addition of surgical terms. Cynthia Kendall, BMET, was kind enough to offer comments on the third edition that helped shape the fourth. Jennifer Parker, Director of ARBO/COPE wrote to alert me about their Web site, which I have added. Irena Prikhodko, Customer Service at AAO, helped me when I was trying to track down the elusive Esterman Grid. Debbie

McCall, RN, of The Franklin Eye Center of Carolina Ophthalmology was kind enough to let me use their 2004 edition of the PDR for Ophthalmology one afternoon. Dr. Charles Kirby, of Eyesight Associates of Western North Carolina, suggested new terms worthy of addition. Other colleagues of assistance were Ken Daniels, OD; Russell Edwards, MD; Jenean Carlton, ABOC, NCLC; and Norma Garber, COMT. Stephen Findlay, Reference Assistant at the Macon County Library, rescued me at the last minute by finding a reference I really needed. Then Collin drove over the mountain to pick it up. And Bernie Calaway listened to brainstorming and helped renumber appendices. Thanks, guys. Thanks is due to the awesome team in SLACK's Professional Book Division: John Bond, Amy McShane, Debra Toulson, Michelle Gatt, Lauren Plummer, and Jim Pennewill. Finally, without the support of my family, I could not spend so many hours at the computer doing work such as this. Thank you to my husband, Jim, whose medical knowledge is helpful but whose support is essential. And thanks to Collin, our 19 year old, who knows exactly how to fix my computer complaints and enjoys spending his percentage. To Munchkin, Boonie, Angel, Josey Dee, and Nadia, a heartfelt meow and a promise of catnip.

Jan Ledford, COMT
October, 2004
Franklin, NC

ACKNOWLEDGMENTS, THIRD EDITION

Taking on the third and subsequent editions of this book meant that I will forever build on the work of Joe Hoffman. I thank him for establishing the foundation. Thank you to SLACK Incorporated employees Amy McShane, Debra Toulson, and John Bond for handing me this project. Others who helped are Tiffany K. Spooner, Paraoptometric Section of the AOA, for providing updated information on paraoptometric assistants; Art Giebel, MD, Loma Linda University Medical Center, a contact of Joe's, for providing abbreviations; Bernie Calaway for proofreading assistance and general encouragement; Jim Ledford, my husband, who understands; and Collin Ledford, our teenaged son, who also understands and even does some writing of his own.

Jan Ledford, COMT

About The Authors

For over 25 years now, *Janice K. Ledford, COMT* has been using her skills both in the ophthalmic exam room and on the printed page. While she is probably best known for her certification review books and editorship of *The Basic Bookshelf for Eyecare Professionals*, she is also a published novelist (search Jan Roadarmel Ledford on the Internet). She is currently employed as a fee-basis technologist with Dr. Charles Kirby as well as the Asheville Veterans Administration Eye Clinic. Jan has two sons, a daughter-in-law, and a granddaughter and grandson. She lives in Franklin, NC with her two cats.

Joseph Hoffman has worked in medical publishing since 1985 and was the editor-in-chief of the *Ocular Surgery News* publication group from 1996 to 2001. He has won writing awards from the American Society of Business Publication Editors and Apex. He is currently the proprietor of Hoffman Health Care Communications.

PREFACE

I am way past grammar school, believe me, but the words "Go look it up" still strike terror in my heart. Not because I do not like to look up new terms—far from it. The problem is that I cannot look up just one! I get sidetracked right away by intriguing entries that I just might want to use someday. In the interest of expediency, it is much easier to have someone tell me the meaning.

Medicine has its own unique breed of terms, founded from Greek, Latin, and who knows where else. The current *Stedman's Medical Dictionary* is a 2-volume set… a place where I could easily get lost and spend many happy hours, if I just had the time.

Many of you in eyecare share my delight; others do not. Here is a single volume containing all things optic (well, lots anyway) plus a smattering of general medical terms to get you by. If you are new to the field, there is a lot to learn. If you are an old-timer (might we coin a new term here: presbytech?), there is something new right around every optic, ophthalmic, and optometric corner.

The task of taking on SLACK Incorporated's ophthalmic dictionary, like most projects, turned out to be bigger than I thought. Not the least of these is a simple difference of opinion on some of the words themselves: Is it Grave disease, Graves disease, or Grave's disease? I found references that confirmed each and every one, and doubtless some of you will not agree with the spelling I selected. Then there are your personal pet obscure terms that I left in (*spiral of Tillaux* is one of mine, so it got in) and obsolete words that made the cut (such as *squint*). Others might argue that the inclusion of some general medical terms takes the book needlessly beyond the realm of eyecare. In the final analysis, all I can offer is one of my favorite (and original) axioms regarding publishing: There is no such thing as a perfect book.

Regardless, a lot of people worked really hard to make this one come as close as possible. Meanwhile, I am starting on the sixth edition, and I would appreciate your input. Please email me at bookspublishing@slackinc.com to share your ideas on what terms should be added and deleted, what new appendices would be most helpful, those definitions that need improvement, alternate spellings and pronunciations, typos—whatever! Together, we will continue to make *The Quick Reference Dictionary of Eyecare Terminology* the most turned-to word reference book in the field.

Jan Ledford, COMT
April 2, 2007

How to Use This Book

As a general rule, the most commonly encountered form of the word (eg, cystoid macular edema) is given as the main entry (rather than edema, cystoid macular). Some groups of related terms, however, have been gathered under a unifying concept (for example, laser or nystagmus). Thus, if you cannot locate a term by a beginning adjective, then see the key word. For example, acquired cataract does not have an entry at all; one would look under cataract to find its meaning.

In addition to regular entries, some of the more important combining forms for ophthalmologic terms (such as phac- and kerat-) have been included.

Cross referencing directs the reader by the word *see*, to synonyms by *another term for*, to antonyms with the word *compare*, and to related terms with the phrase *see also*.

With the fifth edition, we have provided pronunciations for many of the entries. We acknowledge that some terms may have more than one pronunciation. If a single entry offers several endings to the word, the first one is given in pronunciation:

deuteranopia, -opsia (DOO-tur-uh-NOH-pee-uh)

If an entry contains more than one word and one is a common term, the common term will not be given a pronunciation:

afferent nerve (AF-ayr-uhnt)

A *see* entry will not pronounce the referred-to term, which will be pronounced at its entry:

annular scotoma (AN-yuh-ler): *See* scotoma.
scotoma (skuh-TOH-mah)

We continue to add some general medical terms appropriate to the field. A good medical dictionary such as *Stedman's Medical Dictionary, 28th Edition* (Lippincott Williams & Wilkins) will fill in any gaps.

A

A-constant: 1. Number assigned to an intraocular lens (IOL) by the manufacturer based on the lens design; used in formulas for calculating power of IOL needed in a given patient; 2. number derived from actual visual results of IOL implantation by a particular surgeon; used as part of subsequent IOL power calculations to "personalize" the formula and better reflect the influence of surgeon technique.

"A" measurement: The horizontal eye size of a pair of spectacles, measured in millimeters from one side of the eyewire to the other; *see also* boxing system.

A pattern: *See* esotropia, exotropia.

A-scan: As used in ophthalmology, an ultrasound examination to determine the axial length of the eye (distance from the front of the cornea to the back surface of the retina at the macula) and possibly the depth of various intraocular structures; most commonly used in calculating the power of intraocular lenses; *also called* biometry; the "A" stands for amplitude, as the echoes are judged by their relative height; **diagnostic A.** ultrasound used to differentiate tissue (eg, melanoma versus hemangioma); *also called* standardized A-scan.

A-V (arteriovenous) crossing: Situation in which the retinal arterioles press down on the underlying veins that they cross over, reducing blood flow and causing A-V nicking; *also called* crossing changes.

A-V (arteriovenous) nicking: Situation in which the retinal arterioles and veins exhibit areas of compression, giving the appearance that a "nick" has been taken out of them; associated with hypertension.

a-wave: In electroretinography, the first part of the wave-form, generated by the retinal photoreceptor cells; *see also* b-wave, c-wave.

ab externo (ab EX-tern-oh): General medical term meaning from the outside; in ophthalmic usage, describing surgical procedures in which the approach to an anatomic structure is made from outside the globe.

Abbe value (ab-BAY): A rating (from 1 to 100) that indicates the amount of chromatic aberration present in a lens material; a higher number indicates less likelihood of aberration; *also called* Nu value.

abducens nerve (ab-DU-senz): Sixth cranial nerve (CN VI); supplies the lateral rectus muscle.

abduct: General medical term for inducing motion away from the center of the body; in ophthalmic usage, muscles that move an eye toward the temple are called abductors; *compare* adduct.

abduction: Act of moving a body part away from the midline; in ophthalmology, moving the eye outward, toward the ear; *compare* adduction.

abductor: In ophthalmology, any extraocular muscle that acts to move the eye outward; *compare* adductor.

aberration (ab-ur-AY-shun): Uneven refraction by an optical system of the wavefront of transmitted light, resulting in distortion of the image; *see also* chromatic aberration, spherical aberration; aberrations can be chromatic (affecting the colors of the image) or monochromatic (affecting only the focus of the image); in refractive surgery, monochromatic aberrations are usually divided into the lower-order aberrations (astigmatism and defocus, which includes myopia and hyperopia) and higher-order aberrations (coma, spherical aberration, quadrafoil, secondary astigmatism, trefoil, etc); *see also* wavefront, Zernike polynomials.

aberrometer (ab-ur-AHM-uh-ter): In ophthalmic usage, device that measures the optical aberrations of the eye; growing in use among refractive surgeons to create "customized" or "wavefront-guided" correction patterns for the excimer laser to apply to the cornea; *see also* wavefront-guided ablation; *also called* wavefront analyzer.

aberrometry (ab-ur-RAHM-uh-tree): In ophthalmic usage, process of measuring the optical aberrations of the eye and representing them numerically or graphically; *also called* wavefront analysis; *see also* Shack-Hartmann a., Tscherning a.

ablation (ab-LAY-shun): General medical term for destruction of tissue, usually as part of a surgical procedure; in refractive surgery, removal of corneal tissue by a laser (usually the ArFl excimer laser) to reshape the eye to correct ametropia; *see also* customized ablation, photoablation.

ablation zone (ab-LAY-shun): In photorefractive surgery, the portion of the cornea under the flap that is removed with the laser.

abnormal retinal correspondence (ARC): *Another term for* anomalous retinal correspondence.

abrasion: General medical term for a wound in which the layers of tissue are scraped away; in ophthalmic usage, often used as a synonym for corneal abrasion.

Acanthomoeba **(Ay-kan-tho-MEE-buh):** Protozoan known for contaminating homemade saline and hot tubs, and thus a problem to some contact lens wearers; can cause severe corneal infection.

accommodation: Adjustment of focal power of the eye from distance to near vision achieved by contraction of the ciliary muscle, which causes a thickening of the crystalline lens and a slight forward shift in its position, both of which increase its refractive power; **absolute a.** accommodation of either eye independently; **binocular a.** uniform accommodation of both eyes together in convergence (ie, the inward turning of both eyes in viewing a near object); **convergence a.** accommodation that occurs in either eye upon convergence; **far point of a.** distance from the eye to the farthest point clearly visible when accommodation is relaxed; **near point of a.** distance from the eye to the nearest point clearly visible when accommodation is at its maximum; **negative a.** relaxation of accommodation for distance vision; **positive a.** exercise of accommodation for near vision; **range of a.** the distance between the near and far points of accommodation.

accommodative amplitude (AA): The amount of accommodation (measured in diopters) required at the near point of accommodation; *also called* amplitude of accommodation.

accommodative convergence (AC): Inward turning of both eyes that normally occurs in response to accommodation.

accommodative convergence/accommodation (AC/A): The relationship (a ratio) between the amount that the eyes turn inward (accommodative convergence, measured in prism diopters) and the increase in their focusing power (accommodation, measured in diopters) that occurs when viewing a near object, calculated as accommodative convergence divided by accommodation; *see also* accommodation, convergence.

accommodative insufficiency (AI): Abnormal weakening of the accommodation reflex; may be due to injury, disease, or the effects of medication.

accommodative miosis (my-OH-sis): Normal constriction of pupils associated with accommodation.

accommodative reflex: The triad of lens accommodation, convergence, and miosis that occurs during near vision; however, it is not a true reflex.

accommodative spasm: Accommodation without subsequent relaxation of the ciliary muscle, resulting in a prolonged state of near focus (rendering distant objects unclear); *also called* ciliary spasm.

accommodative target: Object or optotype held at close distance to the patient in order to stimulate accommodation.

accommodative tone: State in which the eye is constantly accommodating, occurring where there is substantial accommodative capacity (as in children, especially hyperopes).

acetylcholine (uh-see-til-KOH-leen): Biochemical (neurotransmitter) that activates the parasympathetic nervous system; in the eye, it stimulates the ciliary muscle and the sphincter muscle of the iris; *see also* cholinergic, neurotransmitter; *compare* epinephrine, norepinephrine.

achromatic lens (ak-roh-MAT-ik): An ophthalmic lens that is free from chromatic aberration (ie, it does not break light into its component colors).

achromatism/achromatopsia (uh-KROH-muh-tiz-um/ uh-kroh-muh-TOH-see-uh): Rare condition in which all three visual pigments are absent; total color vision loss where only shades of gray, black, and white are perceived; *also called* rod monochromatism; *compare* dichromatism, monochromatism, trichromatism.

acorea (a-KORN-ee-a): Absence of the pupil.

acquired: Characteristic or disorder that is not inherited but rather occurs separately from the genetic makeup of the individual; *compare* hereditary.

acrylic (uh-KRIL-ik): Of or relating to acrylic acid or its many derivative compounds; in eyecare, usually an optically clear polymer used in the manufacture of lenses.

acrylic lens implant (uh-KRIL-ik): *See* intraocular lens.

acuity: Clarity of vision; specifically, the ability to distinguish fine details; often expressed as a score on Snellen's, Jaeger's, or other vision-testing charts.

acute: In medical usage, denoting the immediate or severe; *compare* chronic, subacute; *see* entries under main word (eg, *see* glaucoma for acute angle-closure glaucoma, etc).

adaptation: General medical term for adjustment to changing conditions; specifically in ophthalmic usage:

color a. adjustment of vision to bright colors such that the color intensity diminishes with time; **dark a.** adjustment of vision in dim light, primarily by increasing levels of rhodopsin (visual purple) in the rods of the retina, making the eye more sensitive to light; *see* scotopia; **light a.** adjustment of vision in bright light by decreasing levels of light-sensitive pigments of the retina; *see* photopia; **photopic a.** *another term for* light a.; **retinal a.** general term for adjustment of vision to varying light conditions; **scotopic a.** *another term for* dark a.

add: 1. Amount of additional refractive power needed in spectacles or contact lenses (prescribed for distance vision correction) to correct a presbyopic eye for near (ie, "reading") vision; 2. the portion of a lens that is designed to provide that additional near corrective power; *see also* segment (definition 2).

adduct: General medical term for inducing motion toward the center of the body; in ophthalmic usage, muscles that move an eye toward the nose are called adductors; *compare* abduct.

adduction: Act of moving a body part toward the midline; in ophthalmology, moving the eye inward, toward the nose; *compare* abduction.

adductor: In ophthalmology, any extraocular muscle that acts to move the eye inward; *compare* abductor.

adenovirus (ad-ne-o vie-russ): The virus that causes epidemic keratoconjunctivitis; *see also* virus.

Adie's pupil or **syndrome (AE-deez):** Uneven contraction of the pupils of each eye upon accommodation (in near vision) in which the affected pupil reacts poorly to light and slowly to near; *also called* myotonic pupil, pupillotonia, tonic pupil.

adjustable suture: Suture placed in glaucoma, refractive, or other surgery to allow tightening or loosening in the postoperative period to modify the results of surgery.

adnexa (ad-NEX-uh): General anatomic term for the structures surrounding an organ; the ocular adnexa are usually considered to include the eyelids, lacrimal apparatus, orbits, and other tissues within the orbits.

adrenaline (ah-DREN-a-lin): *Another term for* epinephrine.

adrenergic (ad-ruh-NER-jic): Substance or system that stimulates the sympathetic nervous system; phenylephrine (a mydriatic) is an adrenergic drug; *compare* cholinergic.

advancement: In ophthalmic usage, operation (usually for correction of strabismus) in which an extraocular muscle or tendon is detached and repositioned more anteriorly to increase its action; **capsular a.** surgical manipulation of Tenon's capsule in order to achieve advancement of an extraocular muscle.

afferent pupillary defect (APD) (A-fair-rent or AFF-er-ent): *Another term for* Marcus Gunn pupil.

afferent nerve (A-fair-rent or AFF-er-ent): Nerve that conducts a sensory impulse (ie, information) from the peripheral point of origin into the central nervous system; *another term for* sensory nerve (*see* entry); *compare* efferent nerve.

after-cataract: *Another term for* capsular opacification.

afterimage: Perception of an image that persists after the visual stimulus ends; *also called* persistence of vision; **complementary a.** afterimage in which the persisting colors are complementary to the colors of the original visual stimulus; **negative a.** afterimage in which bright elements of a visual stimulus persist as dark and dark elements become light; **positive a.** afterimage in which light elements persist as light and dark elements remain dark.

"against" motion: 1. In retinoscopy, the pupillary reflex is said to be "against" when it moves in the opposite direction of the intercept reflex; *compare* neutrality, "with" motion (definition 1); 2. In optics, the illusion that an object viewed through a lens moves in the opposite direction the lens is moved; *compare* "with" motion (definition 2).

against-the-rule astigmatism (ATR): *See* astigmatism.

age-related macular degeneration (ARMD or AMD): *See* macular degeneration.

agonist (AG-on-ist): The muscle receiving primary innervation to contract (eg, the lateral rectus in abduction); *compare* antagonist.

air-fluid exchange: *Another term for* gas-fluid exchange.

air-puff tonometer: *See entry under* tonometer.

akinesia (a-ki-NEE-zuh): General term for lack of motion or inability to move; most often in ophthalmic usage, referring to the lack of voluntary movement of the eye following retrobulbar or peribulbar anesthesia.

alacrima (a-LAK-ri-mah): Absence of tears.

albinism (AL-bin-ism): A genetic disorder in which there is a general lack of melanin (pigment), including in the retinal pigment epithelium, iris, and choroid; ocular manifestations can include nystagmus, photophobia, and subnormal vision; **ocular a.** X-linked disorder in which the ocular manifestations of albinism are present but there is melanin in the skin.

albino (al-BI-no): An individual exhibiting characteristics of albinism.

alexia (al-EX-ia): The inability to understand written language; *also called* word blindness; *compare* dyslexia.

allele (uh-LEEL): An alternative (contrasting) form of a gene that occurs at the corresponding locus in paired chromosomes (eg, the gene for brown eyes is an allele of the gene for blue eyes and vice versa).

Allen cards, chart, or **test:** Visual acuity test employing pictures to assess the vision of young children and the mentally challenged.

allergen (AL-er-jen): Any substance that causes an allergic response.

allergic conjunctivitis: *See* conjunctivitis.

allergic response: A collective term used to describe the body's response to an allergen; typical ocular allergic response could include rash, itching, tearing, and redness.

allergy: Hypersensitivity (acquired or induced) to an allergen such that an allergic response occurs; **contact a.** hypersensitivity to an allergen when coming into direct physical contact (eg, poison ivy, cosmetics, etc); **drug a.** hypersensitivity to medication (eg, penicillin, sulfa, codeine, etc).

alloplastic corneal implant (AL-oh-PLAS-tik): Plastic lens or ring placed into a corneal stromal pocket, usually as a refractive measure.

alpha angle: *See* angle.

alpha chymotrypsin (ky-moh-TRIP-sin): Enzyme injected into the anterior chamber to dissolve zonular fibers and facilitate intracapsular cataract extraction.

alternate cover test: *See entry under* cover test.

alternate prism and cover test (APCT): *Another term for* prism and alternate cover test; *see that entry under* cover test.

alternating amblyopia: *See* amblyopia.

alternating strabismus: *See* strabismus.

amacrine cells (AM-a-krin): Nerve cells that are found in the inner nuclear layer of the retina; *see also* retina.

amaurosis (am-uh-ROH-sis): General term for blindness, usually referring to blindness caused by some defect apart from the tissues of the eyeball; **central a.** temporary blindness resulting from disease or defect of the central nervous system; **hysterical a.** temporary blindness resulting from neurosis; **sympathetic a.** blindness in one eye occurring because of disease in the other eye.

amaurosis fugax (am-uh-ROH-sis FOO-jaks): A temporary state (about 10 minutes or so) of partial or full blindness in one eye often associated with carotid artery disease.

amaurotic nystagmus (am-au-ROT-ik nuh-STAG-muhs): Rapid involuntary movements of a blind eye.

amaurotic pupil (am-au-ROT-ik): Pupil that does not respond to direct light stimulation but does dilate and constrict when the fellow eye receives light stimulus; an eye with an amaurotic pupil is blind, usually because of damage to the optic nerve or retina.

amblyogenic (am-blee-oh-JEN-ik): Causing amblyopia.

amblyope (AM-blee-ope): One who suffers from amblyopia.

amblyopia (am-blee-OH-pee-uh): Impaired vision in one or both eyes that cannot be remedied with corrective lenses and has no obvious organic cause in the structures of the eye or visual pathway (colloquially known as lazy eye); **a. of disuse** *see* suppression a.; **alcoholic a.** amblyopia caused by alcohol toxicity (*also called* amblyopia crapulosa); **alternating a.** diminished vision occurring in the nonfixating eye in alternating strabismus; **ametropic a.** *see* refractive a.; **anisometropic a.** amblyopia arising from a significant difference in the refractive power of the 2 eyes in which the eye requiring the greatest accommodation to achieve clear vision becomes disused; **astigmatic a.** refractive amblyopia occurring because of uncorrected astigmatism; **color a.** general term for impairment of color vision; **crossed a.** amblyopia in one eye with loss of feeling in the opposite side of the face (*also called* amblyopia cruciata); **deprivation a.** *see* suppression a.; **functional a.** amblyopia that can be corrected with eyeglasses or occlusion of the opposite eye in childhood, *also called* reversible a.; **nocturnal a.** *see* nyctalopia; **occlusion a.** type of suppression amblyopia in which central fixation was intentionally obstructed (as with an eye patch); **reflex a.** amblyopia resulting from some insult or injury to the eye; **refractive a.** due to a high uncorrected refractive error; *also called* ametropic amblyopia; **reversible a.** *see* functional a.; **strabismic a.** amblyopia arising from strabismus in which one eye becomes preferred over the other, which then falls into disuse; **suppression a.** amblyopia resulting from deprivation of sight in an eye by ptosis, cataract, corneal opacity, etc; *also called* amblyopia ex anopsia, deprivation amblyopia, amblyopia of disuse.

amblyoscope (AM-blee-uh-skohp): Instrument used to evaluate strabismus and binocular vision; *also called* a troposcope.

ametropia (am-i-TROH-pee-uh): General term for conditions in which the eye does not focus properly but can be corrected with eyeglasses or other vision aids; *also called* a refractive error (*see* astigmatism, hyperopia, myopia, presbyopia); *compare* emmetropia; **axial a.** ametropia attributable to the length of the eyeball (too long in myopia or too short in hyperopia); **curvature a.** ametropia attributable to corneal curvature (too steep in myopia or too flat in hyperopia); **position a.** ametropia attributable to the position of the crystalline lens of the eye (too far forward in myopia or too far back in hyperopia); **refractive a.** general term for any ametropia attributable to an error in the eye's system for focusing light rays on the retina.

amplitude of accommodation: *Another term for* accommodative amplitude.

amplitude of convergence: Maximum angle to which the eyes can turn inward (from parallel lines of sight in distance vision) toward the nose to fix upon a nearby object.

Amsler chart or **grid (AG) (AM-zler):** Visual field testing grid consisting of evenly spaced horizontal and vertical lines, typically white lines on a dark background with a central dot to mark the point of fixation; used as a simple test for detecting defects or distortions in the central 20 degrees of the visual field.

amyloid body (AM-uh-loyd): Deposit of abnormal starch-protein compound seen in amyloidosis.

amyloidosis: Condition in which deposits of amyloid accumulate in various body tissues, including the vitreous humor, ocular nerves, and blood vessels.

anaglyph (AN-uh-glif): Vision test target consisting of two similar images with different portions printed in red, green, and sometimes black; subject views each image separately with each eye, and a red filter is placed before one eye and a green filter before the other; patient reports the image seen, providing a measure of fusion and stereoscopic function.

analgesic (an-uhl-JEE-zik): Drug that relieves pain without rendering the patient unconscious.

anatomic equator: In ophthalmic usage, imaginary line around the circumference of the eyeball placed equidistant from the front and back surfaces (anterior and posterior poles) of the eyeball.

anesthesia: Substance (*see* anesthetic) or condition (eg, disease, injury) that blocks or reduces sensation; **general a.** complete loss of sensation with unconsciousness; *also called* surgical a.; **local a.** loss of sensation in a specific area of the body; **surgical a.** *another term for* general a.; **topical a.** loss of sensation in a specific area by applying an agent directly to the part to be anesthetized; in ophthalmology, use of proparacaine or other "numbing drop" applied directly to the external globe.

anesthetic: Drug that reduces or eliminates sensation, usually so that a surgical procedure may be performed without pain; **general a.** eliminates sensation by rendering the patient unconscious; usually administered systemically by intravenous injection or inhalation; **local or regional a.** eliminates sensation in one area, usually administered by injection to either numb the tissue directly or to block the sensory nerves (called a block); **topical a.** eliminates sensation in one area; usually administered by applying directly to the skin/tissue; tetracaine is a commonly used topical anesthetic in eyecare.

angiogenesis (an-jee-oh-JEN-uh-sis): Process by which new blood vessels are generated; in ophthalmology, usually referring to neovascularization as found in diabetic retinopathy, etc.

angiogenic (an-jee-oh-JEN-ik): Substance or condition that stimulates growth of new blood vessels; *see also* angiogenesis.

angiography (an-gi-OG-ruh-fee): Evaluation of blood vessels following an injection of dye or radiopaque substance; in ophthalmology, generally referring to the examination of iris or retinal blood vessels; *see* fluorescein angiography, indocyanine green angiography.

angioid streaks (AN-jee-oyd, an-JEE-oyd): Red to brown streaks visible on the retina originating from the optic disk.

angioscotoma (an-gi-o-sko-TOH-ma): Visual field defect caused by the shadow of a retinal blood vessel.

angle: 1. The point at which the upper and lower eyelids meet; *see also* canthus; 2. the area of the anterior chamber of the eye where the iris and cornea join (*also called* iridocorneal angle); aqueous humor exits the eye through the angle, thus this structure is *also called* filtration angle; specific tissues and structures that comprise the angle include the iris processes, corneoscleral junction, scleral sulcus, ciliary body, trabecular meshwork, and Schlemm's canal; 3. any one of several standard dimensions used to describe the optical system of the eye, specifically **alpha a.** angle formed at the eye's optical center by the optical and visual axes; **biorbital a.** angle formed by the axes of the two orbits; **gamma a.** angle formed at the eye's center of rotation by the optical and fixation axes; **kappa a.** *see* angle kappa (below); **lambda a.** angle formed at the center of the eye's pupil by the optical and the visual axes. *See also* axis, optical center.

angle-closure glaucoma: *Another term for* closed-angle glaucoma; *see entry under* glaucoma.

angle kappa (KAP-uh): Angle formed at the eye's optical center by the intersection of the pupillary and visual axes; **negative a.k.** the visual axis is temporal to the pupillary axis and falsely creates the impression of esotropia; **positive a.k.** the visual axis is nasal to the pupillary axis and falsely creates the impression of exotropia.

angle of anomaly: *Another term for* angle of deviation.

angle of convergence: Angle formed by the eye's visual axis and a line drawn from the target object to a midpoint between the two eyes.

angle of deviation: Degree to which one eye is shifted from straight-ahead fixation when the fellow eye is fixed straight ahead; *also called* angle of anomaly, squint angle.

angle of incidence: Angle formed by a ray of light that strikes (is "incident" to) an interface between two media, as measured from a line drawn perpendicular to the interface at the point where the light ray strikes.

angle of reflection: Angle formed by a ray of light reflected from the interface of two media, as measured from a line drawn perpendicular to the interface at the point from which the light ray is reflected.

angle of refraction: Angle formed by a ray of light that has crossed an interface between two substances and a line drawn perpendicular to the interface at the point where the light ray crosses.

angle-recession glaucoma: *See* glaucoma.

anhydrosis (an-hi-DROH-sis): Lack of perspiration; in Horner's syndrome, there is no perspiration on the affected side of the face; *see also* Horner's syndrome.

aniridia (an-ah-RID-ee-uh): The absence (sometimes congenital, though in adults more frequently due to trauma) of most or all of the iris.

aniseikonia (an-i-suh-KOH-nee-uh): Unequal retinal image sizes, especially as seen in corrected anisometropia; the eye with the most plus (least minus) lens perceives a larger image than does the eye with the least plus (most minus) eye, resulting in distorted spacial perception; *see also* anisometropia; *compare* iseikonia.

anisoaccommodation (an-i-soh-uh-kahm-uh-DAY-shun): General term for uneven accommodation in the two eyes.

anisoacuity (an-i-soh-ah-CUE-it-ee): Unequal acuity; a problem sometimes related to anisometropia, which can cause difficulty with binocular fusion.

anisochromatic (an-i-soh-kroh-MAT-ik): Color difference either between two or more objects or between different parts of the same object (as in an iris that is not of a uniform color); *see also* heterochromic; *compare* isochromatic.

anisocoria (an-i-suh-KOHR-ee-uh): Uneven size of pupils in the two eyes, usually reserved to describe more than a 1-mm difference in diameter; *compare* isocoria.

anisometropia (an-i-sum-uh-TROH-pee-uh): A difference between the refractive power of the two eyes, usually defined as more than a 1-diopter difference; the condition can affect motility, acuity, and image size; *see* aniseikonia, anisoacuity, anisophoria; *compare* isometropia.

anisophoria (an-i-suh-FOHR-ee-uh): Unequal motility, generally as related to spectacle-corrected anisometropia and antimetropia; prism is induced when the lenses are of sufficiently unequal power; *see also* anisometropia, antimetropia.

anisopia (an-uh-SOH-pee-uh): General term for unequal vision in the two eyes.

ankyloblepharon (ang-kil-oh-BLEF-uh-rahn): Adhesion of the upper and lower eyelids; *also called* blepharosynechia.

annular (AN-yuh-ler): Ring shaped.

annular cataract (AN-yuh-ler): *See* cataract.

annular keratitis (AN-yuh-ler): *See* keratitis.

annular scotoma (AN-yuh-ler): *See* scotoma.

annulus (AN-yuh-luhs): General anatomic term for a ring-shaped structure.

annulus ciliaris (AN-yuh-luhs sil-ee-AIR-us): The outer portion of the ciliary body attached to the ora serrata.

annulus of Zinn (AN-yuh-luhs): The ring of connective tissue attached to the orbit near the optic nerve, anchoring the rectus muscles of the eye; *also called* aponeurosis, circle of Zinn.

anomaloscope (uh-NAHM-uh-luh-skohp): Color matching test that identifies color vision abnormalities (usually for red/green defects) and quantifies them (ie, mild, moderate, severe).

anomalous or **abnormal retinal correspondence (ARC) (uh-NAHM-uh-luhs):** Condition in which parts of the images on each retina come to be linked in the brain's interpretation of the fused image even though they do not correspond to the same point in space, often occurring as a result of untreated strabismus; *compare* harmonious retinal correspondence.

anomalous trichromatism (uh-NAHM-uh-luhs try-KROH-ma-tiz-im): *See* trichromatism.

anophthalmia, -os, -anopia (an-op-THAL-me-uh): Congenital condition in which the eyeball is absent or only partially developed.

anopsia (an-AHP-see-uh): Loss or suppression of vision, usually of only part of the visual field in just one eye.

anorthopia (an-or-THO-pi-a): General term for distortion of vision.

anoxia (an-AHK-see-uh): *Another term for* hypoxia.

ANSI standards (AN-see): Guidelines set forth in a document published by the American National Standards Institute (ANSI) that establish legal requirements for safety eyewear and other eyewear parameters.

antagonist: Muscle that opposes the contracting (agonist) muscle's action (eg, when the lateral rectus abducts the eye, the medial rectus is the antagonist); *compare* agonist.

anterior basal membrane: *Another term for* Bowman's capsule/membrane.

anterior chamber (AC): Area within the eye formed by the structures in front of the iris and filled with aqueous humor; *compare* posterior chamber (which also contains aqueous humor); **AC intraocular lens** (ACIOL) *see* intraocular lens; **AC tap** *another term for* keratocentesis.

anterior hyaloid membrane: *See* hyaloid membrane.

anterior ischemic neuropathy: *See* ischemic optic neuropathy.

anterior pole (of the eye): Imaginary point on the front surface of the cornea centered over the pupil; *compare* posterior pole (of the eye).

anterior pole (of the lens): Point at the front and center of the crystalline lens; *compare* posterior pole (of the lens).

anterior segment (of the eye): General term usually describing structures of the eye, including the lens and all structures anterior to the lens (thus including the anterior and posterior chambers); ophthalmic surgery is roughly divided into the categories of anterior segment (cornea, glaucoma, and cataract procedures) and posterior segment (retina and vitreous procedures); *compare* posterior segment (of the eye).

anterior synechia: *See* synechia.

anterior uveitis: *See* uveitis.

anterior vitrectomy: *See* vitrectomy.

antiangiogenic (an-tee-an-jee-oh-JEN-ik): Treatment or process that stops the formation of blood vessels.

antibacterial: Any substance/drug that destroys or inhibits bacteria.

antibiotic: Drug (derived from bacteria or fungi) used to destroy or inhibit microorganisms, and thus the disorders they cause.

antibody: Protein that forms in response to an antigen; part of the immune system in that it destroys antigens and bestows immunity.

anticholinesterase (an-tee-koh-luh-NES-tuh-rayz): Any substance or system that prevents cholinesterase from "cleaning" acetylcholine from receptor sites; they have a parasympathetic effect; an example is the drug eserine, which constricts the pupil and stimulates the ciliary muscle; *see also* cholinesterase, neurotransmitter.

anticoagulant (an-tee-koh-AG-yuh-luh-nt): Substance that thins the blood, reducing the ability to form clots.

antifungal: Substance/drug that destroys or inhibits fungi.

antigen (AN-tih-jen): Substance that is foreign to the body and causes an immune response after an initial contact; *see also* immune response.

antihistamine (an-ti-HISS-tuh-meen): Substance that blocks the release of histamine from mast cells, thus counteracting an allergic response; *see also* histamine, mast cell.

anti-inflammatory agent: Substance/drug that acts to reduce inflammation; steroids are common anti-inflammatories.

antimetropia (an-ti-mah-TROH-pee-uh): Condition in which one eye is hyperopic while the fellow eye is myopic; *also called* heterometropia; *see also* anisometropia, anisophoria.

antimydriatic (an-tahy-mid-ree-AT-ik): Drug that prevents the pupil from dilating.

antiviral: Any substance/drug that destroys or inhibits viruses.

anomaly (ah-NOM-o-lee): General term denoting any unusual occurrence; departing from the normal.

apex: The tip of a structure or object; in ophthalmology, usually referring to a prism (the tip opposite the base; *compare* base), the globe, or the cornea.

aphake (A-fake): Eye in which the lens is absent, either congenitally or following surgery; compare pseudophake.

aphakia (a-FAY-kee-uh): Absence of the lens of the eye; *see also* cataract extraction; compare pseudophakia.

aphakic (a-FAY-kik): Adjective describing contact lenses or spectacles (*also called* "cataract glasses") prescribed after removal of the crystalline lens of the eye; *see also* cataract extraction; *compare* phakic, pseudophakic.

aphakic glaucoma (a-FAY-kik): *See* glaucoma.

aphasia (a-FAY-zee-uh): The inability to verbalize.

aphotesthesia (a-fot-es-THEE-see-zhuh): Diminished response of the retina following excessive exposure to bright light.

apical clearance: 1. Distance between the back surface of a contact lens and the cornea; *also called* vault; 2. less commonly, distance between the cornea and the crystalline lens.

aplanatic, -ism (ap-lah-NAT-ik): Property of an optical system such that it is free of the aberrations normally associated with spherical lenses.

aponeurosis (ap-oh-noo-ROH-sus): General term for the tendon that anchors a muscle; in the eye, the tendinous bundle that anchors the rectus muscles to the orbit (*also called* annulus of Zinn).

apoptosis (a-pahp-TOH-sis): General medical term for programmed cell death, a process by which cells continue to degenerate and cease functioning long after the initial injury or insult; in ophthalmic usage, usually referring to the progressive loss of retinal cells in glaucoma.

apostilb (abs) (AP-uh-stilb): Unit of brightness; in ophthalmology, a measure of the brightness of a visual field test object.

apotripsis (ap-oh-TRIP-sus): Surgical excision of a corneal opacity.

applanation: Flattening of a normally rounded area, such as the cornea.

applanation tonometer: *See entry under* tonometer.

applanometer (ap-luh-NAHM-uh-tur): *Another term for* applanation tonometer.

aqueous flare: *See* flare.

aqueous fluid or humor: Clear, watery liquid (typically referred to simply as the aqueous) that fills the anterior and posterior chambers of the eye.

aqueous outflow: Process by which the aqueous humor is filtered out of the eye through the angle of the anterior chamber; *see also* angle (definition 2).

aqueous tap: Process of removing some aqueous from the anterior chamber through a needle.

arachnoid sheath (ah-RAK-noid): One of the membranes that surround the optic nerve.

arcuate keratotomy (AK) (AHR-kyoo-it kehr-uh-TAH-tuh-me): *See* keratotomy.

arcuate scotoma (AHR-kyoo-it skuh-TOH-muh): *See* scotoma.

arcus juvenilis (AR-kus joo-vah-NIL-us): Ring of fatty deposits around the edge of the cornea but not quite extending to the limbus appearing in young or middle-aged patients with unusually high blood cholesterol levels or some systemic diseases.

arcus senilis (AR-kus suh-NILL-is): Ring of fatty deposits around the edge of the cornea but not quite extending to the limbus appearing in elderly patients.

Arden index or ratio (AR-din): On electro-oculogram testing, a comparison between the maximum light potential to the minimum dark potential; *see also* dark trough, light peak.

ArFl laser (argon fluoride): *See* laser.

argon laser/argon fluoride (AR-gahn): *See* laser.

argon laser trabeculoplasty (ALT) (AR-gahn): *See* trabeculoplasty.

Argyll Robertson pupil (ARP) (ar-GILL RAH-bert-suhn): Condition in which a pupil constricts upon accommodation but does not react to varying direct or consensual light; usually associated with syphilis.

arrangement tests: Color vision tests that require the subject to organize colors in a regular progression; *see also* Farnsworth-Munsell Test.

arterial circles of the iris (ar-TEER-ee-uhl): Two ring-shaped bands of vascular tissue in the iris: the inner or lesser circle is near the pupil and the major or greater circle is adjacent to the ciliary body.

arterial phase (ar-TEER-ee-uhl): Segment of fluorescein angiography (at about 11 seconds after dye injection) where the arteries of the retina fill with dye; *see also* fluorescein angiography.

arthro-ophthalmopathy (AR-thro-OP-thal-MOP-ah-thee): Degenerative disease that affects the joints and eyes; *see also* Sjögren's syndrome.

artificial tears: Man-made liquid formulated to simulate the composition of tear fluid; used in treating dry eye conditions.

aspheric, -al lens (a-SFEER-ik, a-SFEER-ik-uhl): Lens that focuses light along a meridian rather than to a point; aspheric lenses are used in spectacles, contact lenses, and intraocular lenses to correct astigmatism to reduce peripheral distortion or to provide a range of focusing power from near to far; *see also* cylinder (definition 1), toric lens; *compare* spherical lens.

aspiration: In ophthalmic usage, suction applied by a surgical instrument usually to remove fluid or particulate matter from the eye; *see* irrigation and aspiration.

aspiration flow rate: In phacoemulsification, the instrument setting that determines the maximum amount of fluid per unit of time (usually described in cubic centimeters per minute) that will flow through the eye into the instrument hand piece.

asteroid hyalosis (AS-ter-oyd hi-uh-LOH-sis): *See entry under* hyalosis.

asthenopia (as-thuh-NOH-pee-uh): Impairment of function such that the eye is weak and/or tires easily, possibly accompanied by ocular pain, diminished vision, and/or headache; *also called* eye strain; **accommodative a.** asthenopia resulting from prolonged periods of accommodation (during reading or close work);

muscular a. asthenopia attributable to tiring of the external ocular muscles; **nervous a.** asthenopia resulting from neurosis, characterized by eye fatigue and possibly constriction of the visual field; **tarsal a.** asthenopia attributable to pressure of the eyelids on the eye, which induces astigmatism.

astigmatic clock/dial (ay-stig-MAT-ik): Vision test target consisting of straight radial lines (like the spokes of a wheel); the patient reports which lines, if any, appear darker. (If using plus cylinder, the axis is parallel to the dark lines as the patient sees them; if using minus cylinder, the axis is perpendicular to the dark lines as the patient sees them.) *Also called* clock dial, fan dial, sunburst dial.

astigmatic or **arcuate keratotomy (AK) (ay-stig-MAT-ik kehr-uh-TAH-tuh-me):** Surgical correction of astigmatism by making partial-thickness arcing incisions into specific areas of the cornea; *see also* keratotomy.

astigmatism (astig) (ah-STIG-mah-tiz-um): Visual defect attributable to the presence of an elliptical (ie, egg or football shaped) rather than spherical shape in the refracting surfaces of the eye, resulting in the diffusion of light rays along a particular line (axis); **acquired a.** astigmatism resulting from some injury or insult to the eye; **against-the-rule a. (ATR)** astigmatism in which the steep axis is within 30 degrees of the horizontal; *also called* inverse a.; *compare* with-the-rule a. (below), oblique a. (below); **asymmetrical a.** astigmatism in which the steepest and flattest meridians are not 90 degrees from one another; **complex a.** combination of corneal and lenticular astigmatism in the same eye; **compound a.** astigmatism in which the flat and steep axes are either both hyperopic (**compound hyperopic a.**) or myopic (**compound myopic a.**); **corneal a.** astigmatism attributable to the shape of the refractive surface of the cornea; **direct a.** *another term for* with-the-rule a.; **hypermetropic** or **hyperopic a.** astigmatism in which both axes are hyperopic (compound) or one focal line falls on the retina and the other behind (simple); **inverse a.** *another term for* against-the-rule a.; **irregular a.** astigmatism in which the flat and steep axes are not at right angles or astigmatism resulting from variable curvature along a given meridian of the eye; **lenticular a.** astigmatism attributable to the shape of the refractive surfaces of the crystalline lens; **mixed a.** astigmatism in which one axis is hyperopic and the other is myopic; **myopic a.** astigmatism in which both axes are myopic (compound) or one focal line falls on the retina and the other in front (simple); **oblique a.** astigmatism occurring along the 45-degree or 135-degree meridians; *compare* against-the-rule a., with-the-rule a.; **pathological a.** astigmatism that results from some disease; **physiologic a.** small degree of astigmatism occurring normally in virtually all eyes, usually unnoticed; **regular a.** astigmatism in which the curvatures of the flat and steep axes are uniform across the width of the eye and lie approximately at right angles to each other; **residual a.** amount of astigmatism left uncorrected by a contact lens; **secondary a.** in optics, the higher-order aberration that distorts an image across two axes: one axis where the central area of each half has focus that is too strong and a peripheral area where it is too weak, and the other axis in which the pattern is reversed; this often causes monocular diplopia; **simple a.** astigmatism in which one focal line falls on the retina and the other falls behind the retina (**simple hyperopic a.**) or in front of the retina (**simple myopic a.**); **symmetrical a.** astigmatism in which the steepest and flattest meridians in opposite halves of the eye lie on a straight line through the center of the eye; **with-the-rule a. (WTR)** astigmatism in which the steep axis is within 30 degrees of the vertical (so named because it is the most common type of astigmatism found in the human eye); *also called* direct a.; *compare* against-the-rule a. (above), oblique a. (above).

astringent (uh-STRIN-jent): Substance used to shrink tissues and stop any discharge.

asymptomatic (ay-simp-toh-MAT-ik): Having no symptoms; *compare* symptomatic; *see* symptom.

atonic (a-TAHN-ik): General term for lack of muscle tone.

atonic ectropion (a-TAHN-ik ek-TROH-pee-uhn): Condition in which weakness of the eyelid muscles results in the lid turning outward from the eye, exposing the conjunctiva.

atopic conjunctivitis: *See* conjunctivitis.

atopy (AT-uh-pee): General term for condition marked by unusually high allergic sensitivity of many tissues throughout the body to a number of allergens.

atrophy (AT-roh-fee): General medical term referring to the degeneration of a body structure.

attention reflex of the pupil: Change in the size of the pupil when fixation takes place.

audito-oculogyric reflex (AUD-i-oh-toh-oc-u-lo-JY-nik): Turning of the eye in the direction of startling noises.

autogenous keratoplasty (ah-TAH-juh-ness KEHR-uh-toh-plas-tee): Keratoplasty in which only the patient's own corneal tissues are used; *also called* autokeratoplasty; *compare* homogenous keratoplasty.

autoimmune disease: Disorder in which the body reacts to and attacks its own tissues (eg, AIDS and lupus erythematosus).

automated lamellar keratoplasty (ALK or LK) (luh-MELL-er): Surgical procedure in which a microkeratome is used to make a corneal flap; the underlying cornea is then flattened by removing tissue with a microkeratome or laser (LASIK).

automated perimetry: *See* perimetry.

automated vitrectomy: *See* vitrectomy.

autonomic nervous system (ah-toh-NAHM-ic): Division of the nervous system that regulates the automatic processes of the body; its two branches are the sympathetic and parasympathetic nervous systems.

autorefractor or **automated refractor (AR):** Computerized instrument for objectively measuring the refractive power of the eye; *see also* refractor.

autosomes (AH-tuh-sohms): The chromosomes other than those that determine the sex of the individual; in the human, the 22 non-sex chromosomes of the 23 pairs of chromosomes.

Axenfeld loops (AKS-en-feld): *See* loops of Axenfeld.

axial hyperopia: *See* hyperopia.

axial length of the eye: Distance from the cornea's anterior to the macula along the principal axis of the eye; *see also* A-scan.

axial myopia: *See* myopia.

axis: General term for the imaginary line passing through a solid body, representing a hypothetical axis around which the object could be rotated; any one of several standard reference lines used to describe the anatomy and optical system of the eye, specifically: **cylinder a.** term denoting the orientation of a cylindrical lens where the image is formed; *compare* meridian (definition 3); **external a.** axis from the anterior pole of the eye to the posterior pole; **internal a.** axis from the anterior pole of the eye to the point on the retina just opposite the posterior pole; **lens a.** axis from the anterior pole to the posterior pole of the crystalline lens; **optical** or **principal a.** axis passing through the optical center of the eye and perpendicular to the plane of the crystalline lens; **pupillary a.** axis centered on and perpendicular to the plane of the pupil; **visual a.** axis along which light rays travel from an object to the macula (*also called* line of sight).

axometer (ak-SAHM-it-ur): Instrument used for finding optical axes, especially as used in adjusting glasses.

axon (AKS-ahn): Filament extending from a nerve cell along which impulses are conducted away from the cell body toward the synapse; *see also* dendrite (definition 1), neuron, synapse.

B

"B" measurement: The vertical eye size of a pair of spectacles, measured in millimeters from the top of the eyewire to the bottom; used in describing placement of the optical center or add position; *see also* boxing system.

B-scan: As used in ophthalmology, an ultrasound examination to create a real-time, two-dimensional cross-section view of the eye; most commonly used to evaluate eyes with opaque media and orbital structures; the "B" in B-scan is for brightness as echoes are judged by their relative intensities.

b-wave: In electroretinography, the second part of the waveform; generated primarily by the Muller and bipolar cells; *see also* a-wave, c-wave.

bacillary layer (BASS-eh-lair-ee): Layer of column-like cells (rods and cones) in the retina; *also called* columnar layer.

bacillus (buh-SIL-us): Bacterium that is rod-shaped; plural: bacilli.

back surface toric: *Another term for* posterior toric.

back vertex power (BVP): Portion of the total refractive power imparted by the rear surface of a lens; *compare* front vertex power.

background diabetic retinopathy (BDR): *See* diabetic retinopathy.

bacteria: Single-celled organisms, some of which cause disease; classified by shape (*see* bacillus, coccus, spirillum) and staining characteristics (*see* gram stain); of special interest in ophthalmology are *Staphylococcus*, *Streptococcus*, and *Pseudomonas*, among others; singular: bacterium.

bacterial conjunctivitis: *See* conjunctivitis.

bacterial endophthalmitis: *See* endophthalmitis.

bactericidal (bak-truh-SIDE-uhl): Having the property to kill bacteria; *compare* bacteriostatic.

bacteriostatic (bak-teer-ee-o-STAT-ik): Having the property to inhibit growth of bacteria; *compare* bactericidal.

bag: *Another term for* capsular bag.

Bagolini lens (bag-oh-LEEN-ee): Lens with fine parallel lines across its width used to evaluate retinal correspondence.

balanced salt solution: Mixture of water and salts (added to prevent electrolyte imbalance) used as an irrigating fluid in surgery.

balancing: Binocular refractometric technique used to ensure that accommodation is equally relaxed in each eye.

ballast: *See* prism ballast.

band keratopathy/keratitis: *See* keratopathy.

bandage contact lens: *See* contact lens.

bar reader: Device placed between the reader and the page to block out different portions of a page for each eye; used in binocular vision diagnosis and divergence training.

Bard's sign: Phenomenon used to distinguish various types of nystagmus; patient with nystagmus is directed to follow finger motion across the field of view: in congenital nystagmus the rapid eye motions will decrease as the gaze shifts, while in organic nystagmus the motions increase.

barrel distortion: Bowed-out distortion of images that results from the steep curvature of spectacle lenses used to correct severe nearsightedness (ie, strong minus lenses); *compare* pincushion distortion.

barrier filter: In ophthalmic photography, a membrane that removes unwanted light; in fluorescein angiography, a filter that absorbs blue light.

basal cell carcinoma (BAY-zuhl): Common malignant skin lesion, most notably on sun-exposed areas of the face; this carcinoma is invasive, but rarely metastasizes; *compare* melanoma, squamous cell carcinoma.

basal tearing (BAY-zuhl): *See* tearing.

base: Bottom, foundation, or broad area of a structure; **prism b.** broad end of a prism, opposite the apex; *compare* apex.

base curve (BC): General term for the curvature of the standard surface of a lens by which it is described; in spectacle and contact lenses, the base curve is measured on the less steep surface, most commonly the surface of the lens nearest the eye.

base-down (BD), base-in (BI), base-out (BO), and base-up (BU) prism: *See* prism.

basement membrane: General medical term for the layer of tissue underlying some epithelial cell layers.

basement membrane (of choroid): *Another term for* Bruch's membrane.

basement membrane (of corneal epithelium): Thin membrane lying above Bowman's membrane to which the corneal epithelium adheres.

basophil (BAY-soh-fil): *Another term for* mast cell.

BAT: Acronym for brightness acuity test; *see* glare test.

beam splitter: Optical device that uses a partially reflective mirror to divide light into two beams similar in appearance but of reduced intensity, typically to create two images for viewing or two laser beams for delivery.

bedewing (beh-DOO-ing): Appearance of dew-like deposits on the cornea (which is said to be "bedewed"); *see* guttata.

Behr's pupil (bahrz): Dilation of the pupil resulting from a lesion far along the path of the optic nerve; because the two optic nerves cross, the dilated pupil will be on the opposite side of the body from the lesion.

Bell's palsy: Paralysis of the muscles of one side of the face due to inflammation of the facial nerve (CN VII), resulting in an inability to completely close the eyelids on that side; *also called* facial palsy, seventh nerve palsy.

Bell's phenomenon: Normal outward and upward rotation of the eyes that occurs when the lids are closed.

benign (bi-NYN): 1. Not cancerous; used to describe tissue that is localized and noninvasive; *compare* malignant; 2. with no life-threatening significance; harmless.

benign essential blepharospasm (bi-NAHYN): *See* blepharospasm.

Benson's disease or **sign:** *Another term for* asteroid hyalosis; *see* hyalosis.

benzalkonium chloride (ben-zel-KOHN-ee-um KLOOR-ide): Preservative often used in contact lens care solutions and topical ophthalmic medications.

Berlin's edema: Severe swelling of the macula following a blow to the head, resulting in permanent loss of part of the visual field; *also called* commotio retinae.

Berry's circle: Vision test target used to evaluate stereopsis.

best corrected visual acuity (BCVA): Maximum visual acuity that can be achieved using corrective lenses to compensate for any refractive error; *see also* corrected visual acuity; *compare* uncorrected visual acuity.

beta blockers (BEY-tuh): Class of drugs (adrenergic antagonists) used to treat glaucoma by reducing aqueous production (eg, timolol, betaxolol, levobunolol).

bichrome test (BYE-krome): *Another term for* duochrome test.

biconcave lens: Lens that is concave (ie, hollow like a bowl) on both surfaces; a type of minus lens.

biconvex lens: Lens that is convex (ie, bulging outward) on both surfaces; a type of plus lens.

Bielschowsky test (beelz-KOW-skee): *Another term for* head tilt test.

bifocal lens: Lens with two principal focal lengths (*see also* multifocal lens); a variety of such optical systems have been invented for vision correction (eg, bifocal spectacles or contact lenses used to correct presbyopia); there have also been bifocal intraocular lenses, but these represent only a small portion of the lenses in use; *see also* trifocal lens; **executive b.** bifocal in which the segment runs the entire width of the frame; **invisible/no-line b.** *another term for* progressive addition lens.

bifoveal fixation: *See* fixation.

bilateral: Anatomic term meaning on both sides or, in its specific ophthalmic use, both eyes of an individual; *compare* contralateral, ipsilateral, unilateral.

binasal: Occurring nasally in both eyes; *compare* bitemporal.

binocular: Said of visual properties or processes that involve both eyes working together; *compare* monocular; for binocular diplopia, binocular fixation, etc, *see* definitions under main words.

binocular microscope: Microscope that has two oculars (ie, eyepieces) for both the viewer's eyes, thus providing a three-dimensional view.

binocular ophthalmoscope: *See* ophthalmoscope.

binocular vision: A way of expressing the manner in which the two eyes work together; **grade 1 b.v.** vision in which there is simultaneous perception; **grade 2 b.v.** vision in which there is simultaneous perception as well as fusion; **grade 3 b.v.** highest quality of vision in which there is simultaneous perception, fusion, and stereopsis.

bioadhesive (bi-oh-add-HE-siv): "Glue" that is compatible with human tissue and used instead of sutures; *also called* tissue adhesive.

biocompatible (bi-oh-kahm-PAT-uh-buhl): Material or substance that is harmonious with living tissue or organisms.

biohazard: Material or substance that is dangerous to humans or the environment.

biometry (bye-AHM-uh-tree): In ophthalmology, usually referring to ultrasonic measurements, especially A-scan; *see also* A-scan.

biomicroscope: *Another term for* slit lamp.

bioptics (bye-AHP-tiks): 1. Spectacles incorporating a telescopic lens system for use by low-vision patients; 2. in refractive surgery, the combination of two procedures to correct a large refractive error (eg, LASIK and phakic lens implantation).

bipolar cells: Retinal cells that bridge the light-perceiving bacillary layer and underlying nerve cells; *see also* retina.

biprism: 1. Measuring tip in Goldmann tonometry that splits the mires into two half-circles that are then aligned properly when measuring intraocular pressure; 2. base-to-base prisms used to measure cyclodeviations.

bitemporal: Occurring temporally in both eyes; *compare* binasal.

bitoric lens (bye-TOHR-ik): Contact lens that has a toric front surface to correct astigmatism and a toric back surface to prevent the lens from rotating, thus keeping it oriented in the proper axis.

Bitot's spots (BEE-toh): Tiny, dull, grayish lesions on the bulbar conjunctiva caused by vitamin A deficiency.

Bjerrum's area (beh-JEHR-uhms): Area of retinal nerve fibers corresponding to the area between 12 degrees and 20 degrees of the visual field; this is the most vulnerable area to damage by glaucoma.

Bjerrum's scotoma or **sign (beh-JEHR-uhms):** *See* scotoma.

black cataract: *See* cataract.

blanching of sclera: Whitening of the sclera.

blank: Unfinished spectacle or contact lens that has not yet been ground to its final refractive power.

blank size: Millimeter measurement of the lens blank required for a pair of spectacles; calculated by adding the effective diameter (ED) of the eyewire (with decentration, if any), plus 2 mm to allow for edging; *see also* effective diameter.

bleb: Soft-tissue space filled with fluid, most commonly in ophthalmic usage referring to a space created to receive drainage of aqueous fluid in glaucoma-filtering surgery.

blend: Smoothing of the junctions between the zones of a contact lens to increase comfort and reduce prismatic aberration.

blephar-, -o-: Combining form meaning eyelid.

blepharitis (blef-uh-RI-tis): Inflammation of the eyelid, most often referring to the edge of the lid along which the eyelashes are located; **angular b.** blepharitis with inflammation mainly of the canthi; **anterior b.** type of chronic blepharitis attributed to staphylococcus or seborrhea; **marginal** or **posterior b.** type of chronic blepharitis due to meibomian gland disorders; **seborrheic b.** blepharitis associated with seborrhea, thus marked by scaling and sometimes redness and itching.

blepharochalasis (blef-uh-roh-kuh-LAY-sis): Condition in which the skin of the eyelid sags, sometimes enough to overlap the lid margin and block vision; *see also* dermatochalasis.

blepharoconjunctivitis (blef-uh-roh-con-junk-tiv-AHY-tis): Inflammation of the conjunctiva and eyelid.

blepharophimosis (blef-uh-ro-fuh-MO-sis): Hereditary condition involving marked ptosis, epicanthal folds, and ectropion.

blepharoplasty (BLEF-uh-roh-plas-tee): General term for plastic surgical procedure of the eyelid(s) that can be reconstructive or cosmetic; usually referring to correction of blepharochalasis; *also called* lid lift; *see* blepharochalasis.

blepharoplegia (blef-uh-roh-PLEE-gee-uh): Paralysis of the eyelids.

blepharoptosis (blef-uh-rahp-TOH-sis): *Another term for* ptosis.

blepharorrhaphy (blef-uh-ROHR-uh-fee): Suturing the eyelids together; *also called* tarsorrhaphy.

blepharospasm (BLEF-uh-roh-SPAZ-uhm): Uncontrollable muscle spasm of the eyelid that can vary from a slight twitch (tic) to being strong enough to shut the eye; *see also* spasm, tic; **benign essential b. (BEB)** bilateral, involuntary spasms of the orbicularis oris muscle; the spasms tend to increase in strength and frequency (ie, progresses from a simple tic to a spasm), sometimes to the point of debilitation; *also called* essential b.

blepharostat (BLEF-uh-ro-stat): *See* speculum.

blepharosynechia (blef-uh-roh-suh-NEE-kee-uh): *Another term for* ankyloblepharon.

blind spot: Area in which the retina is joined to the optic nerve such that it forms a "funnel" of nerve cells that is not sensitive to light at its center; not usually noticed subjectively but readily detected even with the most simple visual field test; more properly called the physiologic blind spot to distinguish it from damaged areas of the retina; *also called* the physiologic scotoma; **baring of the bs.** visual field defect involving nerve fiber bundles emanating from the optic nerve and creating an arcuate scotoma arising from the blind spot.

blindism(s): Repetitive motions (eg rocking, rubbing, or pressing on the eyes) exhibited by some blind children; *see also* entopic phenomena.

blindness: Partial (as in the following terms) or total lack of the visual sense, more properly referred to as amaurosis; *see also* count-finger vision, hand-motion vision, light perception vision, light projection vision, no light perception vision, visual acuity; **color b.** colloquial term for impaired visual function at certain wavelengths of light (*see also* specific type of color vision loss [eg, deuteranopia, protanopia, etc]); **cortical/cerebral b.** visual loss caused by pathology in the visual cortex or an interruption to the blood flow in these areas; *see also* visual cortex; **eclipse b.** central scotoma and decreased vision resulting from direct viewing of a solar eclipse and resultant exposure to ultraviolet radiation; recovery may take months, if it occurs at all; **flash b.** usually temporary loss of vision due to an intense flash of light; **hysterical b.** state of visual impairment that has an emotional rather than physical or physiological cause; **legal b.** state of visual impairment defined by public law or legal contract (eg, an insurance policy) precluding certain activities such as driving, and qualifying individuals for certain tax or social service benefits; legal blindness is usually defined as best corrected Snellen's acuity of 20/200 or less in the better-seeing eye or visual field of 20 degrees or less; **night b.** *see* nyctalopia; **river b.** *see* onchocerciasis; **snow b.** temporary decreased vision usually accompanied by corneal epithelium damage resulting from exposure to solar radiation reflected from snow; **word b.** *see* alexia.

blink reflex: Automatic response of eyelids to close; normal blinking (about every 8 seconds) serves to swab the ocular surface with tears; reflex blinking can be caused by ocular irritation, bright light, an object coming toward the eye, or a sudden noise.

blood-aqueous barrier, blood-eye barrier, or **blood-vitreous barrier:** Physiologic mechanisms that generally prevent passage of fluid or cells from the blood into the eye.

blown pupil: Pupil that is fixed and dilated and does not respond to any stimuli; *also called* fixed, dilated pupil.

blowout fracture (of the orbit): Fracture in which the bones comprising the eye socket are disconnected and displaced outward from their normal position; if the fracture occurs in the orbital floor, extraocular muscles may herniate through the opening, limiting range of motion and causing diplopia.

blue cone monochromatism: *Another term for* monochromatism.

blue-yellow perimetry: Colloquial term for visual field test in which the test targets are blue and yellow, which appears to enhance the ability of the test to locate field defects.

blur point: In testing visual acuity, the blur point is reached when the refractive power of a lens or prism can no longer be increased without causing vision to be blurred.

botulin or **botulinum (BTX) (BOCH-uh-lin** or **boch-uh-LIE-num):** Toxic substance produced by *Clostridium botulinum* bacteria; used in ophthalmology for treatment of blepharospasm and certain types of strabismus.

Bowman's capsule, layer, or **membrane:** Layer of the cornea lying above the corneal stroma and beneath the corneal epithelium; *also called* anterior basal membrane.

boxing system: Standardized way of measuring spectacle frames; *see also* "A" measurement, "B" measurement, "C" measurement.

brachytherapy (brack-uh-THAYR-uh-pee): A cancer radiation therapy that involves placing a radioactive source (implant) in or near a tumor.

brain noise: In visual evoked response test results, extraneous waves that look like a response but are instead just brain activity unrelated to the stimulus.

branch retinal artery (BRA): One of the small arteries that branch off the central retinal artery.

branch retinal artery occlusion (BRAO): Blockage of a branch retinal artery, usually in the temporal retina, impairing retinal blood flow but often resulting in no loss of vision or only minor visual field loss.

branch retinal vein (BRV): One of the small veins in the retina that drains into the central retinal vein.

branch retinal vein occlusion (BRVO): Blockage of blood flow in an area where a branch retinal vein is crossed by a branch retinal artery, resulting in retinal hemorrhage and a sudden blurring or loss of vision in part of the visual field.

break point: In ocular motility, the point at which the subject cannot maintain fusion; 1. the near distance at which convergence fails and one eye drifts out; *see* near point of convergence; 2. the initial amount of prism that induces diplopia; *compare* recovery point.

break-up time (BUT): Length of time from the blink of an eye until the tear film evaporates, usually measured at the slit lamp using fluorescein dye; *also called* tear break-up time; *see also* symptomatic tear film break-up time.

bridge: Part of a spectacle frame front that crosses the nose and joins the two eyepieces.

bridle suture: Suture placed through the insertion of an extraocular muscle in order to give the surgeon control over the position of the eye.

brightness acuity test (BAT): *See* glare test.

browlift: Cosmetic surgical procedure to elevate the eyebrows; often paired with blepharoplasty; *see also* blepharoplasty, browplasty.

Brown's syndrome: Condition, usually congenital but possibly as a result of trauma or arthritis, in which fibrous adhesions of the tendon sheath of the superior oblique muscle prevent the eye from looking upward in adduction; *also called* sheath syndrome, superior oblique tendon sheath syndrome.

browplasty: General term referring to any surgery of the eyebrow, usually referring to a browlift; *see* browlift.

Bruch's membrane (brooks): Innermost layer of the choroid to which the retinal pigment epithelium adheres; *also called* basement membrane of choroid.

brunescent (broo-NESS-ent): Brown; descriptive of very mature, dark cataracts; *see also* cataract.

Brushfield's spots: Tiny white, crescent-shaped spots on the iris periphery, often associated with Down syndrome.

buckle: *See* scleral buckle.

buckling procedure: *See* scleral buckling procedure.

bulb: In ophthalmic usage, synonym for the eyeball.

bulbar conjunctiva (BUHL-bar): Portion of the conjunctiva that covers the eyeball, extending almost to the corneoscleral limbus; *see also* conjunctiva; *compare* palpebral conjunctiva.

bullae (BOOL-ee): Plural of bulla, a blister-like lesion.

bullous keratopathy (BUHL-us kehr-uh-TAHP-uh-thee): Degeneration of the cornea; **pseudophakic b.k.** corneal degeneration attributable to implantation of an intraocular lens.

buphthalmia, -os (boof-THAL-mee-uh, boof-THAL-mus): Abnormal enlargement of a child's eye due to congenital glaucoma, in which high intraocular pressure has distended the globe; *also called* hydrophthalmia.

buttonhole: Complication of LASIK in which a thin, oblong hole forms in the center of the corneal flap.

C

C-loop lens: *See* intraocular lens.

"C" measurement: Horizontal measurement across the front of a pair of spectacles, including the "A" measurement of each eyewire plus the width of the bridge; *also called* datum line; *see also* boxing system.

c-wave: In electroretinography, the part of the waveform generated by the retinal pigment epithelium, generally obtained only if the patient is sedated; *see also* a-wave, b-wave.

caloric nystagmus: *See* nystagmus.

canaliculitis (can-uh-lik-yuh-LITE-us): Inflammation of the tear duct, usually a result of infection or operative procedure.

canaliculus (can-uh-LIK-yuh-luhs): Tear duct, more properly called canaliculus nasolacrimalis; plural: canaliculi; **common c.** junction of superior and inferior c. that then joins into the lacrimal sac; **inferior c.** canaliculus running from the lower punctum and to the common canaliculus; **superior c.** canaliculus running from the upper punctum and to the common canaliculus.

canal of Schlemm: *See* Schlemm's canal.

cancer: General term describing cells that destroy tissue and potentially result in death; *see* type of cancer (eg, basal cell carcinoma, etc).

candela (cd): Standard unit used in measurement of the intensity of light; the metric unit that replaced the "candle."

cannula (KAN-yuh-luh): Tube used in surgery to perform irrigation or aspiration of fluids or to introduce smaller instruments into an incision.

can-opener capsulotomy: *See* capsulotomy.

canthotomy (kan-THAW-tuh-mee): Surgical procedure in which an incision is made into the area where the upper and lower eyelids meet.

canthus (KAN-thuhs): Either of two angles formed by the meeting of the upper and lower eyelids; *also called* angle, ocular angle, tarsal angle; the one near the temple is called the lateral canthus and the one near the nose is called the medial canthus; plural: canthi.

capsular advancement: *See* advancement.

capsular bag: Membrane that encases the crystalline lens, attached to the ciliary muscle via zonules; *also called* bag.

capsular opacification: Cloudiness of the lens capsule resulting from the spread of lens epithelial cells across the part of the capsule that remains after cataract extraction; *also called* after-cataract, secondary membrane.

capsular tension ring (CTR): Polymethylmethacrylate device used to stabilize the capsular bag and lens during cataract surgery; it may be left in the eye postoperatively.

capsule: General medical term for the outer membrane surrounding an anatomic structure; most commonly in ophthalmic usage referring to the lens capsule, the transparent round sac containing the lens of the eye, attached at its periphery by the zonules to the ciliary body, often referred to as the capsular bag or simply "the bag"; **anterior c.** front portion of the capsule between the lens and the iris; **Bowman's c.** corneal layer between the stroma and epithelium; **posterior c.** rear portion of the capsule between the lens and the vitreous body; **Tenon's c.** thin, outermost membrane of the eye enclosing the entire globe except for the cornea.

capsulectomy (kap-suh-LEK-tuh-me): General term for surgical removal of a capsule.

capsulorrhexis (KAP-soo-loh-REKS-his): 1. Surgical procedure in which an anterior capsulotomy is made by puncturing, then grasping and tearing a hole in the capsule rather than by simply cutting it with a sharp instrument; *compare* can-opener capsulotomy under capsulotomy; 2. the opening made in the capsule in this manner.

capsulotomy (kap-suh-LOT-uh-me): 1. Surgical procedure to make an opening in a capsule, usually the lens capsule, as the first step in extracapsular cataract extraction; 2. the opening made in the capsule in this manner; **anterior c.** surgical procedure to open the anterior capsule (or the opening itself), most commonly as one step in removal of a cataractous lens (*see also* can-opener c., capsulorrhexis); **can-opener c.** surgical technique in which a series of small cuts are made in a circle around the periphery of the anterior lens capsule, which is then removed; *compare* capsulorrhexis; **posterior c.** surgical procedure to open the posterior capsule (or the opening itself), often referring to the procedure performed with the Nd:YAG laser to open an opacified posterior capsule months or years after cataract extraction.

carbon dioxide (CO$_2$) laser: *See* laser.

carbonic anhydrase inhibitor (CAI) (kahr-BAHN-ik ann-HY-drayz): Class of glaucoma medications that act by reducing aqueous formation (eg, dorzolamide [topical], acetazolamide [oral]).

carcinoma (CA) (kahr-suh-NOH-mah): Malignant growth arising from epithelial tissue.

cardinal fields/positions of gaze: *See* gaze; *also called* fields of gaze.

cardinal points: Six points on the axis of an optical system that are used in describing its properties.

caruncle (CAR-ung-kuhl): *See* lacrimal caruncle.

CAT scan: *See* computerized tomography.

cataract: Area of opacification in ocular tissue that impedes the transmission of light rays to the retina; most commonly, the opacification of the lens that occurs as a natural consequence of aging, which is a leading cause of blindness in many parts of the world but surgically corrected on a wide scale (and with great success) in the developed world where ophthalmologic care is available; **acquired c.** noncongenital juvenile cataract; **after c.** opacification of the posterior lens capsule, following removal of a cataractous crystalline lens; the term is somewhat of a misnomer because the cataract does not actually recur; *see* capsular opacification; **annular c.** ring-shaped opacity of the lens in which the central lens remains clear; **axial c.** opacity located in the optical axis of the crystalline lens; **black c.** very mature (ie, advanced stage) cataract that is opaque black, very dense, and hard; **brunescent c.** very mature cataract that has a brownish appearance, often very dense and hard; **capsular c.** *see* capsular opacification; **complicated c.** *another term for* secondary c.; **congenital c.** cataract present at birth; **cortical c.** opacification of the lens cortex, usually in radial streaks or spokes, rather than the nucleus; **degenerative c.** opacification of ocular tissue that results from a degenerative change; *compare* developmental c.; **developmental c.** opacification of ocular tissue that results from a disturbance of normal development; *compare* degenerative c.; **hypermature c.** progression of mature cataract to a state in which the lens begins to shrink and eventually soften, with harmful leakage of lens proteins; **immature/incipient c.** faint lenticular changes that do not affect vision; **intumescent c.** opacified lens that has swelled with absorbed fluid; **juvenile c.** cataract occurring in childhood; **lamellar c.** most common type of congenital cataract, with opacity occurring between the nucleus and outer lens fibers; *also called* zonular cataract; **lenticular c.**

opacification of the crystalline lens; **mature c.** crystalline lens that has become opaque and exceedingly hard over a prolonged period of time; **morgagnian c.** progression of hypermature cataract in which the lens cortex is completely liquefied and the hard, opaque nucleus is no longer held stationary in the lens capsule; **nuclear c.** or **nuclear sclerosis (NS) c.** opacification of the center (nucleus) of the crystalline lens; **peripheral c.** opacification that is out of the optical axis and thus only minimally impairs vision; **polar c.** opacification located at the anterior or posterior pole of the crystalline lens; **posterior subcapsular c. (PSC)** opacification of the posterior part of the lens nucleus; **presurgical c.** cataract that does not yet warrant removal; **secondary c.** cataract associated with intraocular disorders, such as uveitis; the term is sometimes mistakenly applied to capsular opacification; *also called* complicated c., **senile c.** cataract occurring in an elderly individual as a natural part of aging; **subcapsular c.** opacification of the inner surfaces of the lens capsule caused by overgrowth of epithelial cells; **traumatic c.** opacification of ocular tissue (especially the crystalline lens) resulting from a blow or penetrating injury to the eye, often quite rapid in onset and profound in extent; **zonular c.** *another term for* lamellar cataract.

cataract extraction (CE): General term for surgical procedures to remove the opacified crystalline lens of the eye; all such procedures have in common an incision into the anterior chamber of the eye, but there are many variations in the size of the incision, its location, and the instrumentation and technique used to remove the lens material; the eye immediately after cataract extraction is in a state known as aphakia (ie, without a lens), and an eye in which an intraocular lens has been implanted is said to be pseudophakic (ie, "false" lens); *see also* cryoextraction, extracapsular cataract extraction, intracapsular cataract extraction, phacoemulsification.

cataract glasses: *Another term for* aphakic spectacles; *see* aphakic.

cataractogenic (kat-uh-rak-toh-JEN-ik): Causing or facilitating the formation of a cataract.

cataractous (kat-uh-RAK-tus): Ocular tissue that is like or affected by cataract.

catarrh (kuh-TAHR): General term meaning inflammation of a mucous membrane; in ophthalmology, generally referring to vernal conjunctivitis; **spring c.** *another term for* vernal conjunctivitis; *see* conjunctivitis.

catch trial: In visual fields, the presentation of a target brighter than the subject previously responded to at that point or an interval where no target is presented in order to help determine subject reliability.

cat's eye pupil: Condition in which the pupil is a narrow, vertical slit.

cautery: Use of heat to burn or scar tissue; can also refer to similar use of electric current, cold (*see* cryo-), or chemicals.

cavitation (kav-uh-TAY-shun): In ophthalmic usage, a phenomenon in which the ultrasonically vibrating phacoemulsification tip creates microscopic areas of intense turbulence that pulverizes lens material.

cell: In ophthalmic usage, the appearance of white blood cells in the anterior chamber as a result of inflammation, most often following surgery or trauma; *see also* flare.

cell and flare (C/F): In ophthalmic usage, usually the appearance of white blood cells in the anterior chamber accompanied by the presence of protein particles in the aqueous humor, indicating intraocular inflammation, usually after surgery or trauma.

cellophane maculopathy/retinopathy (mac-u-LOP-uh-thee): Wrinkling of an epiretinal membrane associated with distorted vision; *see also* epiretinal membrane.

cellulitis (sel-yuh-LIE-tus): Infection of a diffuse nature, generally of tissue just under the skin; **orbital c.** infection involving the contents of the orbit, including the globe, producing redness, swelling, pain, and exophthalmos; **pre-septal c.** infection of the subcutaneous tissues around the orbit.

cellulose acetate butyrate (CAB) (SEL-yuh-lohs AS-uh-tayt BYOO-tuh-rayt): One of several plastics from which rigid gas permeable lenses are made.

cellulose sponge: A widely used surgical instrument consisting of a wedge of absorptive cellulose material mounted on a short handle.

central fixation: *See* fixation.

central fusion: *See* fusion.

central nervous system (CNS): The half of the nervous system controlled by the brain and spinal cord.

central retinal artery: One of the main blood vessels bringing blood into the retina from the ophthalmic artery.

central retinal artery occlusion (CRAO): Blockage of the central retinal artery resulting in sudden, permanent loss of vision across a wide area of the visual field.

central retinal vein: Major vein that drains blood from the retina, exiting the eye in the area of the optic nerve.

central retinal vein occlusion (CRVO): Blockage of the central retinal vein resulting in retinal hemorrhage and sudden loss of vision, usually involving the central visual field.

central scotoma: *See* scotoma.

central serous chorioretinopathy (CSC) (SEER-uhs KOH-ree-oh-ret-in-OP-uh-thee): Condition similar to central serous retinopathy, except with greater involvement of the choroid; *see* central serous retinopathy.

central serous retinopathy (CSR) (SEER-uhs ret-in-OP-uh-thee): Condition in which there is swelling and elevation of retinal tissues in the area of the macula, sometimes progressing to the point of detachment, that causes a perceptible but usually not permanent visual field loss.

central suppression: Action of the brain to ignore the portion of the image in the center of the visual field.

central vision: Vision obtained with the macula/fovea.

central visual acuity: That level of vision when an image is focused directly on the fovea, as opposed to peripheral vision.

centrocecal scotoma (sen-troh-SEE-kul): *See* scotoma.

cerebrum (suh-REE-bruhm): Largest part of the brain, made up of four lobes (frontal, parietal, temporal, occipital).

chalazion (kuh-LAY-zee-uhn or shuh-LAY-zee-uhn): Chronic granuloma of the eyelid resulting from blockage and inflammation of a meibomian gland; *see also* meibomian cyst; *compare* hordeolum.

chalcosis (kal-KOH-sis): Copper deposits, generally in the cornea.

chatter: In ophthalmic usage, undesirable phenomenon in phacoemulsification in which the crystalline lens rapidly vibrates on the instrument tip as it is simultaneously attracted by aspiration and repelled by the vibration of the tip.

chemodenervation (kee-moh-dee-ner-VAY-shun): Use of a compound (eg, botulinum A toxin) to block the impulse from a nerve to the muscle; used in the treatment of strabismus and blepharospasm and for cosmetic purposes; *see also* botulin.

chemosis (kee-MOH-sis): Swelling of the conjunctiva; adjective: chemotic.

cherry-red spot: Descriptive term referring to the condition in which the macula is bright red due to retinal ischemia; often associated with central retinal artery occlusion.

chiasm (KY-az-uhm): General anatomic term for an intersection (from the Greek letter chi, which is written as X); in ophthalmology, referring to the optic chiasm; *see* optic chiasm.

chief complaint: The main reason that the patient has sought medical care; features include onset, duration, location, and degree; *see also* history.

***Chlamydia* (kluh-MID-ee-uh):** An unusual bacteria that requires a host for reproduction like a virus; of concern in ophthalmology is the chlamydial disease trachoma; *see* trachoma.

chlorolabe (KLOHR-oh-layb): Visual pigment present in the "green" retinal cones that absorbs light in the green frequencies (around 540 nm); one of three visual pigments; *see also* cyanolabe, erythrolabe, trichromatism.

choked disk: *Another term for* papilledema.

cholinergic (koh-luh-NUR-jik): Refers to substances that activate the parasympathetic nervous system; pilocarpine (a miotic) is a cholinergic drug; *see also* acetylcholine; *compare* adrenergic; **c.-blocking** *another term for* parasympatholytic.

cholinesterase (koh-luh-NES-tuh-rase): Enzyme that "cleans up" the neurotransmitter acetylcholine; blocking its action allows the neurotransmitter to have a prolonged effect; *see also* anticholinesterase, neurotransmitter.

chondroitin sulfate (kahn-DROIT-un SUHL-fayt): Component of some viscoelastic materials.

choriopathy (koh-ree-OHP-uh-thee): Noninflammatory disease of the choroid.

chorioretinal (KOHR-ee-oh-RET-in-uhl): Of or involving the choroid and retina.

choroid (KOHR-oyd): Highly vascular tissue layer lying under the retina, merging at the angle of the anterior chamber with the ciliary body and the iris (all three structures comprise the uvea).

choroidal detachment (kohr-OYD-ul): Separation of the choroid from the sclera, usually as a result of injury.

choroidal flush or **phase (kohr-OYD-ul):** Initial phase of fluorescein angiography in which dye first enters the retinal vasculature, causing a glow in the choroid; may not always be visible as a separate phase; *see also* fluorescein angiography.

choroidal neovascular membrane (kohr-OYD-ul nee-oh-VAS-cu-lar): Network of vascular tissue resulting from choroidal neovascularization.

choroidal neovascularization (CNV) (kohr-OYD-ul nee-oh-vas-cu-lar-i-ZAY-shun): Condition in which new, abnormal blood vessels grow into the choroid beneath the retinal pigment epithelium.

choroidal nevus (kohr-OYD-ul NEE-vus): Small, well-defined area of benign pigmentation or vascularization in the choroid.

choroideremia (KOHR-oyd-er-EE-me-uh): Sex-linked hereditary condition in which the retinal pigment epithelium and choroid begin to degenerate in the first few months or years after birth; in males it eventually leads to blindness but in females it rarely causes significant vision loss.

choroiditis (KOHR-oyd-I-tus): Inflammatory disease of the choroid; type of posterior uveitis; *see also* uveitis.

chromatic aberration: Uneven focusing of an optical system such that white light is partially or completely broken down into its component colors; *see also* aberration.

chromosomes: Thread-like structures made up of genes and found in the nucleus of every body cell; chromosomes occur in pairs, half contributed by the mother and half by the father at conception; collectively they determine the genetic make-up of an individual; *see also* gene; **sex c.** the chromosomes responsible for determining sex (ie, the X [female] or Y [male] chromosome).

chronic: In medical usage, denoting long-term or a non-emergency; *compare* acute, subacute.

cicatrix (SIK-uh-triks): Scar tissue; adjective: cicatricial; some cases of ectropion and entropion are described as cicatricial, and some glaucoma operations construct what is known as a cicatricial filter.

cilia: Plural of cilium.

ciliaris (sil-ee-AYR-uhs): *Another term for* ciliary muscle.

ciliary: 1. Of or related to the eyelashes; 2. of or related to the ring-shaped structure joining the iris and choroid; *see* ciliary body.

ciliary arteries: Several branches of the ophthalmic artery that carry blood to every anatomic structure of the eye except the inner part of the retina.

ciliary body: Ring-shaped structure joining the iris to the choroid and containing the ciliary muscle and ciliary processes.

ciliary muscle: Ring-shaped muscle in the ciliary body; it contracts when stimulated by a near target; *also called* ciliaris; *see also* accommodation.

ciliary nerves: Any of several nerve fiber bundles that carry nerve impulses to the pupillary sphincter and ciliary muscle as well as from the cornea (short ciliary nerves) or that carry impulses either to the pupillary dilator muscle or sensory impulses from the cornea, iris, and ciliary body (long ciliary nerves).

ciliary processes: Finger-shaped extensions of the ciliary body that produce aqueous humor and provide an attachment for the zonules that support the lens capsule.

ciliary spasm: Painful contractions of the ciliary body due to some pathologic condition (eg, iritis), drug (eg, pilocarpine), or sustained accommodation (*also called* accommodative spasm).

ciliary sulcus: Groove formed by the junction of the ciliary body and iris; posterior chamber intraocular lenses are sometimes placed into the sulcus when implantation into the lens capsule is not possible.

ciliary veins: Any of several veins that drain blood from the major structures of the eye.

ciliary zonules: *Another term for* zonules.

cilium (SIL-ee-um): Proper term for an eyelash; plural: cilia.

circle of least confusion: In optics, area of the conoid of Sturm that represents the least-distorted portion of an image that is transmitted by an optical system that is spherical along one axis and cylindrical along another; *see also* conoid of Sturm.

circle of Zinn: *Another term for* annulus of Zinn.

circumduction: In ophthalmic usage, circular "rolling" of the eye, applicable to voluntary and involuntary movement.

clear lensectomy or **clear lens removal:** Refractive surgical procedure to correct large degrees of nearsightedness by removing the crystalline lens.

clock dial: *Another term for* astigmatic clock.

closed-angle glaucoma: *See* glaucoma.

CMV (cytomegalovirus) retinitis (si-toh-MEG-uh-loh-VI-rus): *See* retinitis.

cobalt blue filter: Light filter placed on the slit lamp light source to induce fluorescence of topical fluorescein dye for corneal examination; *see also* exciter filter.

coccus (KOK-us): Bacterium that is round shaped; may occur singly or in pairs, clusters, or strands; plural: cocci.

Cogan's microcystic dystrophy (KOH-gunz): *Another term for* map-dot-fingerprint dystrophy; *see* corneal dystrophy.

coherent light: Light in which all of the component waves are in phase as in a laser beam; *see also* laser, phase (definition 1).

collagen shield: Protein-based contact lens used as a temporary corneal bandage; enzymes in the tears dissolve the shield within hours or days.

collarette: 1. *Another term for* cylindrical dandruff; 2. border between the pupillary and ciliary zones of the iris, visible on the anterior surface of the iris as a line of transitional color about 1.5 mm from the edge of the pupil.

collyrium (kuh-LEER-ee-um): General term for an eyewash.

coloboma (kohl-uh-BOH-mah): Partial absence of or gap in ocular structures, as in retinal coloboma, iris coloboma, etc, usually in the lower half of the eye and usually as a result of incomplete fusion of fetal tissue; **atypical c.** coloboma in the upper half of the eye.

color: Subjective perception of the varying wavelengths of light.

color adaptation: *See* adaptation.

color blindness: *See* blindness, type of defect (eg, deuteranopia, protanopia, etc).

color vision test: Any of several tests designed to identify and/or quantify color blindness; *see also* specific tests such as anomaloscope, Ishihara's test, etc.

columnar layer: *Another term for* bacillary layer.

coma (KOH-ma): In optics, the higher-order aberration that distorts an image across one axis so that it is focused too strongly on one side of the axis and too weakly on the other side of the same axis, often resulting in blurring and "ghosting" of images.

comitant (strabismus): *See* strabismus.

commotio retinae (kuh-MOH-shee-oh RET-in-ee): *Another term for* Berlin's edema.

compliance: Meeting guidelines; may refer to the patient (as in compliance with treatment programs) or to the physician/practitioner (as in compliance with laws and other specifications).

compound astigmatism, compound hyperopic astigmatism, or **compound myopic astigmatism:** *See* astigmatism.

computerized tomography (CT or **CAT) scan (tuh-MAH-gruh-fee):** Imaging technique using ionizing radiation to visualize inner structures of the body; in ophthalmology, used to evaluate fractures, inflammation, or tumors; *compare* magnetic resonance imaging.

concave: Having a curved, indented surface, like the inside of a bowl; *compare* convex.

concave lens: Lens with a concave surface that causes parallel rays of light to diverge and thus can be used to correct myopia; *see also* minus lens; *compare* convex lens; **double c.l.** lens that has two concave surfaces.

concavoconvex lens: Lens that has one concave and one convex surface; *also called* meniscus lens.

concomitant (strabismus): *See* strabismus.

conductive keratoplasty (CK): Refractive surgical procedure to correct hyperopia and presbyopia in emmetropes and hyperopes in which radiofrequency energy is applied to the peripheral cornea; usually referring to a proprietary treatment employing a radiofrequency probe; *compare* laser thermal keratoplasty.

cone: Term used in ophthalmic applications to geometrically describe anatomic structures and optical properties; **distraction c.** white crescent-shaped area sometimes seen on funduscopy in myopic eyes; **myopic c.** staphyloma at the posterior pole of the eye; **ocular c.** the eyeball and its sheath of muscle, blood vessels, and nerves, approximately conical in shape.

cone cells or **retinal cones:** One of two types of light-sensitive cells in the retina (rods are the other type); often simply referred to as cones, they are concentrated in the macula and function in the discrimination of color and fine detail mainly in the central field of view under lighted conditions; *compare* rod cells.

cone dystrophy: Hereditary degenerative disorder of cone cells with progressive loss of central and color vision.

conformer: Plastic insert placed in the eye after enucleation, over the implant and conjunctiva, to maintain the conjunctival cul-de-sac until a prosthesis can be fit.

confrontation field test: Gross method for measuring the approximate extent of the visual field; the examiner sits facing the test subject and holds a target far to the subject's side, then brings it slowly into the field of view; the subject reports when the object becomes visible; eyes are tested singly; **simultaneous c.f.t.** the examiner holds a hand peripherally on each side of the midline and wiggles the fingers of one or both hands; the patient must identify on which (or both) side there is movement; eyes are tested singly.

congenital: Present at birth; *compare* infantile, juvenile, senile.

congruous (KAHN-groo-us): Similar in form.

congruous field defect (KAHN-groo-us): *See* visual field defect.

congruous hemianopia (KAHN-groo-us hem-mee-uh-NOH-pee-uh): Loss of half the visual field in each eye in which the field defects are the same size, shape, and location.

conjugate movement: *Another term for* version; some references specify parallel movements of the eyes.

conjunctiva (conj) (con-junk-TY-vuh): Ocular tissue lining the inner surface of the eyelids (ie, **palpebral c.**), which folds in to join with the tissue covering the sclera (ie, **bulbar c.**); the "pocket" of the fold is called the cul de sac; **limbal c.** edge of the conjunctiva overlying the sclera near its transition zone into the cornea.

conjunctival impression cytology (CIC) (con-junk-ty-val): A method of determining the concentration of goblet cells in the conjunctiva; goblet cell loss is observed in certain disorders.

conjunctival injection (con-junk-ty-val): Condition in which the conjunctiva is red, swollen, and engorged with dilated blood vessels.

conjunctival sac (con-junk-tahy-vahl): *Another term for* fornix.

conjunctivitis (con-junk-ti-VAHY-tus): General term for inflammation of the conjunctiva; colloquially known as pink eye; **allergic c.** conjunctivitis resulting from an allergic reaction, either to airborne allergens or substances (such as topical medications) placed into the eye; **atopic c.** conjunctivitis occurring as one manifestation of systemic allergy (atopia); **bacterial c.** conjunctivitis resulting from an infection of the surface tissues of the eye; **c. of newborn** purulent conjunctivitis of an infant less than 2 weeks old; **follicular c.** appearance of tiny clear or yellow sacs of lymphocytes and inflammatory cells on the conjunctiva after prolonged irritation, often as a result of viral infection; **giant papillary c. (GPC)** condition in which wart-like protrusions (ie, papillae) appear on the inside of the eyelid accompanied by mucus discharge; *also called* papillary c.; **herpetic c.** conjunctivitis resulting from an infection with herpes virus; **inclusion c.** inflammation of the conjunctiva due to presence of *Chlamydia* organisms; **neonatal c.** conjunctivitis in the newborn; *see also* ophthalmia neonatorum; **papillary c.** *another term for* giant papillary c.; **vernal** or **seasonal c.** chronic allergic conjunctivitis that occurs in both eyes during warm weather; *also called* spring catarrh, vernal catarrh, warm weather c.; **viral c.** conjunctivitis resulting from an infection with a virus.

conoid of Sturm (KOH-noid uv STERM): Geometric representation of light refracted through a lens that is spherical along one axis and cylindrical along another; *see also* circle of least confusion.

consecutive: In ophthalmic usage, describing a condition (usually unwanted) that results after surgery (eg, consecutive hyperopia is an adverse result of radial keratotomy to correct myopia); *also called* induced (definition 1).

consensual pupillary reflex: *See* pupillary reflex.

consent: *See* informed consent.

constant exotropia: *See* exotropia.

constriction: 1. Referring to abnormally closed-in isopters on a visual field map; 2. decrease in pupillary size as a reaction to light, accommodation, injury, or drugs; *see also* miosis; 3. narrowing of an opening (eg, punctum, etc).

contact angle: *Another term for* wetting angle.

contact dermatitis: Reaction (often allergic) to a substance that has come into contact with the skin.

contact lens (CL): 1. Hand-held lens system, usually incorporating prisms and/or mirrors, placed on the cornea to provide a view inside the eye or to focus laser energy for delivery into the eye; 2. vision-correcting lens placed directly on the cornea of the eye; **bandage c.l.** lens used for therapeutic purposes (usually to protect the cornea or deliver medication following surgery or trauma) rather than to correct vision; **corneal c.l.** contact lens designed to rest upon the cornea rather than extending onto the sclera; **daily wear (DW) c.l.** contact lens that is approved for wear during waking hours only and is to be removed every day; **disposable c.l.** soft contact lens that is worn for a specified time then discarded and replaced with a fresh lens; **extended wear (EW) c.l.** contact lens that is approved for wear during sleep; **fitting c.l.** lens used to check for correct fit on patient before a contact lens prescription is given or lenses dispensed; *also called* trial c.l.; **gas-permeable (GP) c.l.** modern contact lens composed of polymers formulated to transmit oxygen; **hard c.l.** contact lens composed of polymethylmethacrylate (rarely used now); **keratoconus c.l.** rigid contact lens designed to correct and retard keratoconus;

piggyback c.l. technique in which two contacts are placed on top of each other in the same eye, most usually a soft lens with a rigid lens on top; **rigid c.l.** contact lens made of relatively inflexible material (versus "soft"); term usually refers to gas-permeable contacts; **scleral c.l.** contact lens designed so that its periphery rests on the sclera rather than the cornea; **soft (S) c.l.** modern contact lens made from silicone or water-containing hydroxyethylmethacrylate (HEMA); **toric c.l.** contact lens that incorporates cylinder power to correct astigmatism; **trial c.l.** *another term for* fitting c.l.

contraindication: Reason(s) why a treatment or procedure should not be done.

contralateral: Anatomic term meaning on opposite sides; *compare* bilateral, ipsilateral, unilateral; **c. synergists** *another term for* yoke muscles.

contrast: Property of an image such that it has bright and dark areas; the relative brightness of the various components can be measured in comparison to each other or against a reference gray scale.

contrast sensitivity: The ability to distinguish fine gradations of brightness, often diminished under conditions of glare, especially in the presence of a cataract and other ocular pathology.

contrast sensitivity test (CST): Vision test target consisting of patterns of lines (sine-wave gratings) of various densities: the test subject is asked to describe the orientation of the lines (vertical, horizontal, oblique); acuity is the most closely spaced lines that the subject can correctly discern; the basis for the test is that the traditional eye chart is high contrast, giving a measurement of better acuity than actually exists, especially in the presence of cataracts and other pathology.

contusion: General medical term referring to bruising.

converge: General term meaning coming together; *see also* convergence; *compare* diverge; 1. in ophthalmic usage, the turning of both eyes inward; 2. in optics, the bending of light rays such that they come together.

convergence: 1. In optics, the gathering together of parallel light rays to a point of focus after passing through a plus lens; 2. in ophthalmic usage, coordinated action of ocular muscles that draws both eyes inward to fixate upon the same point in space; the processes of convergence and accommodation normally are linked; *compare* divergence; **accommodative c.** convergence stimulated by and working in conjunction with accommodation; **fusional c.** convergence operating to keep an image focused upon the foveae of both eyes; **maximum c.** or **near point of c.** point at which the eyes can no longer maintain fixation together on an approaching near object and one eye drifts out; **proximal c.** convergence generated by the perception that an object is near; **tonic c.** degree of convergence maintained by the tone of the ocular muscles.

convergence amplitudes: Measurement of break and recovery points of convergence using base-out prism; increased prism power is introduced until the subject reports diplopia (break point), then decreased until there is again one image (recovery point).

convergence excess: Condition in which the eyes "overshoot" (ie, move inward too much) during near vision.

convergence insufficiency: Condition in which the eyes fail to turn inward enough to achieve or maintain fusion during near vision.

convergent deviation or **strabismus:** *Another term for* esotropia.

convergent lens: *Another term for* plus lens.

convex: Having a rounded, protruding surface, like a globe; *compare* concave.

convex lens: Lens with a convex surface that causes parallel rays of light to converge and thus can be used to correct hyperopia; *see also* plus lens; *compare* concave lens; **double c.l.** lens that has two convex surfaces.

convexoconcave lens (kahn-VEKS-oh-kahn-KAYV): Lens that has one convex and one concave surface; *also called* meniscus lens.

core-, -o-: Combining form meaning pupil.

corectopia (kohr-ek-TOH-pee-uh): Condition in which the pupil is not in the center of the iris.

cornea (K): Clear structure at the front of the eye overlying the iris; it imparts the greatest focusing power of all the ocular media; composed (from outer- to innermost) of the epithelium, Bowman's membrane, the stroma, Descemet's membrane, and the endothelium; the cornea joins the sclera at the limbus and consists of similar tough, fibrous tissue; *see also* words beginning with the root kerat-, meaning cornea.

corneal abrasion: Injury in which tissues are scraped from an area on the surface of the cornea, usually involving the corneal epithelium but possibly extending more deeply.

corneal astigmatism: *See* astigmatism.

corneal bedewing: Dew-like beads on the surface of the cornea, usually visible only under magnification; *see* guttata.

corneal button: Piece of corneal tissue, either full thickness (for penetrating keratoplasty) or partial thickness (a lamellar keratoplasty), intended for use as a graft.

corneal cap: Complication of LASIK surgery in which the corneal flap detaches; *see also* flap.

corneal decompensation: Condition in which chronic failure of the corneal endothelium to maintain the proper water content of the corneal stroma results in swelling, clouding, and degeneration of the cornea.

corneal dellen: Small concavities at the outer edges of the cornea that sometimes appear after ocular surgery.

corneal dystrophy: General term for hereditary condition in which there is defective development or degeneration of corneal tissue; **Cogan's microcystic c.d.** *another term for* map-dot-fingerprint c.d.; **endothelial c.d.**

condition, possibly worse in one eye than the other but always present bilaterally, in which guttata appear in the corneal endothelium, eventually resulting in loss of vision due to corneal edema as normal endothelial function is impaired; *see also* guttata; **epithelial basement membrane c.d.** *another term for* map-dot-fingerprint c.d.; **Fuchs' c.d.** progressive degeneration of the cornea related to dysfunction of the corneal epithelium; *also called* Fuchs' endothelial dystrophy (FED); **lattice d.** progressive condition, usually beginning around puberty, in which lines of opacification appear through the corneal stroma and slowly increase in thickness and number; *also called* lattice keratitis; **map-dot-fingerprint (MDF) c.d.** condition in which small concentric dots and lines with the appearance of a map or fingerprint appear in the corneal epithelium; *also called* Cogan's microcystic c.d., epithelial basement membrane dystrophy, fingerprint c.d.

corneal ectasia (ek-TAY-zee-uh): *Another term for* keratectasia.

corneal edema: Condition in which the cornea swells with water and becomes cloudy; almost always a result of damage to the corneal endothelium; *also called* steamy cornea.

corneal endothelium: Innermost layer of the cornea, only one cell thick, that acts to pump excess water out of the cornea; these cells are quite delicate and do not regenerate if damaged.

corneal epithelium: Outermost layer of the cornea, only one cell thick, that regenerates rapidly if damaged or even if the whole layer is removed (as in certain ophthalmic procedures).

corneal erosion: Loss of the corneal epithelium over some or all of the area of the cornea; **recurrent c.e.** chronic condition in which erosion periodically occurs due to inadequate adhesion of regenerated epithelium to its basement membrane.

corneal graft: *See* keratoplasty.

corneal guttata: *See* guttata, endothelial corneal dystrophy *under* corneal dystrophy.

corneal hydrops (HY-drahps): Accumulation of aqueous fluid within the cornea as a result of the loss of tissue integrity of the corneal endothelium and Descemet's membrane.

corneal lathing: *Another term for* keratomileusis.

corneal map: *Another term for* corneal topography.

corneal melting: Condition in which layers of the cornea degenerate and slough off due to an inflammatory process.

corneal reflection pupillometer (CRP): Device used to measure pupillary distance by using the reflection of the instrument's light on the cornea; gives binocular and monocular measurements; *also called* pupillometer; *see also* pupillary distance.

corneal reflex: 1. Reflection of light from the cornea's surface; 2. reflex blinking caused by corneal irritation; *see also* blink reflex.

corneal refractive therapy (CRT): Use of rigid contact lenses during sleep to reshape the cornea and correct myopia and small amounts of astigmatism, enabling the user to go without glasses or contacts during the day.

corneal staining: Method of evaluating the cornea (usually with the slit lamp) using dye; fluorescein dye will pool into any corneal defects or under contact lenses and glow bright green when observed with a cobalt blue light; the pattern of fluorescein staining often assists in diagnosis; rose bengal stains any degenerated or dead corneal epithelium.

corneal stroma: Transparent connective tissue making up the central layer of the cornea.

corneal tattooing: *Another term for* keratopigmentation.

corneal topography: Technique in which an image projected onto the cornea is analyzed by a computer to obtain a representation of the shape of the corneal surface and thus an indication of its refractive power; *also called* corneal mapping, videokeratography.

corneal transplant: *See* keratoplasty.

corneal ulcer: Loss of tissue from the surface of the cornea due to a disease process, often an infection, and usually painful; *see also* ulcer.

corneoscleral (KOHR-nee-oh-SKLAR-ul): Of or involving the cornea and sclera.

corneoscleral junction: *Another term for* limbus.

corneoscleral spur: *Another term for* scleral spur.

corrected visual acuity (VA$_{cc}$): Visual acuity measured with the patient's current corrective lenses in place (ie, no attempt is made to further improve vision optically); *compare* best corrected visual acuity, uncorrected visual acuity.

correction: In ophthalmic usage, spectacles or contact lenses prescribed to counteract myopia, hyperopia, astigmatism, or any other ametropia.

correspondence: *See* retinal correspondence.

cortex: In ophthalmic usage, the soft outer portion of the crystalline lens of the eye; **visual c.** area of the occipital lobe of the brain that receives visual input.

cortical attachments: Areas in which the nucleus and cortex of the crystalline lens adhere together.

cortical blindness: *See entry under* blindness.

corticosteroids: Substances used to reduce inflammation; topical steroid drugs used in ophthalmology include prednisone, dexamethasone, and fluorometholone; topical steroids are sometimes combined with antibiotics to fight infection as well; side effects in the eye can include increased intraocular pressure; *also called* steroids; *compare* nonsteroidal anti-inflammatory drugs.

cotton-wool spots (CWS): Small areas of the retinal nerve fiber layer that have lost their blood supply and become wispy white spots with no clear borders; *also* *called* soft exudates (although technically they are not exudates); *see also* retinal exudates.

couching: Obsolete treatment for cataract in which the whole lens of the eye was detached and pushed out of the visual axis, usually accomplished with a needle inserted into the anterior chamber of the eye.

count-finger vision: Very low level of visual acuity in which no greater detail can be perceived than the number of fingers held before the eyes; *see also* hand-motion vision, light perception vision, light projection vision, no light perception vision, visual acuity.

coupling agent: In ophthalmology, a clear, thick substance used to cushion a lens (eg, goniolens) or ultrasound probe (eg, B-scan) where it contacts ocular tissues; in ultrasound, it also acts to facilitate transmission.

cover test: Test to determine the presence of phoria or tropia; there are several types but all involve having the subject fixate on a target while the examiner covers an eye and observes for any movement; if there is no movement, the patient is orthophoric; **alternate c.t.** or **cross c.t.** cover test performed by quickly moving the occluder from one eye to the other so that there is no time for binocular fixation to occur; used to detect the presence and direction of deviation but cannot distinguish between phoria and tropia; **cover-uncover test** cover test performed by covering then uncovering one eye; used to distinguish between tropia and phoria and to determine the direction of deviation; **prism and alternate c.t. (PACT)** or **prism and c.t.** use of prisms in conjunction with alternate cover test in order to measure the amount of deviation.

cover-uncover test: *See* cover test.

CPT© (Current Procedural Terminology) codes: System of designating medical procedures and services, developed by the American Medical Association to facilitate billing and care review by providing uniformity in communication.

cranial nerve(s) (CN): Twelve pairs of nerves (motor, sensory, and mixed) that originate in the brain, designated both by Roman numerals (I to XII) and names; six of them affect vision either directly or indirectly; the optic nerve is CN II; *see* Appendix 5.

crazing: In ophthalmic usage, the appearance of a network of fine lines or cracks on a lens, most often a contact lens.

cribiform plate/cribrosa: *See* lamina cribrosa.

cross cover test: *Another term for* alternate cover test; *see that entry under* cover test.

cross cylinder: Lens composed of two cylindrical components of the same power, one plus and one minus, superimposed at right angles to each other, used to measure astigmatism; *also called* Jackson cross cylinder.

cross-eyed: Lay-term for strabismus, especially esotropia; *see also* wall-eyed.

cross fixation: Condition in which the left eye becomes dominant in gaze toward the extreme right and the right eye becomes dominant in gaze toward the extreme left.

crossed diplopia: *Another term for* heteronymous diplopia.

crossing changes: *Another term for* A-V crossing.

crowding phenomenon: Tendency for an amblyopic eye to have finer acuity if the optotypes are presented alone rather than as a row or group; *also called* separation difficulty.

cryo- (KRY-oh): Combining form meaning cold; used in medical terminology to describe treatments or surgical procedures involving very low temperatures (usually several hundred degrees below zero).

cryoextraction: Technique of intracapsular cataract extraction in which the lens capsule and its contents are frozen to the tip of a surgical instrument (ie, cryoprobe) and removed as a unit; now largely abandoned in the United States but still performed by many surgeons around the world; *see also* cataract extraction, extracapsular cataract extraction, intracapsular cataract extraction, phacoemulsification.

cryopexy (KRI-oh-PEK-see): Surgical procedure that attempts to fix a tissue into place by application of extreme cold (most commonly in ophthalmic usage, a detached retina against the choroid).

cryophake (KRI-oh-fake): Instrument used in cataract cryoextraction.

cryoprobe: General term for instrument used in cryosurgery.

cryoretinopexy (KRI-oh-ret-no-pex-ee): *See* retinopexy.

cryosurgery or **cryotherapy:** General term for application of extreme cold to tissue.

crystalline lens: Proper term for the natural lens of the eye (usually called simply the lens), consisting of a soft outer cortex and hard nucleus in the center; use of the full term *crystalline lens* is helpful as a distinction from manufactured lenses for vision correction.

CT scan: *See* computerized tomography.

cul de sac: General anatomic term for a sac with only one opening (from French for "bottom of the bag"); in ophthalmic usage, the sac formed by the bulbar and palpebral conjunctivae; *also called* fornix, conjunctival sac; *see also* conjunctiva.

culture: 1. A method of growing bacteria and fungi in the laboratory; **c. medium** a substance formulated for growing microorganisms in the lab; 2. technique whereby a sample of infected tissue or exudate is placed into growth medium.

cup: General term referring to a depression; **"bean pot" c.** glaucomatous cup where there is no visible neural rim; **glaucomatous c.** *see* cupping; **physiologic c.** in ophthalmic usage, the normal slight depression at the center of the optic nerve.

cup-to-disk ratio (c/d): Measure of the proportion of damaged area (ie, cup) to visually functional area (ie, disk) of the retina, representing the relative progression of glaucomatous damage; *see also* glaucoma.

cupping: Sign of glaucomatous damage in which the optic disk is affected by an area of increasing concavity, representing nonfunctioning retinal cells.

customized ablation: General term in refractive surgery to describe an excimer laser procedure that has been modified to fit the needs of a particular patient, most often referring to a highly individualized pattern of laser treatment designed to correct not only myopia, hyperopia, and astigmatism, but also higher-order optical aberrations; *see also* wavefront-guided ablation.

cyanolabe (sy-AN-oh-layb): Visual pigment present in the "blue" retinal cones that absorbs light in the blue frequencies (around 440 nm); one of three visual pigments: *see also* chlorolabe, erythrolabe, trichromatism.

cyanopsia (sy-uh-NAHP-see-uh): Visual disturbance in which everything appears blue; *compare* erythropsia, xanthopsia.

cycl-, -o-: Combining form meaning circle or ring; in ophthalmic usage, the iris and/or ciliary body.

cyclitic membrane: Formation of fibrous tissue in the anterior part of the vitreous body as a result of severe inflammation of the ciliary body.

cyclitis (sy-KLIH-tis): Inflammation of the ciliary body; *also called* intermediate uveitis; *see* uveitis.

cyclocryotherapy (sy-cloh-cry-oh-THAYR-oh-pee): Application of very low temperatures to the ciliary body performed in an attempt to decrease the production of aqueous fluid by the ciliary processes as a treatment for glaucoma.

cyclodestruction: General term for glaucoma surgical procedures that destroy portions of the ciliary body (as with extreme cold, laser energy, or other means) in order to decrease the production of aqueous fluid.

cyclodialysis: Largely abandoned glaucoma surgical procedure in which the root of the iris is detached from the ciliary body so that aqueous fluid may pass more easily out of the anterior chamber and thus reduce intraocular pressure.

cyclodialysis cleft: Detachment of the ciliary body, often from trauma, causing hypotony.

cycloduction: Rotation of one eye around its visual axis (anterior-posterior pole); *also called* cyclotorsion; *compare* cyclovergence.

cycloplegia (sy-kluh-PLEE-jee-uh): Paralysis of the ciliary muscle in which the eye does not accommodate in response to the usual stimuli.

cycloplegic (sy-kluh-PLEE-jik): In ophthalmology, a drug that causes cycloplegia (eg, tropicamide, cyclopentalate, etc).

cycloplegic refraction (sy-kluh-PLEE-jik): Determin-ing the refractive error of a cyclopleged eye that cannot accommodate or focus, used especially in children; compared to manifest refraction to determine presence and amount of any latent hyperopia; *see also* hyperopia, manifest refraction.

cyclotorsion: *Another term for* cycloduction.

cyclovergence: Rotation of both eyes around their visual axes (anterior-posterior poles); if the right eye rotates clockwise, the left eye rotates counterclockwise and vice versa; *compare* cycloduction.

cylinder (cyl): 1. In optics, a lens that is flat along one axis and circularly curved along the perpendicular axis or the property of a lens that is relatively flat along one axis and more curved along the perpendicular axis; *compare* sphere; **minus c.** refracting surface of a lens in which the lens material is fashioned into the concave reverse of a cylindrical shape (ie, as if a cylinder had been carved out of the lens and discarded); **plus c.** refracting surface of a lens in which the lens material is fashioned into the convex shape of a cylinder; 2. in refraction, the component of refractive error that can be corrected with a cylindrical lens (roughly synonymous with astigmatism).

cylinder axis: Direction in which correcting cylinder is placed to correct a refractive error.

cylinder power: A measurement of the strength of a cylindrical lens, given in diopters; cylinder power may be designated as plus or minus, and the axis must be given; *see also* transposition.

cylindrical dandruff (CD): Crusting at the base of an eyelash in blepharitis; *also called* collarette.

cyst: A blister-like, fluid- or air-filled lesion, generally benign.

cystoid macular edema (CME): Swelling of the central focusing area of the retina, typically as a result of trauma or as a complication of ophthalmic surgery.

cystotome (SIS-tuh-tohm): Surgical instrument for cutting a sac; most often in ophthalmic usage, instrument for cutting into the lens capsule.

cytomegalovirus (CMV) retinitis (sy-toh-MEG-uh-loh-VY-rus): *See* retinitis.

D

dacry-, -o-: Combining form meaning tear fluid; *see also* lacri-.

dacryocyst (DAK-ree-oh-sist): *Another term for* nasolacrimal sac.

dacryocystitis (DAK-ree-oh-sis-TIE-tus): Inflammation of the nasolacrimal sac, usually because of an infection and blocked nasolacrimal duct.

dacryocystorhinostomy (DCR) (DAK-ree-oh-SIS-toh-ry-NAHS-tuh-mee): Procedure in which an opening between the dacryocyst and the nasal passage is created or reopened.

dacryostenosis (DAK-ree-oh-stuh-NOH-sis): Blockage of the nasolacrimal passages.

Dalrymple's sign (DAL-rim-pulz): Lid retraction specifically related to Graves' disease; *see also* Graves' disease.

dark adaptation: *See* adaptation; *also called* scotopic adaptation.

dark adaptometry: Measurement of the eye's ability to dark-adapt over time; used in cases of night vision problems; *see also* Goldmann-Weekers dark adaptometer; **d.a. curve** plot line showing a patient's responses to dark adaptometry testing.

dark room provocative test: The patient is placed in a dark room to ascertain if this will cause angle closure due to pupillary dilation; *see also* mydriatic provocative test, provocative test.

dark trough: In electro-oculography, the response with the least width during the dark-adapted phase of testing; *compare* light peak; *see also* Arden ratio.

datum line: *Another term for* "C" measurement.

débride (duh-BREED): To remove foreign material and/ or dead tissue from a wound.

decentration: General term for misalignment; in ophthalmic usage, usually referring to displacement of a lens (spectacle, contact, or intraocular) or prism out of the visual axis.

decibel (dB): In ophthalmology, a measurement of the intensity of a visual field stimulus.

decongestant: Substance used to reduce swelling and blood accumulation in an area; in ophthalmic usage, a drug that reduces ocular redness.

defocus: In optics, the lower-order optical aberration that focuses an image too strongly or weakly, resulting in myopia or hyperopia, respectively.

degenerative cataract: *See* cataract.

degenerative myopia: *See* myopia.

degree: 1. In history taking, the extent to which a problem exists; 2. in strabismus, a measurement that indicates the amount of crossing; 1 degree equals approximately 2 prism diopters.

dehiscence (dee-HIS-uhns): General medical term for a splitting open of tissue, often as a result of fibrosis in the course of healing of a traumatic or surgical wound; in ophthalmic usage, typically referring to splitting of retinal tissue or breakage of the lens zonular fibers.

dellen (DEL-en): *See* corneal dellen.

dendrite: 1. Short filaments of a nerve cell body that receive impulses from other nerve cells (via the axons of those cells); *see also* axon, neuron, synapse; 2. branching corneal ulcer caused by the herpes simplex virus.

dendritic (den-DRIT-ik): Describing a tree-like shape; used often in ophthalmic terminology to describe lesions on the cornea that have a branched appearance (eg, as in dendritic keratitis), usually referring to a herpes simplex ulcer.

deorsumversion (dee-OR-sum-ver-zhun): Downward turning of both eyes; *compare* supraversion.

deoxyribonucleic acid (dee-OX-ee-RIYBO-noo-KLAY-ic): *See* DNA.

depression: Turning down of the eye; *also called* infraduction; *compare* elevation.

depressor: 1. Extraocular muscle that acts to move the eye downward (ie, the inferior rectus and superior oblique); *compare* elevator; 2. instrument used to apply pressure; **scleral d.** instrument applied externally to the globe in order to push the retina into view of an ophthalmoscope.

depth of field: Space in front of and behind an object of regard in which other objects can also be clearly seen; the depth of field is typically very shallow for nearby objects and deeper for very distant objects; typically of consideration in photography.

depth perception: The ability to discern the relative distance of objects within the field of view, made possible by the varying degrees of convergence necessary to focus upon objects at varying distances from the observer; present even when binocular vision and fusion are not achieved; *compare* stereopsis.

dermatochalasis (DER-muh-toh-kuh-LAY-sis): General term referring to loose, baggy skin; *see* blepharochalasis.

desaturated 15 panel: Color matching test that employs 15 very pale colored caps that the patient arranges; results differentiate between protan, deutan, and tritan even if the defect is subtle; *compare* Farnsworth-Munsell D-15; *also called* Lanthony desaturated D-15 panel.

Descemet's membrane (DES-uh-mayz): Inner tissue layer of the cornea to which the corneal endothelium adheres.

detachment: Separation of tissue layers that are normally attached; in ophthalmic usage, most commonly referring to the retina or choroid; *see also* choroidal detachment, retinal detachment, posterior vitreous detachment.

deutan (DOO-tan): Color vision defect involving the green color mechanism and linked to the X chromosome; this is the most common form of color blindness; *see* deuteranomaly, deuteranopia.

deuteranomaly (DOO-tur-uh-NAH-muh-lee): Partial impairment of the green color mechanism resulting in poor red/green discrimination, although red is normally vivid.

deuteranopia, -opsia (DOO-tur-uh-NOH-pee-uh): Severe or total lack of the green color mechanism; red and yellow-green both look orange; red-orange, orange, and yellow are all the same strong red-orange color; magenta and green are gray tones; blue-green to purple are various confusing shades of blue.

deviation: In ophthalmic usage, a turning of the eye from the point of fixation; **convergent d.** *see* esotropia; **dissociated vertical d.** deviation in which either eye drifts upward when it is occluded; **divergent d.** *another term for* exotropia; **primary d.** where an ocular muscle is paralyzed, the deviation that exists when the nonparalyzed eye is fixating; **secondary d.** where an ocular muscle is paralyzed, the deviation that exists when the affected eye is forced to fixate (typically the primary d. is less than the secondary d.); **skew d.** a vertical strabismus caused by an anomaly in the brainstem or cerebellum.

dextro-: Prefix describing structures or processes appearing or occurring toward the right; referring to the right eye in ophthalmic usage, as in the phrase oculus dexter (OD); *compare* sinistro-.

diabetic retinopathy (DR): Ocular effect(s) of diabetes mellitus, characterized by edema, bleeding, and neovascularization of the retina, with progressive loss of vision if left untreated; laser therapy is currently used in treatment; **background d.r. (BDR)** earlier stage of DR characterized by small hemorrhages and macular edema; **proliferative d.r. (PDR)** severe stage of DR in which neovascularization, large hemorrhages, and ischemia occur.

diagnosis: A determination of the cause of an illness/disorder/complaint; **differential d.** the determination of which diagnosis, out of two or more possibilities, is the one causing the illness/complaint.

diagnostic: Referring to diagnosis; providing information leading to a diagnosis; **d. A-scan** ultrasound used to evaluate intraocular masses and other pathological conditions (as opposed to measuring axial length); gives a one-dimensional scan; *also called* standardized A-scan; **d. B-scan** ultrasound used to differentiate tissues and evaluate intraocular pathology; gives a two-dimensional scan; **d. fields/positions of gaze** *see* gaze.

dialysis: In ophthalmic usage, the separation of connected tissues or structures.

dichromatism (die-KROH-muh-tiz-um): Condition in which only two of the three retinal cone pigments are present; *see* specific condition deuteranopia, protanopia, tritanopia; *compare* achromatism, monochromatism, trichromatism.

differential diagnosis: *See* diagnosis.

diffraction: Property of light attributable to its wave-like nature; light passing through a very narrow opening (about the same width as the wavelength of the light) is bent from its original path; theoretically, diffraction provides an alternative optical system to refraction for artificial lens design.

diffractive multifocal lens: Optical system that attempts to use diffraction in order to impart two or more focal points to incoming light, one "fundamental" focus provided by conventional refractive optics and the other(s) provided by diffraction.

diffuse: General term meaning spread out and not concentrated in one area.

diffuse illumination: In slit lamp biomicroscopy, the use of nonfocused, scattered light to provide a view of the whole eye and its adnexa, often for photography.

diffuse lamellar keratitis: *See entry under* keratitis.

diffuser: Filter for the light source of an optical instrument that scatters light without changing its color, thereby reducing reflections that can occur with point sources of illumination.

digital tonometry: *See* tonometry.

dilation or **dilatation:** General term for widening of an opening; in ophthalmic usage, the widening of the pupil in dim light or as a result of pharmaceuticals (more properly called mydriasis); dilation must be induced in order to perform certain intraocular examinations and surgical procedures.

dilator: 1. *Another term for* pupillary dilator muscle; 2. instrument used to increase the size of an opening.

dimer (DY-mur): A compound that is formed by the joining of two like molecules; *see also* excimer laser *under* laser.

diode laser: *See* laser.

diopter (D): 1. Measure of the focusing power of a lens, defined as the reciprocal of the focal length measured in meters; for example, a lens that focuses light from a very distant object ("infinity") to a point 1 m behind the lens has a power of 1 D, whereas a lens that focuses light at 2 m has a power of 0.5 D; 2. by analogy, degrees of myopia (designated as minus diopters) or hyperopia (designated as plus diopters), as well as astigmatism, are described by the dioptric power of the lens needed to correct the defect (resulting in descriptions like "the patient is a 4 diopter myope"); 3. measure of the refracting power of a prism; *see* prism diopter.

dioptric: Adjectival form of diopter.

diplopia: Perception of two images where there is only a single object (colloquially known as double vision); *see also* polyopia; *compare* triplopia; **binocular d.** double vision resulting from the lack of fusion of the images from each eye; **crossed d.** double vision in which the image from one eye is seen on the opposite side of the image from the fellow eye; **horizontal d.** doubled images are side-by-side; **monocular d.** double image seen with only one eye rather than both, resulting from some abnormality of the ocular media or a neurological problem in processing the image from the retina; **vertical d.** double vision in which the two images are one above the other.

direct illumination: In slit lamp biomicroscopy, method of viewing by shining light from the slit lamp upon the ocular structures to be viewed; *compare* indirect illumination.

direct light/pupillary response: *See* pupillary response.

direct ophthalmoscopy: Process of viewing a magnified image of the inside of the eye; it is called direct because the image is seen right-side-up; most often referring to the use of a hand-held ophthalmoscope through which the examiner looks with one eye (thus obtaining only a two-dimensional image with no depth); *compare* indirect ophthalmoscopy; *see also* ophthalmoscope.

disability: The extent to which a person cannot meet normal social, emotional, occupational, physical, or other demands due to impairment; *compare* impairment.

disciform keratitis (DIS-kuh-form): *See* keratitis.

disjunctive movements: *Another term for* vergence (definition 2).

disk (or, less preferred, **disc) (d):** General anatomic term for flat, circular structures; in ophthalmic usage, portion of the retina where nerve fibers converge to form the optic nerve (more properly called the optic disk or the optic nerve head); **choked d.** *another term for* papilledema.

disk diameter (dd): Subjective evaluation of the size or location of entities in the fundus, designated by number (ie, 1 disk diameter, 2 disk diameters, etc).

disk drusen: *See* drusen.

dispensing: In ophthalmic usage, the business of selling spectacles and/or contact lenses, including fitting, adjusting, and educating the customer.

dispensing optician: Optician who fits glasses and contact lenses from a prescription generated by a licensed eye care practitioner.

dissociated vertical deviation (DVD): *See* deviation.

distance between centers (DBC): Distance, in millimeters, between the optical centers of lenses mounted in a pair of spectacles; usually equal to the patient's pupillary distance.

distance between lenses (DBL): Width of the bridge of a pair of spectacles at its narrowest point, in millimeters.

distance vision: Vision of objects relatively far from the eye, approaching infinity; the distance at which visual tasks such as driving are considered to be performed, generally defined to be a minimum of about 20 feet; *compare* near vision; *see also* vision.

distichiasis (dis-tuh-KIE-uh-sis): Growth of extra eyelashes, sometimes from the meibomian glands.

distometer (dis-TAHM-uh-ter): Rotating conversion chart used to properly change lens power for varying vertex distances.

diverge: General term meaning moving away; *see also* divergence; *compare* converge; 1. in ophthalmic usage, the turning of both eyes outward, away from the midline; 2. in optics, the bending of light rays such that they move away from each other.

divergence: 1. In optics, the spreading outward of parallel light rays after passing through a minus lens; 2. in ophthalmic usage, outward turning of both eyes; *compare* convergence.

divergent deviation: *See* strabismus.

divergent lens: *Another term for* minus lens.

divergent strabismus: *See* strabismus.

Dk: Unit of measure of the oxygen transmission of contact lens materials, given as the product of the material's oxygen diffusion coefficient (D) times oxygen solubility (k) in the material at a given thickness, temperature, and hydration.

DNA (deoxyribonucleic acid): The molecular material containing the genetic design of each cellular organism.

Doctor of Osteopathy (DO): A practitioner of osteopathy; *also called* osteopath; *see* osteopathy.

documentation: Permanent recording of the elements of a patient exam, including the history, the results of any tests, findings, proposed and recommended treatment, discussions with the patient, and other items; may be written, entered in a computer system, or tape recorded; may not be erased but may be corrected by further documentation; *see also* history.

doll's eye sign: Turning of the eyes in the opposite direction from which the head is moved; it is an attempt by the vestibular system to maintain fixation.

dominance: In genetics, the state of a gene's being expressed, if it is present; *see also* dominant, recessive.

dominant: 1. In ophthalmology, usually referring to the preferred eye (*see* dominant eye); 2. in genetics, a gene that, if present, obscures the expression of a recessive gene at that locus; *see also* allele; *compare* recessive.

dominant eye: The eye that is subjectively preferred for use by an individual (eg, the eye the patient uses to sight with a camera or rifle) much the way one hand or the other is preferred; *compare* nondominant eye.

Donders' law (DAHN-derz): In any tertiary (oblique) eye position, the extraocular muscles exert the same torsion, regardless of how the eye was moved to attain that direction of gaze.

donor: Person who designates that his or her tissues and/or organs be used after death for implantation or research; **d. tissue** tissue that is taken from a donor postmortem; in ophthalmology, most often referring to corneal tissue.

Doppler ultrasound: Imaging technique in which the reflection of high-frequency sound waves from a moving object is analyzed to create a representation of the movement; used in ophthalmic applications to study ocular blood flow, especially in the retina and optic nerve, as well as intraocular and orbital tumors.

dot-and-blot hemorrhage: Appearance of small hemorrhages in the tissues of the retina, usually associated with diabetic retinopathy but also seen with other conditions.

double concave lens: *See* concave lens.

double convex lens: *See* convex lens.

double vision: *Another term for* diplopia.

drusen (DROO-zen): Circular, yellowish bodies that appear on the choroid as a consequence of aging or in some retinal degenerations; vision is rarely affected.

dry eye syndrome: Common condition in which a defect in the composition or production of the tears or incomplete closure of the eyelids results in corneal dryness, discomfort, and possible risk to the cornea; *see also* keratoconjunctivitis sicca.

dry macular degeneration: *See* macular degeneration.

Duane's retraction syndrome: Inherited abnormal function of the rectus muscles wherein the eye retracts into the orbit and the upper eyelid drops when the eye is moved in toward the nose; usually monocular; *also called* retraction syndrome.

duction: Movement of an eye by the extraocular muscles; *see also* forced duction test; *compare* vergence.

duochrome test: Projector slide that is green on one half and red on the other (split vertically); used to prevent over-minusing; *also called* bichrome test, red-green test.

duration: In history taking, the patient's report of how long a specific symptom lasts.

duty cycle: In cataract surgery, length of time that a phaco-emulsification needle is actually vibrating during any setting that calls for ultrasound power to switch on and off automatically (usually measured in hundreds of milliseconds); *see also* pulsed phaco power.

dye laser: *See* laser.

dynamic stabilization: Method of stabilizing toric contact lenses by thinning the upper and lower edges of the lens, which offers the least resistance to the lids during blinking and thus helps to prevent rotation and maintain the orientation of the lens to correct astigmatism in the proper axis; *compare* posterior toric, prism ballast, truncation.

dyslexia (dis-LEX-ee-ah): Difficulty reading, writing, and spelling even though the letters are known, intelligence is normal, and there is no sensory deficit; *compare* alexia.

dystrophy (DIS-troh-fee): General medical term meaning a degeneration of tissues due to defective nutrient supply; *see also* corneal dystrophy.

E

"E" test: A visual acuity test that uses only the letter E, which is turned up, down, and to the right or left; used to test children and other illiterates; *also called* illiterate E, tumbling E.

Eales' disease (eelz): Condition predominantly of young adult males characterized by repeated retinal hemorrhage.

eccentric fixation: State in which an eye fixates upon an object in such a way that the image of the object does not fall on the fovea, most often as compensation for damage in the area of the fovea.

ecchymosis (ek-uh-MOH-sis): General medical term for discoloration due to hemorrhage within a tissue; bruising.

echography (ek-OG-ruh-fee): *Another term for* ultrasonography.

ectatic corneal dystrophy (ek-TAT-ik): *Another term for* keratoconus.

ectopic (ek-TAH-pik): General medical term describing a dislocated organ or part, as in an ectopic lens or pupil.

ectropion (ek-TROH-pee-un): General medical term for the twisting inside-out of a structure, most commonly in ophthalmic usage referring to a condition in which the lid turns outward from the eye, exposing the conjunctiva; *compare* entropion; **cicatricial e.** caused by scarring; **involutional e.** caused by age-related atrophy of the eyelid muscles and tissues, *also called* senile ectropion; **mechanical e.** caused when lid(s) are displaced, as in by a tumor; **paralytic e.** most frequently caused by paralysis of CN VII; **senile e.** *another term for* involutional e.

edema: General medical term referring to swelling due to fluid collection/retention.

edge glare: Unwanted scattering of light striking the edge of a contact lens or intraocular lens, perceived as streaks or other visual disturbances that reduce visual acuity.

edger: Machine used to trim lenses to fit into spectacle frames.

effective diameter (ED): The diagonal size of the eyewire (lens opening) in a pair of spectacles, measured in millimeters.

effective power (of a lens): Perceived power of an ophthalmic lens, which varies with the distance of back surface of the lens from the eye (more critical in lenses of higher power); for example, a plus power lens decreases in effective power the farther it is moved away from the eye, although the literal (nominal) power of the lens has not changed; *compare* nominal power (of a lens); *see also* vertex distance.

efferent nerve (EF-ayr-uhnt): Nerve that conducts a central nervous system response to a sensory impulse, causing a reaction; *another term for* motor nerve; *compare* afferent nerve.

electroencephalography (EEG) (eh-LEK-tro-en-SEF-uh-LAHG-ruh-fee): Method of recording electric potentials in the brain.

electromagnetic spectrum: The range of energy waves conducted through the electrical fields present throughout space, from long-wavelength energy (eg, radio waves) to short-wavelength energy (eg, cosmic radiation); visible light includes the wavelengths from about 3800 to 7600 angstroms, recognized as colors from violet to red, respectively.

electro-oculography (EOG) (eh-LEK-troh-ahk-yoo-LAH-gruh-fee): Technique for analyzing the function of the retinal pigment epithelium via electrodes placed on the test subject's face; changes in electrical potential are recorded as the subject alternates looking from one fixation point to another in a Ganzfeld bowl; *see also* electrophysiology.

electrophysiology: Assessment of a structure's health by evaluating its electrical activity. In ophthalmology, such tests include the electroretinogram, the electro-oculogram, and the visual evoked response/visual evoked potential; *see also* electro-oculography, electro-retinography, visual evoked response.

electroretinography (ERG) (eh-LEK-troh-ret-uh-NAH-gruh-fee): Technique for measuring the response of the retina to light stimuli in a Ganzfeld bowl through electrodes placed on the surface of the globe; **flicker fusion ERG** performed with lighted Ganzfeld bowl using 30 flashes per second to elicit a cone-isolated response; **focal ERG** *another term for* macular ERG; **full-field ERG** determines the response of the entire retina to a quick flash of light; tests both rods and cones; **macular ERG** determines the response of a very small area of the retina (usually the macula); *also called* focal ERG; **mesopic ERG** performed in dark with a stimulus that activates both rod and cone cells; **pattern ERG** determines the response of the retinal ganglion cells using an alternating checkerboard pattern; **photopic ERG** performed with lighted Ganzfeld bowl using one or several flashes to elicit a cone-dominated response; **scotopic ERG** performed in the dark with a stimulus that activates the rod cells; *see also* electrophysiology.

elevation: Turning up of the eye; *also called* supraduction, sursumduction; *compare* depression.

elevator (muscle): Extraocular muscles (ie, the superior rectus and inferior oblique) that move the eye upward; *compare* depressor.

Elschnig's pearls (EL-shnig): Small whitish nodules of lens epithelium that sometime appear on remnants of the lens capsule after cataract extraction.

Elschnig's spots (EL-shnig): Small pale areas of dead choroidal tissue often associated with hypertension.

emmetrope (EM-uh-trohp): One who has no refractive error and does not need corrective lenses to see well.

emmetropia (em-uh-TROH-pee-uh): Condition in which the unaided eye properly focuses light onto the retina; *compare* ametropia.

emmetropization (em-uh-TROH-peh-ZAY-shun): Resolution of refractive error, usually referring to the resolution of hyperopia as a child grows.

emulsion: 1. In pharmacology, suspension of liquid droplets of medication in a vehicle with which it does not mix; *compare* solution, suspension; *see also* vehicle; 2. in ophthalmology, may refer to a chemical used in photo processing.

encircling band: *Another term for* scleral buckle.

endocapsular (en-doh-KAP-suh-ler): Appearing or occurring within the lens capsule; *see also* phacoemulsification.

endolaser: Laser where the beam is delivered to the treatment area via endoscopy (ie, a tube inserted into the body/organ).

endolenticular (en-do-len-TIK-yuh-ler): Appearing or occurring within the crystalline lens; *see also* phacoemulsification.

endophthalmitis (en-dop-thal-MY-tis): Inflammation of the internal ocular tissues, occasionally an infection after surgery or penetrating injury that can lead to loss of vision and of the eye itself if not controlled; **bacterial e.** endophthalmitis caused by infection; **endogenous e.** endophthalmitis caused by infection elsewhere in the body; **sterile e.** endophthalmitis caused by some agent other than infection.

enophthalmos (en-op-THAL-mus): Condition in which the eyeball recedes into the orbit; **senile e.** enophthalmos that occurs with age, usually caused by loss of orbital fat.

endoscope: Instrument used to look inside the body or an organ (including the eye) for medical purposes.

endothelial camera: *Another term for* specular microscope.

endothelial cell count/density (ECD): Evaluation of the endothelium to estimate cell number and integrity, usually prior to intraocular surgery.

endothelium: In general, a thin cell layer that lines blood and lymph vessels as well as serous cavities; *see also* corneal endothelium.

endpiece: Part on either side of a spectacle frame front to which the temples are attached.

enhancement: Euphemism for a repeat of treatment; the term has become well-established in ophthalmology, especially among refractive surgeons.

entopic phenomena (en-TAHP-ik): Visual perceptions that originate from within the eyeball or visual cortex, resulting from pressure or other atypical stimulation; can include seeing an image of corpuscles moving through one's own retinal blood vessels, an image of the vessels themselves, dark or light spots (*see* phosphene), flashes, and "seeing stars" when rising too quickly; blind children sometimes press on their eyeballs to elicit entopic phenomena; *see also* blindisms.

entopic test (en-TAHP-ik): Rough estimation of macular function where a light is held against the closed eyelid to elicit entopic phenomena; *also called* Purkinje entopic test.

entropion (en-TROH-pee-un): General term for an inward twisting of a structure, most commonly in ophthalmic usage a folding inward of the lid, resulting in the lashes rubbing against the globe; *compare* ectropion; **involutional** or **senile e.** caused by atrophy of the lower lid muscles; **spastic e.** intermittent entropion caused by squeezing of the lids or irritation.

enucleation: Removal of the whole eyeball after severing the muscle, nerve, and vascular attachments.

enucleation implant: *Another term for* orbital implant.

eosinophil (ee-uh-SIN-uh-fil): Inflammatory white blood cell that appears as a reaction to allergy and parasitic invasion.

epicanthal fold or **epicanthus (ep-eh-KAN-thahl** or **ep-eh-KAN-thuhs):** Fold of skin overlying the inner canthus, especially common and prominent in persons of Asian descent; **e. inversus** the epicanthus runs into the lower lid; **e. tarsalis** the epicanthus runs into the skin fold of the upper lid.

epidemic keratoconjunctivitis (EKC): *See* keratoconjunctivitis.

epikeratophakia (EP-ee-KEHR-uh-toh-FAY-kee-uh): Epikeratoplasty performed as part of a cataract extraction procedure.

epikeratoplasty (EP-ee-KEHR-uh-toh-plas-tee): Refractive surgical procedure in which donor corneal tissue is sutured over the patient's cornea (after removal of the corneal epithelium) to correct myopia, hyperopia, or astigmatism; somewhat unpredictable but reversible.

epilation (ep-uh-LAY-shun): General term referring to removal of hair/cilia at the root.

epinephrine (ep-uh-NEF-run): One of two biochemicals (neurotransmitters) that conducts messages for the sympathetic nervous system (the other is norepinephrine); *also called* adrenaline; *see also* norepinephrine; *compare* acetylcholine.

epinucleus (ep-uh-NOO-klee-us): Tissue surrounding the relatively harder crystalline lens nucleus.

epiphora (i-PIF-er-uh): Excessive tear flow due either to overproduction of tears or insufficient drainage by the lacrimal system.

epiretinal membrane (ERM): Detachment of the internal limiting membrane of the retina from the retina and vitreous body, occurring for a variety of reasons (eg, pathology, surgery, or trauma) and sometimes progressing to cellophane maculopathy (ie, wrinkling of the membrane) and macular pucker (ie, contraction of the membrane in the area of the macula).

episclera (ep-ee-SKLAYR-uh): Outermost layer of the sclera containing fine connective tissue and blood vessels.

episcleritis (ep-ee-sklehr-I-tus): Inflammation of the episclera; *see* episclera.

epithelial basement membrane dystrophy: *Another term for* map-dot-fingerprint dystrophy; *see entry under* corneal dystrophy.

epithelial ingrowth: Undesirable healing of corneal wounds or incisions in which the corneal epithelium invades the internal surfaces of the healing wound.

epithelial punctate keratitis: *Another term for* superficial punctate keratitis; *see entry under* keratitis.

epithelium: The avascular outer layer of a tissue; *see also* corneal epithelium.

equator: General term for an imaginary line midway between two poles of a sphere; often used to describe the location of points on the eyeball or crystalline lens (eg, equatorial staphyloma or equatorial cataract).

erosion: General medical term referring to gradual decomposition of a tissue.

erythema (er-uh-THEE-muh): General medical term meaning redness.

erythrocyte (uh-RITH-ruh-site): *Another term for* red blood cell.

erythrolabe (uh-RITH-roh-layb): Visual pigment present in the "red" retinal cones that absorb light in the red frequencies (around 570 nm); one of three visual pigments; *see also* chlorolabe, cyanolabe, trichromatism.

erythropsia (er-ah-THROP-see-uh): Visual disturbance in which everything appears red; *compare* cyanopsia, xanthopsia.

esodeviation: A deviation of the eyes in which one eye turns inward; may be latent (phoria) or manifest (tropia); *compare* exodeviation.

esophoria (E) (ee-soh-FOR-ee-uh): Heterophoria in which one eye turns inward when deprived of the visual stimulus for fusion; *compare* exophoria.

esotropia (ET) (ee-soh-TROH-pee-uh): Type of strabismus in which one eye turns in toward the nose (*also called* convergent deviation, convergent strabismus, internal strabismus); *compare* exotropia; **A pattern e.** esotropia in which the eyes are more converged in up-gaze; **accommodative e.** esotropia usually appearing in the first few years of life in which excessive turning inward of the eye occurs during near vision; **acquired e.** esotropia that occurs after age 1; **congenital (infantile) e.** large esotropia occurring in the first 6 months of life without significant refractive error; **intermittent e.** esotropia that is not present all the time (ie, the subject is sometimes able to fuse); **nonaccommodative e.** esotropia that measures the same even when fully corrected for hyperopia, including the latent component; *see also* hyperopia; **V pattern e.** esotropia in which the eyes are more converged in down-gaze.

essential blepharospasm: *See* benign essential blepharospasm *under* blepharospasm; *also called* benign essential blepharospasm.

Esterman grid: A transparent grid that is placed over a visual field test to evaluate field loss for disability ratings.

ethmoid bone: One of the bones of the orbit.

ethylenediaminetetraacetic acid (EDTA) (ETH-uh-leen-DYE-uh-meen-TEH-trah-uh-SEE-tik): Preservative used in some fluid medications.

etiology: General medical term referring to the cause of a disease or disorder.

eversion: General medical term for turning inside out; in ophthalmic practice, to evert the eyelid is to turn the lid inside out so the palpebral conjunctiva can be examined.

evisceration (ee-vis-er-AYE-shun): Removal of the eyeball's contents.

evoked potential: *See* visual evoked response.

excavation of optic disk: *See* cupping.

excimer laser: *See* laser.

excise: General medical term meaning to surgically remove tissue; *compare* incise.

excision: General medical term referring to the surgical removal of tissue.

exciter filter: Blue filter placed on the light source of the fundus camera to induce fluorescence of injected fluorescein dye for retinal photography and examination.

excycloduction/extorsion (ex-si-clo-DUC-shun/ex-TOR-zhun): Rotation of the eye away from the midline of the face around the visual axis, generally seen when the head is tilted; *compare* incycloduction/intorsion.

executive bifocal: Classic spectacle design in which the near (reading) segment of the lens extends across the entire width of the bottom of the lens with a clearly visible line dividing it from the upper far (distance) segment.

exenteration (ek-SEN-tuh-RAY-shun): Surgical removal of the globe in addition to orbital contents (eg, muscles, lids, etc).

exfoliation (ex-foe-lee-AY-shun): General term for the process in which tissue flakes apart in scale-like pieces.

exfoliation syndrome (XFS) (ex-foe-lee-AY-shun): Condition in which flakes of ocular and somatic material appear on structures in the anterior chamber, including the trabecular meshwork, where they may block aqueous outflow and cause a rise in intraocular pressure (pseudoexfoliative glaucoma); while "true" exfoliation in the eye is considered to occur within the crystalline lens itself, in ophthalmic usage, this term usually describes exfoliation/pseudoexfoliation syndrome, where flakes appear on the lens; *also called* pseudoexfoliation syndrome.

exodeviation (eks-oh-dee-vee-AY-shun): A deviation of the eyes in which one eye turns outward; may be latent (phoria) or manifest (tropia); *compare* esodeviation.

exophoria (X) (ek-soh-FOR-ia): Heterophoria in which an eye turns outward when deprived of a visual stimulus that stimulates fusion; *compare* esophoria.

exophthalmia, -os (eks-op-THAL-mia): Protrusion of the eye(s); *also called* proptosis.

exophthalmometer (ex-op-THAL-mah-me-ter): Instrument used to measure eye protrusion.

exotropia (XT) (ek-suh-TROH-pee-uh): Type of strabismus in which one eye is turned outward (*also called* divergent deviation, divergent strabismus, external strabismus); *compare* esotropia; **A pattern e.** exotropia in which the deviation is greater in down-gaze; **constant e.** exotropia that is present all the time; **intermittent e.** exotropia that is not present all the time (ie, the subject is sometimes able to fuse); **V pattern e.** exotropia in which the deviation is greater in up-gaze.

exposure keratitis: *See* keratitis.

expression (expressivity): In genetics, the characteristic demonstrated by the combination of corresponding genes (alleles) at a given locus; eg, if both alleles for eye color are blue (recessive), the expressivity in that individual will be blue eyes.

expulsive hemorrhage: Sudden, heavy bleeding from the choroid and retina of the eye, most often occurring during a surgical procedure and having the potential to force ocular tissues out of the incision; it is the most dramatic and potentially most devastating intraoperative complication of ophthalmic surgery.

extended wear lens: Contact lens intended to be worn overnight or, in some cases, up to several weeks without removal; the cornea beneath the lens receives oxygen via the tears as well as through the lens material itself.

external hordeolum: *See* hordeolum.

external limiting membrane (of retina): Zone of the retina intermingling with and directly under the photoreceptors (ie, rods and cones), forming a border with the outer nuclear layer; *also called* outer limiting membrane; *see* retina.

external rectus muscle: *Another term for* lateral rectus muscle.

external strabismus: *Another term for* exotropia.

extort: To induce motion of an eye so that the "north pole" of the globe tilts outward away from the other eye; *compare* intort.

extracapsular cataract extraction: General term for surgical techniques in which the anterior lens capsule is partially or completely removed in order to facilitate cataract extraction, usually referring to procedures in which a lens loop is used to remove the lens as an intact unit; *see also* cataract extraction, phacoemulsification; *compare* intracapsular cataract extraction.

extraocular muscles (EOMs): Rectus and oblique muscles attached to the outside of the eye and the inside of the bony orbit; responsible for movements of the eyeball.

exudate (EKS-yoo-dayt): *See* retinal exudates.

exudative retinitis (eks-yoo-DAY-tiv): *See* retinitis.

eye bank: Organization that serves as a clearing house for donated eyes, most importantly to provide corneas for penetrating keratoplasty but also to distribute eyes unsuitable for transplantation for use in research and training.

eye popping: In most infants, the reflex of opening the eyes wide in response to decreased light levels.

eye shield: Protective, rigid cover (usually plastic or metal) that fits over the eye and rests against the facial bones; *see also* Fox shield.

eye strain: *Another term for* asthenopia.

eyeball: Common term for the globe; *see* globe.

eyebrow: Row of hairs above the orbit at the brow, properly called supercilium.

eyelash: Fine, short hair arising from the margin of the eyelid; properly called cilium; plural: cilia.

eyelid: Either of two flaps of skin that cover the eye during blinking; *see also* combining forms beginning with blephar-, palpebr-, and tars-; **e. eversion** turning the eyelid inside out as when checking for a foreign body; **e. speculum** *see* speculum.

eyewire: Part of a spectacle frame front that holds the lens; each frame has a left and right eyewire joined by a bridge.

facial nerve: Central nerve seven (CN VII); motor and sensory nerve associated with blinking, facial expression, and reflex tearing.

facial palsy: *Another term for* Bell's palsy.

facility of outflow: *See* outflow facility.

facultative hyperopia: *See* hyperopia.

facultative suppression: Mental "blocking out" of the image produced by one eye in order to prevent double vision, occurring only when the eye is deviated; *compare* obligatory suppression.

faint: *Another term for* syncope.

falciform fold (FAL-suh-fohrm): Fold of connective tissue where extraocular muscles attach to the globe.

false negative: Response to a stimulus that is not present; in ophthalmic usage, most commonly referring to visual field testing.

false positive: Failure to respond to a stimulus that is present and within the threshold of causing a response; in ophthalmic usage, most commonly referring to visual field testing.

family history: That part of the patient history that records any relevant disorders in the patient's genetic relatives; *see also* history.

fan dial: *Another term for* astigmatic clock.

far point of accommodation: *See* accommodation.

Farnsworth test: *Another term for* Farnsworth-Munsell Test.

Farnsworth-Munsell Test: Any one of several tests of color vision; *also called* Farnsworth test; **F-M. D-15** employs 15 brightly-colored caps that the patient arranges; results differentiate between protan, deutan, and tritan color defects unless these are subtle; **F-M. 100-Hue** employs 85 colored caps that the patient arranges; results differentiate between protan, deutan, and tritan color defects as well as give an "error score" for quantifying the defect.

farsighted/farsightedness: *Another term for* hyperopia.

fascia (FASH-ee-uh): General medical term for sheet of fibrous tissue covering an anatomic structure and providing it with attachment, support, and protection during movement.

fascia bulbi (FASH-ee-uh BUHL-bye): *Another term for* Tenon's capsule.

FDA grid: Data from clinical studies of US Food and Drug Administration-approved intraocular lenses compiled in the 1980s for evaluating future intraocular lenses (IOLs); it includes rates of sight-threatening complications as well as postoperative visual acuity.

fenestration (fen-uh-STRAY-shun): In rigid contact lenses, putting a tiny hole in the lens to increase tear fluid exchange; **optic nerve f.** surgically created "window" in the sheath of the optic nerve to drain subarachnoid fluid, reducing papilledema in patients with pseudotumor cerebri.

field: *Another term for* visual field.

field defect: *See* visual field defect.

field of view: The area in which one can see without turning the head or eyes.

field of vision: *Another term for* visual field (definition 1).

fields of gaze: *See* gaze; *another term for* cardinal fields of gaze.

fifth cranial nerve (CN V): *Another term for* trigeminal nerve.

filamentary keratitis: *See* keratitis.

filariasis (fil-uh-RY-uh-sis): Parasitic infestation with threadworms, possibly affecting the eyes; *see also* onchocerciasis.

filter: In optics, a membrane that absorbs unwanted light, making certain structures or dyes more visible; *see also* barrier filter, cobalt blue f., exciter f., red-free f.

filtering bleb: *See* bleb, filtering operation.

filtering implant or **valve:** Device implanted to control intraocular pressure by allowing aqueous fluid to drain from the anterior chamber.

filtering operation: Surgical procedure used in the treatment of glaucoma in which an opening is created through which aqueous fluid may pass from the anterior chamber into a sac (ie, bleb) created beneath the conjunctiva, thus lowering the pressure within the eye.

filtration angle: *See* angle (definition 2).

finger counting vision: *See* count-finger vision.

fingerprint corneal dystrophy: *Another term for* map-dot-fingerprint corneal dystrophy; *see* corneal dystrophy.

fish-mouth: Undesirable postoperative condition in which the edges of a wound or incision fail to close but instead curl and gape open.

fissure: General medical term for a natural slit-like opening; in ophthalmology usage, referring to the opening between the upper and lower lids or to openings in the bony orbit.

fitting triangle: Desirable method of adjusting and fitting spectacles so that the frames touch the patient only on the bridge of the nose and the top of each ear.

fix: 1. In ophthalmology, sometimes used in place of the word fixation; 2. in microbiology, any method of preserving tissue/cells on a microscope slide; sometimes called fixation.

fixation: Looking directly at an object so that its image falls on the macula; requires that the eyes be steady (*compare* nystagmus) and have a measure of visual function depending on the target; *also called* central fixation; **binocular** or **bifoveal f.** ability to bring both eyes to bear upon the same object; requires coordination of ocular muscles; *see also* fusion; **central f.** *another term for* fixation; **eccentric f.** image does not fall on the macula but rather some peripheral retinal point, generally associated with long-standing amblyopia; **monocular f.** fixation of one eye (versus binocular f.).

fixation object/target: Device at which the patient looks to assist in maintaining fixation during an examination or treatment; also called object of regard.

fixed, dilated pupil: *Another term for* blown pupil.

flap: In ophthalmic surgery, a piece of tissue dissected away from the eye but left attached at one edge so that it can be repositioned over the site of the operation.

flare: Presence of protein particles in the aqueous humor, indicating intraocular inflammation, usually after surgery or trauma; *see also* cell.

flare and cell: In ophthalmic usage, usually the appearance of protein particles and white blood cells in the aqueous humor/anterior chamber, indicating intraocular inflammation.

flash visual evoked response: *See* visual evoked response.

flashes: Perception of sudden bursts of light in the absence of external stimuli, usually a symptom of retinal traction; *also called* light/lightning flashes.

flat: In ophthalmic usage, usually describing the surface curvature of a lens or ocular medium that imparts relatively low refractive power; *compare* steep.

flat axis: The least curved (and thus least refractive) of the principal meridians of a curved surface, either of the ocular media (cornea or lens) or a prescription lens; *compare* steep axis.

flat chamber: Collapse of the anterior chamber as a result of insufficient intraocular pressure, typically because of loss of aqueous humor due to trauma or surgical complication.

flat top spectacles: Bifocal spectacles in which the top of the bifocal segment is a straight line (as opposed to round).

flattening: In refractive surgery, decreasing the curvature of the cornea to correct myopia; *compare* steepening.

Fleischer ring (FLY-shur): A brownish iron deposit in the corneal epithelium around the base of the cone in keratoconus.

flicker fusion electroretinography: *See* electroretinography.

flicker fusion test: Measure of retinal cone function in which the frequency of a flashing light is increased until the flashes are perceived as one continuous light; *see also* electroretinography.

Flieringa ring (fly-uh-RING-uh): Metal ring placed on the sclera during ophthalmic surgery to maintain the shape of the eye and prevent loss of vitreous humor.

floaters: Dark specks or strands in the field of view caused by cells or other nontransparent material in the vitreous.

floppy eyelid syndrome (FES): Disorder in which there is loss of elasticity in the eyelid tissue and tarsal plate (to the point where the upper lid is easily everted), resulting in exposure of the globe during sleep and subsequent chronic irritation.

flow: In ophthalmic surgery, the passing of irrigation fluid through the eye; *see also* aspiration flow rate.

fluence: In optics, the rate of delivery of light energy over time, usually used to describe the amount of laser energy being delivered to a treatment area.

fluid-gas exchange: *Another term for* gas-fluid exchange.

fluorescein (FLOHR-uh-seen): Yellowish fluorescent dye used in many ophthalmic diagnostic procedures; for examination of corneal surface defects it is used topically; for evaluation of the retinal vasculature it is injected intravenously.

fluorescein angiography (FA) (FLOHR-uh-seen anj-ee-OG-ruh-fee): Imaging technique in which fluorescein dye is injected into a vein in the arm (or hand); the dye fluoresces when exposed to blue light, revealing the circulatory system of the choroid and retina in vivo; *see also* specific phrases: arterial, choroidal flush, laminar flow, late.

fluorescein clearance test (FLOHR-uh-seen): Assessment of the lacrimal system by applying fluorescein drops to the eye and timing how long it takes to drain away with the tear fluid.

fluorescein stain (FLOHR-uh-seen): Topical application of fluorescein to assess the condition of the corneal surface or the fit of a rigid contact lens.

fluorescence: Excitation of a material's electrons caused by light energy such that photons of light are emitted when the electrons fall back into their original orbits; this property is used in imaging techniques; *see also* fluorescein angiography.

fluorophotometry (flohr-oh-foh-TAHM-uh-tree): Method of assessing fluid flow (eg, the flow of aqueous humor through the anterior chamber) by measuring the concentration of fluorescein over time using a slit lamp fluorometer.

focal distance or length: Distance from a lens to the point at which rays of light converge to a focal point; if the power of a lens in diopters (D) is known, focal length in meters (F) is calculated using the formula $F = 1/D$.

focal electroretinography (eh-lek-troh-ret-un-AHG-ruh-fee): *See* electroretinography.

focal point: The point at which the rays of light converge; *also called* focus (definition 2); *see also* image.

focometer (foh-KAHM-uh-ter): Portable instrument used to determine a patient's refractive error; the patient adjusts the instrument until the target image is clear, the measurement is then read off a scale.

focus: 1. To bring together rays of light with an optical system so as to obtain an image of an object; 2. *another term for* focal point.

fogging: Purposely blurring vision by the addition of plus lenses either to eliminate accommodation (in refractometry) or to semiocclude the fogged eye.

foldable intraocular lens: *See* intraocular lens.

follicles: In ophthalmic usage, tiny clear or yellow sacs of lymphocytes and inflammatory cells appearing on the conjunctiva after prolonged irritation, often as a result of viral infection.

follicular conjunctivitis (fah-LIK-yuh-lur): *See* conjunctivitis.

foot-candle or foot lambert: Measure of the intensity of light falling on a given surface area, defined as 1 lumen per square foot.

foramen (fuh-RAY-mun): General medical term for a short, canal-like natural opening; in ophthalmology, generally referring to the optic foramen; *see* optic foramen.

forced duction test: In ophthalmic usage, test in which an anesthetized eye is physically moved by the examiner to check for mechanical restrictions to movement; the ease with which the eye can be moved and the speed with which it returns to a neutral position are observed; *also called* passive forced duction test, traction test.

foreign body (FB): Any object lodged in ocular tissue, usually as a result of trauma; **inorganic f.b.** object from a nonliving source (such as metal); **intraocular f.b.** object that has entered the globe; **organic f.b.** object from a living source (such as plant or animal matter).

foreign body sensation: Perception that an object is lodged in ocular tissue, either because such an object is actually present or because of an abrasion, inflammation, trichiasis, or other condition.

fornix (FOHR-niks): General medical term for an arch-like anatomic structure; in ophthalmic usage, *another term for* cul-de-sac, conjunctival sac; plural: fornices.

fourth cranial nerve (CN IV): *Another term for* trochlear nerve.

fovea (FOH-vee-uh): Small depression in the center of the macula in which cone cells are densely packed; *see also* macula.

foveal avascular zone (FAZ): Central 0.3- to 0.45-mm area of the fovea in which there is no direct vascular supply.

foveola (foh-VEE-uh-luh): Central pit of the fovea.

Fox shield: Perforated metal eye shield, allowing the wearer some vision through the openings; *see also* eye shield.

frame difference: The difference, in millimeters, between the horizontal (ie, "A" measurement) and vertical (ie, "B" measurement) measurements of the eyewires in a spectacle frame; has a bearing on lens thickness and position in that a thick lens has a better cosmetic appearance if the frame difference is small.

frame front: The two eyewires, bridge, and endpieces (where the temples are attached) of a pair of spectacles; *see also* temple.

frame pupillary distance (frame PD): Measurement, in millimeters, from the geometric (versus optical) center of the lenses in a pair of spectacles; taken by measuring from the nasal edge of one eyewire to the temporal edge of the other; *also called* geometric center distance (GCD).

Fresnel lens/prism (fruh-NEL): Lens composed of concentric rings that are sections of simple lenses of varying refractive power; it is thin yet provides great focusing or prismatic power although the optics are not as good as a regular lens; *see also* press-on lens/prism.

front vertex power: Portion of the total refractive power imparted by the front surface of a lens; *compare* back vertex power.

frontal bone: One of the bones of the orbit.

Fuchs' dystrophy (fyooks): The most common type of corneal endothelial dystrophy, characterized by the presence of guttata; also called Fuchs' corneal dystrophy, Fuchs' endothelial dystrophy; *see also* corneal dystrophy.

full-field electroretinography: *See* electroretinography.

fundus: General term for the base of an organ or area; in ophthalmic usage, the retina, macula, optic disk, and retinal blood vessels as seen through an ophthalmoscope.

fundus camera: Camera that is fitted especially for imaging the optic nerve, macula, and surrounding area; used in traditional photography as well as fluorescein angiography.

funduscopy (fuhn-DOSS-kuh-pee): In ophthalmic usage, viewing the retinal fundus.

fungi: A group of parasitic plants that do not produce chlorophyll; some may cause infection, especially in an immunocompromised host; of most concern in ophthalmology are *Candida*, *Fusarium*, and *Aspergillus*.

fusion: Binocular process in which each eye exerts the effort to fixate on the same object; **central f.** situation in which the image of an object falls on the fovea of each eye; **motor f.** action of the oculomotor system to align the eyes to achieve sensory fusion; **sensory f.** action of the brain in combining the slightly disparate images from each eye into one perceived, three-dimensional image; stereopsis cannot exist without fusion, but fusion can exist without stereopsis; *see also* stereopsis.

fusion amplitude: Range between the maximum convergence and maximum divergence that can be tolerated while still maintaining fusion (ie, points at which fusion is lost); measured in prism diopters.

G

Galilean telescope: *See* telescope.

gamma angle: *See* angle.

ganglion (GANG-lee-on): Cluster of nerve cell bodies.

ganglion cell layer (GANG-lee-on): Retinal cell layer consisting of sensory cells whose axons form the fibers of the optic nerve.

Ganzfeld bowl (GANZ-feld): Instrument (similar to a perimeter) used in electro-oculography, electroretinography, and visual evoked response; *see also* electro-oculography, electroretinography, visual evoked response.

gas-fluid exchange (GFE): Surgical procedure in which infusion fluid introduced into the posterior segment as part of retinal detachment repair is removed and replaced with air, a heavy synthetic gas, or a mixture of the two; *also called* air-fluid, fluid-gas exchange.

gas-permeable contact lens (GPCL): *See* contact lens.

gaze: Reference to the direction in which one is fixating, especially in strabismus testing; **cardinal (diagnostic) fields/positions of g.** or **fields of g.** directions of fixation that exhibit the functions of various extraocular muscles; some references list six: they are right, left, up right, up left, down right, and down left, others eight: they are the previous six listed plus straight up and straight down, and yet others list nine: they are the previous eight plus straight-ahead; *see also* range of motion; **primary g.** position of fixating straight ahead; also called primary position.

gene: Individual units of heredity that make up chromosomes and thus determine the hereditary make-up of each individual; each gene occupies a specific place (locus) in the chromosome; genes are composed of DNA; *see also* allele, chromosomes, heredity.

gene map: *Another term for* karyotype.

Geneva lens measure (juh-NEE-vuh): *Another term for* lens clock.

geniculate body (juh-NIK-yuh-lit): Area of the human brain that bridges the optic nerve and the cerebral cortex.

genotype (JEE-noh-typ): The specific combination of genes that causes the unique characteristic make-up of each individual; visual representation of the genotype is generated as a karyotype or gene map.

geometric center distance (GCD): *Another term for* frame pupillary distance.

geometric optics: Branch of optics that studies how light reacts when striking or penetrating a surface or object; *compare* physical optics, physiological optics.

"ghost figures": Hazy, patchy subepithelial scar tissue remaining after a herpes simplex infection of the cornea.

ghost vessels: Empty blood vessels remaining after resolution of corneal neovascularization.

giant papillary conjunctivitis (GPC): *See* conjunctivitis.

giant retinal break or **tear:** Retinal tear extending across three or more clock hours (90 degrees) of the eye.

Giemsa stain (GEEM-zuh): Dye used to detect and identify immune-related/inflammatory cells under the microscope.

glabella (gluh-BEL-uh): Point immediately above the bridge of the nose between the eyebrows, used as a reference point, particularly in reconstructive and plastic surgery.

glare: Distortion in an optical system whereby light from point sources (eg, the sun or automobile headlights) is dispersed across the field of view; glare has been cited as a particular problem for cataract patients; *see also* glare test, halo, starburst.

glare test: Test in which varying amounts of bright light are shown into the subject's eye during visual acuity evaluation; the purpose is to simulate room, outdoor, and full sun lighting; typically, visual acuity decreases in patients with cataracts (especially posterior subcapsular) when glare is added; one widely-used instrument is the brightness acuity tester (BAT).

glaucoma: Group of ocular disorders in which damage to the optic nerve and visual field loss are usually associated with high intraocular pressure; a leading cause of blindness throughout the world, glaucoma causes irreversible vision loss but in its early stages has no symptoms; *see also* glaucoma suspect, ocular hypertension; **acute angle-closure g.** sudden rise in intraocular pressure caused by blockage of the angle of the anterior chamber, marked by painful onset and extremely high pressure; **angle-closure g. (ACG)** *another term for* closed-angle g.; **angle-recession g.** type of secondary glaucoma following ocular trauma that tears the ciliary body, resulting in scarring and diminished outflow of aqueous fluid; **aphakic g.** elevated intraocular pressure after removal of the crystalline lens of the eye; **chronic g.** high intraocular pressure that is sustained over a prolonged time without any critical sudden rises; may be of closed- or open-angle type; **ciliary block g.** *another term for* malignant glaucoma; **closed-angle g.** normal drainage through the angle is blocked off and aqueous fluid rapidly builds up in the anterior chamber, creating high intraocular pressure and nerve damage; may be acute or chronic; *also called* angle-closure g., narrow-angle g.; **congenital g.** rare form of glaucoma that is present at birth; **hemolytic g.** glaucoma caused by blockage of the angle of the anterior chamber by blood cells; **iris-block g.** glaucoma caused when the iris blocks the angle; **juvenile g.** glaucoma occurring in youth; **low-pressure** or **low-tension g.** glaucoma occurring at an intraocular pressure usually considered to be within the normal or low range; *also called* normal pressure g.; **malignant g.** postoperative elevation of intraocular pressure that occurs when the anterior chamber is flattened from behind (ie, the posterior segment's volume is increased), closing the angle; *also called* ciliary block g.; **narrow-angle g.** *another term for* closed-angle g.; **neovascular g.** glaucoma caused by growth of blood vessels into the angle of the anterior chamber, which impairs outflow of aqueous fluid; **normal pressure g.** *another term for* low-pressure glaucoma; **open-angle g.** glaucoma caused by build-up of aqueous fluid in the anterior chamber due to impaired outflow through the tissue spaces of the angle even though the angle is open; **phacolytic g.** glaucoma resulting from leakage of lens proteins in very advanced cases of cataract; **pigmentary g.** glaucoma resulting from iris pigment dispersed into the angle; *compare* pigmentary dispersion syndrome in which no glaucoma occurs; **primary g.** general term for glaucoma unrelated to previous disease (generally divided into primary closed-angle and primary open-angle glaucoma); *compare* secondary g.; **pseudoexfoliation g.** rise in pressure is caused by material blocking the trabecular meshwork; *see* exfoliation syndrome; **pupillary block g.** glaucoma caused when the crystalline lens crowds against the iris, obstructing the pupil and trapping aqueous; **secondary g.** glaucoma resulting from disease or injury; may be open-angle or closed-angle; *compare* primary g.; **steroid-induced g.** glaucoma resulting from steroid use.

glaucoma suspect: Situation in which the patient exhibits symptoms that indicate glaucoma may occur or already exists; *see also* ocular hypertension.

glaucomatous (glah-KOH-muh-tus): Like or of glaucoma.

glaucomatous cataract (glah-KOH-muh-tus): Opacification caused by high intraocular pressure.

glaucomatous cupping (glah-KOH-muh-tus): *See* cupping.

glioma (glee-OH-muh): Tumor that originates from cells associated with brain or spinal cord tissue; in ophthalmology, notably of the optic nerve.

globe: Term referring to the eyeball itself exclusive of the ocular adnexa; *also called* orb.

GMS stain: A dye used to detect and identify fungi under the microscope.

goblet cells: Mucin-producing cells found in mucous membranes; in the eye, goblet cells are located in the conjunctiva and produce the mucin found in tears.

Goldmann applanation tonometer (GOHLD-mahn): *See* tonometer.

Goldmann lens (GOHLD-mahn): *See* goniolens.

Goldmann perimeter (GOHLD-mahn): *See* perimetry.

Goldmann tonometer (GOHLD-mahn): *See* tonometer.

Goldmann-Weekers dark adaptometer (GOHLD-mahn): Instrument used to test dark adaptation; *see* dark adaptometry.

goniolens (GOH-nee-oh-lenz): Lens, typically incorporating several mirrors, that allows one to see or direct laser energy into the angle of the anterior chamber; the lens is placed directly onto the anesthetized eye; many configurations are available, including the Goldmann, Hruby, Karickhoff, Koeppe, and Zeiss lenses; alternate classifications include children's (of smaller size), single-sided, four-sided, three-mirror, and operating goniolenses.

goniophotocoagulation (GOH-nee-oh-FOH-toh-koh-AG-yuh-LAY-shun): Laser procedure for treatment of glaucoma that attempts to lower intraocular pressure by using laser energy (directed by a goniolens) to open the trabecular meshwork; *see also* trabeculectomy.

gonioscopy (goh-nee-AH-skah-pee): Examination of the angle of the anterior chamber using a goniolens.

goniotomy (goh-nee-AHT-o-mee): Surgical procedure in which tissue is removed from the filtration angle of the eye in congenital glaucoma.

grade I, II, III, and IV: Many medical conditions, including ophthalmic entities such as capsular opacification, cataract, corneal haze, etc, are assessed by assigning subjective grades from I (or 1, noticeable) to IV (or 4, severe); although some researchers periodically attempt to define objective criteria for the grades assigned to these various conditions, clinicians prefer to establish their own definitions for use in patient records; *see* Appendix 8.

graft: 1. General medical term for inserting tissue into or over a defect; 2. the tissue utilized in a grafting procedure; *see also* keratoplasty.

gram stain: Dye used to classify bacteria; gram-positive bacteria stain dark blue and gram-negative bacteria stain red.

gram-negative: The property of some bacteria to stain red when gram stain is applied.

gram-positive: The property of some bacteria to stain dark blue when gram stain is applied.

Graves' disease: Thyroid overactivity generally resulting in exophthalmos but sometimes also associated with dysfunction of extraocular muscle and optic nerve as well as corneal involvement; ocular involvement is also called thyroid eye disease; *see also* Dalrymple's sign.

gray line: Faint anatomical line/groove on the lid margin demarcating the openings of meibomian glands to the surface of the lid.

grid: *Another term for* Amsler grid, FDA grid.

growth medium: *Another term for* medium (definition 2).

Gullstrand's schematic/reduced eye (GUHL-strandz): *See* schematic eye (definition 2); *also called* reduced eye.

Gunn's pupil: *See* Marcus Gunn pupil.

guttata (goo-TAH-tuh): General medical colloquialism for a spot or spots with the appearance of water droplets; in ophthalmic usage, referring to the appearance of such spots on the inner surface of the cornea; *see* endothelial corneal dystrophy *under* corneal dystrophy; plural: indeterminable, although guttata as the singular and guttatae as the plural seem to be well accepted; *see also* bedewing.

H

Halberg clip (HAL-burg): Trial lens holder that attaches to the patient's glasses; used for over-refraction.

half-eyes: *Another term for* half-glasses.

half-glasses: Spectacles that have only the correction for near vision; typically they are a small frame set farther down on the nose than conventional glasses so the wearer can look over them for distance viewing; *also called* half-eyes.

halo: Distortion in an optical system that causes a bright "cloud" or ring to be seen around point sources of light such as the sun or car headlights; *see also* glare, starburst.

hand-motion or **hand movement vision (HM):** Very low level of visual acuity in which no greater detail can be perceived other than the motion of a hand waved before the eyes; *see also* count-finger vision, light perception vision, light projection vision, no light perception vision, visual acuity.

haploscope (HAP-luh-skohp): Instrument that presents two separate fields of view to the two eyes for evaluation of binocular vision.

haptic: Portion of an intraocular lens comprised of a thin arm that curves outward from the optic; *also called* loop; *see also* optic.

hard exudates: *See* retinal exudates.

Hardy-Rand-Rittler (HRR) plates: Color vision screening test using pseudoisochromatic plates; test results identify and quantify color vision defects.

harmonious retinal correspondence (HRC): State in which corresponding points from the two images focused on each retina are properly associated in the image created by fusion in the brain; *also called* normal retinal correspondence (NRC); *compare* anomalous retinal correspondence.

Hartmann-Shack aberrometry: *See* Shack-Hartmann aberrometry.

haze: General term in ophthalmic usage for cloudiness of normally clear optical medium, usually referring to the cornea.

head tilt: Abnormal head posture in which the head is tilted toward one shoulder or another, or chin up or chin down to compensate for strabismus, nystagmus, or refractive error; *compare* head turn; *see also* ocular torticollis.

head tilt test: Three-step test to determine what cyclovertical muscle is implicated in a strabismus; *also called* the Bielschowsky test, the three step test (3ST).

head turn: Abnormal head position where the subject turns the head to the right or left to compensate for strabismus, nystagmus, or refractive error; *compare* head tilt; *see also* ocular torticollis.

Health Insurance Portability and Accountability Act (HIPAA): National standard that requires, among other things, that patient privacy be protected.

health literacy: Extent to which a patient comprehends health-related concepts, utilizes communication modalities to gather information, accurately interprets information from the media, moves through the health care system, recognizes and uses local resources, and makes health care decisions based on personal and social knowledge.

heavy fluid or **gas:** Any of several materials used in posterior segment surgery to replace the vitreous humor following vitrectomy, often as part of retinal detachment repair; these materials include perfluorocarbons such as perfluoropropane (C3F8), silicone oil, and sulfur hexafluoride (SF6).

HEMA: Hydroxyethylmethacrylate, polymer from which most soft hydrogel contact lenses are made; *see* hydrogel.

hemangioma (hi-man-jee-OH-muh): A tumor consisting of blood vessels; usually benign.

hemianopia, -opsia (hem-ee-uh-NOH-pee-uh): Partial or total loss of vision in half the visual field in one or both eyes; the upper or lower portions of the visual field, as well as the right and left sides, can be affected; *compare* quadrantanopia; **absolute h.** total loss of all visual perception in half the visual field; **altitudinal h.** loss of the upper or lower half of the visual field; **bilateral h.** partial or total loss of vision affecting the visual field of both eyes (*also called* binocular or true hemianopia); **binasal h.** loss of the half of the visual field on the side nearest the nose in each eye (ie, left field of the right eye and right field of the left eye); **binocular h.** *another term for* bilateral hemianopia; **bitemporal h.** loss of the temporal field in each eye (ie, right field in the right eye, left field of the left eye); **homonymous h.** loss of half the field in both eyes such that the loss is the same (superimposable) in each eye; **incongruous h.** loss of half the field in both eyes such that the loss is not identical in each eye; **quadrant h.** loss of one quarter of the visual field in each eye (*also called* quadrantanopia); **true h.** *another term for* bilateral h.; **unilateral h.** loss of half the visual field of only one eye.

hemorrhage (heme): General medical term for bleeding, but especially when profuse.

HeNe laser: *See* laser (helium-neon).

Henle's fibers (HEN-leez): Nerve fibers that join the rod and cone cells of the retina in the area of the fovea.

hereditary: Any trait or disorder that is genetically transmitted by the individual's progenators; *compare* acquired.

heredity: Any trait (including genetic, personality, emotional, etc) that is transmitted to progeny.

Hering's law of simultaneous innervation: Physiologic principle that the nerve stimulus generated by the oculomotor system to move the fixating eye is duplicated for the yoke muscle of the other eye, resulting in parallel movement of the eyes; *see also* yoke muscle.

Herpes simplex type 1 (HER-peez SIM-plecks): Virus that causes cold sores and dendritic corneal ulcers (herpes keratitis).

Herpes zoster (HER-peez ZOS-ter): Virus that causes shingles; *see* Herpes zoster ophthalmicus.

Herpes zoster ophthalmicus (HER-peez ZAHS-tur op-THAL-muh-kuhs): Herpetic viral infection affecting the trigeminal nerve (CN V) and the eye, generally as a part of shingles (which can occur without ocular involvement).

Hertel exophthalmometer (her-TEL ex-op-thal-MOM-ehter): Instrument that measures ocular protrusion bilaterally; has a calibrated base that increases reliability in repeat measurements.

hetero-: Prefix meaning different.

heterochromic (HET-uh-roh-KROHM-ik): General term describing a tissue or organ that shows a mottling of colors when normally it is of a single hue (eg, a heterochromic iris); *see also* anisochromatic; *compare* isochromatic.

heterometropia   (het-uh-roh-muh-TROH-pee-uh): *Another term for* antimetropia.

heteronymous diplopia (het-uh-RON-uh-mus): Double vision in which the image seen by the right eye is perceived to be to the left of the image seen by the left eye; also known as crossed diplopia; *compare* homonymous diplopia.

heterophoria (het-uh-roh-FOHR-ee-uh): *Another term for* phoria.

heterophthalmia (HET-er-op-THAL-mee-uh): General term for the difference in structure or function between the two eyes.

heteropsia (het-er-AHP-see-uh): State in which one eye has different visual characteristics (eg, degree of myopia) than the fellow eye.

heterotropia (het-er-oh-TROH-pee-uh): *Another term for* tropia.

higher-order aberration: *See* aberration.

HIPAA: *See* Health Insurance Portability and Accountability Act.

hippus: Rhythmic contraction and dilation of the pupils independent of any stimulus, often seen when shining a light into the eye in order to evaluate pupillary reflexes; not usually indicative of pathology.

Hirschberg test (HERSH-burg): Identification of tropia by noting the position of the reflections of a fixation light on the patient's corneas; if both reflections are on the visual axis (slightly nasal), the eyes are orthotropic, but if the reflection is on the axis in one eye but not the other, a tropia may be present; *see also* Krimsky measurement/test.

histamine (HISS-tuh-meen): Chemical released from mast cells (basophils) in response to injury and causing an inflammatory response (eg, constriction of bronchioles, dilation of blood vessels, decreased blood pressure, etc) in the body; *see also* antihistamine, mast cell.

histo spots (HISS-toh): Retinal lesions caused by histoplasmosis; *see* presumed ocular histoplasmosis syndrome.

histoplasmosis (hiss-toh-plaz-MOH-sis): Ocular infection caused by inhalation of the fungus *Histoplasma capsulatum* and usually causing choroiditis; *see* presumed ocular histoplasmosis syndrome.

history: Process of interviewing the patient in order to document his or her medical conditions, past and present, both systemic and ocular; includes family history, social history, medications, allergies, signs, symptoms, aggravating and relieving factors, as well as answers to pertinent questions regarding the patient's complaint(s); *see also* chief complaint, documentation, family history, ocular history, past medical history.

HIV: *See* human immunodeficiency virus.

Hollenhorst plaques (HAHL-en-hohrst): Emboli of cholesterol lodged in the retinal arterioles and causing occlusion; they are sparkly and orange-yellow.

holmium laser thermokeratoplasty (HOHL-me-uhm thur-moh-KEHR-uh-toh-plas-tee): *Another term for* laser thermal keratoplasty.

homogenous keratoplasty (huh-MAJ-uh-nus): Keratoplasty in which the tissue comes from a donor (of the same species); *compare* autogenous keratoplasty.

homonymous diplopia (huh-MAHN-uh-mus): Double vision in which the image seen by the right eye is perceived to be to the right of the image seen by the left eye; *also called* uncrossed diplopia; *compare* heteronymous diplopia.

homonymous field defect (huh-MON-uh-mus): Visual field defect that is the same in each eye (eg, both left halves of each visual field); *compare* incongruous field defect.

Honan balloon (HOH-nan): Device placed on the eye before ophthalmic surgery designed to put pressure on the eye in order to reduce intraocular pressure.

hordeolum (hor-DEE-oh-luhm, hor-dee-OH-luhm): Infection of one of the glands on the edge of the eyelid (external h. or sty) or in the palpebral conjunctiva (internal h.); *see also* meibomian cyst; *compare* chalazion.

horizontal meridian: In ophthalmic use, usually referring to the horizontal line dividing the visual field into upper and lower halves; a field defect that does come to but does not cross the horizontal meridian (such as a nasal step) is said to respect the horizontal, and indicates a problem in the arcuate nerve fiber bundle; *compare* vertical meridian.

horizontal prism bar: *See* prism bar.

horizontal raphe: *See* raphe.

Horner's syndrome: Disorder of the third cranial nerve causing miosis, ptosis, and anhidrosis (lack of sweating) on the affected side.

horopter (hohr-AHP-ter, HOHR-ahp-ter): An imaginary arc that allows correlation of points in space to points on the retina; images in front of or behind the horopter will be perceived as double; *see also* Panum's fusion area.

horseshoe tear: Retinal tear in which a U-shaped flap of retinal tissue (ie, attached on one side) is pulled away from the retina.

host: Organism that provides essential nutrition and/or habitat for a parasite.

HOTV test: Visual acuity test for children in which the letters H, O, T, and V on a chart are matched to the same letters on cards.

HRR plates: *See* Hardy-Rand-Rittler (HRR) plates.

Hruby contact lens (ROO-bee): *See* goniolens.

Hudson-Stähli line (HUHD-suhn STAH-lee): Thin, horizontal band of iron deposits in the cornea where the upper and lower eyelids meet when the eye is closed; generally seen in the elderly.

human immunodeficiency virus (HIV): Virus implicated in acquired immunodeficiency syndrome (AIDS).

humor: General term for a fluid; **aqueous h.** *see* aqueous fluid; **vitreous h.** *see* vitreous body.

hyaline degeneration (HY-uh-lin): Benign, round, clear-grayish area of 2 mm to 3 mm on the sclera near the site of rectus muscle insertion, usually in those over age 60.

hyalitis (hy-uh-LITE-us): Inflammation in the vitreous gel, usually exhibiting cells and haze; *also called* vitreitis/vitritis; *compare* hyalosis.

hyaloid artery (HY-uh-loyd): Fetal blood vessel that supplies the embryonic crystalline lens and generates the central retinal artery and which disintegrates prior to birth; occasionally, a remnant remains on the lens after birth, *see* Mittendorf's dot.

hyaloid membrane (HY-uh-loyd): In ophthalmic usage, the thin membrane that surrounds the vitreous, consisting of the anterior hyaloid membrane (*also called* vitreous face) and the posterior hyaloid membrane; *also called* vitreous membrane.

hyalosis (hy-uh-LOH-sus): Degeneration of the vitreous; *compare* hyalitis; **asteroid h.** small white bodies in the vitreous humor occurring most often in one eye, in the elderly, and in males more than females, usually with little effect on vision; they are composed of lipids and calcium; *also called* Benson's disease/sign.

hyaluronic acid (hy-uh-loo-RAHN-ik): Component of certain viscoelastic substances.

hydrodelamination or **hydrodelineation (hy-droh-dee-lam-uh-NAY-shun** or **hy-droh-dee-LIN-ee-a-shun):** In ophthalmic usage, surgical technique in which fluid is injected into the lens nucleus in order to break it up to facilitate cataract extraction.

hydrodissection (hy-droh-dy-SEK-shun): Most often in ophthalmic usage, surgical technique in which water is injected between tissue layers in order to separate them; usually employed in cataract extraction to separate the lens nucleus from the surrounding cortex; *compare* viscodissection.

hydrogel: Material used to make contact lenses and intraocular lenses; the hydrogel polymer (centered around the hydroxyethylmethacrylate [HEMA] molecule) is hydrophilic, which means that it can absorb large amounts of water and theoretically is more "friendly" to living tissue than hydrophobic materials.

hydrophilic (hy-druh-FIL-ik): Describing a material that readily absorbs water.

hydrophobic (hy-druh-FOH-bik): Describing a material that repels water.

hydrops: General medical term for accumulation of watery fluid in tissue; **corneal h.** aqueous fluid accumulation within the cornea due to decreased tissue integrity of the corneal endothelium and Descemet's membrane.

hydrophthalmia, -os (hy-drop-THAHL-mee-uh): *Another term for* buphthalmia.

hydroxyethylmethacrylate (HEMA) (hy-DROKS-ee-eth-il-meth-ACK-ruh-layt): *See* hydrogel.

hyperemia (hy-per-ee-mee-uh): General medical term denoting presence of excessive blood.

hyperfluorescence (hy-per-floor-ESS-ehns): Area of abnormally increased fluorescence on a fluorescein angiogram, often indicating leakage from blood vessels.

hypermature cataract: *See* cataract.

hypermetropia (hy-per-mi-TROH-pee-uh): *Another term for* hyperopia.

hyperope: Individual with hyperopia; *compare* myope.

hyperopia: Visual defect in which the eye focuses rays of light so that the focal point is behind the retina; commonly known as farsightedness, the hyperopic eye is not able to see objects that are nearby; *also called* hypermetropia; *compare* myopia; **absolute h.** farsightedness that cannot be compensated for by accommodation, measured as the least amount of plus needed to produce clear vision; **axial h.** farsightedness attributable to the length of the eye (ie, the eye is too short for the refractive power of the cornea and crystalline lens); **facultative h.** *another term for* manifest h.; **latent h.** farsightedness that can be overcome by accommodation, generally measurable only during cycloplegia; **manifest h.** the amount of farsightedness that falls between absolute and latent hyperopia; figured as the difference between the measurement for absolute hyperopia and the maximum amount of plus the noncycloplegic patient can accept and still retain clear vision; *also* *called* facultative h.; **refractive h.** farsightedness that is attributable to the refractive power of the eye (ie, the cornea and lens are too weak to bring the incoming rays of light to focus on the retina).

hyperopic: Adjective referring to hyperopia or farsightedness; *compare* myopic.

hyperopic astigmatism: *See* astigmatism.

hyperopic keratomileusis (hy-per-OP-ic KER-uh-toh-ma-LOO-sis): *See* keratomileusis.

hyperosmotics (hy-per-ahs-MAHT-iks): Class of drugs that reduce intraocular pressure by drawing aqueous out of the eye; most commonly used to treat acute angle-closure glaucoma (eg, glycerin, isosorbide, mannitol).

hyperphoria (hy-per-FOR-ee-uh): Phoria in which one eye drifts upward when fusion is broken (generally by occluding the eye); *compare* hypophoria.

hypertelorism (hy-per-TEL-uh-rizm): General medical term for an abnormally large distance between two anatomic structures; in ophthalmic usage, an abnormally large distance between the eyes, a congenital condition usually accompanied by problems with ocular alignment and motility.

hypertensive retinopathy: *See entry under* retinopathy.

hypertropia (hy-per-TROH-pee-uh): Strabismus in which the nonfixating eye turns upward relative to the fixating eye; *compare* hypotropia.

hyphema (hy-FEE-muh): Bleeding into the anterior chamber of the eye.

hypophoria (hy-poh-FOR-ee-a): Phoria in which one eye drifts downward when fusion is broken (generally by occluding the eye); *compare* hyperphoria.

hypoplasia (hy-po-PLAY-zee-uh): Failure of an organ or body part to develop properly.

hypopyon (hy-POH-pee-ahn): Collection of pus in the anterior chamber of the eye.

hypotelorism (hy-poh-TEL-uh-riz-um): General medical term for an abnormally small distance between two anatomic structures; in ophthalmic usage, an abnormally small distance between the eyes.

hypotony (hy-POT-uh-nee): In ophthalmic usage, abnormally low intraocular pressure (usually <5 mm Hg); *see also* intraocular pressure.

hypotropia (hy-puh-TROH-pee-uh): Strabismus in which the nonfixating eye turns downward relative to the fixating eye; *compare* hypertropia.

hypoxia (hy-POK-see-uh): Abnormal reduction in the amount of oxygen available to a tissue; in ophthalmic usage, most frequently referring to lack of oxygen to the cornea related to contact lens wear; *also called* anoxia, oxygen deprivation.

hysterical: General medical term for a disorder triggered by emotional struggles; in ophthalmic usage, visual disorders due to emotional rather than organic causes; **h. blindness** *see* blindness; **h. visual field** *see* visual field defect.

iatrogenic (disease) (i-a-truh-JEN-ik): Disorder unintentionally caused by a treatment.

ICD codes: *See* International Code of Diseases.

idiopathic (id-ee-uh-PATH-ik): Disorder without a known cause.

illiterate E: *Another term for* "E" test.

illumination: *See* specific type of illumination (ie, direct i., indirect i., retroillumination, etc).

image: The representation of an object that is produced at the focal point of an optical system; *see also* focal point; **real i.** image produced at the focal point of a plus lens; this image is formed behind the lens and can thus be projected onto a screen; **virtual i.** image produced at the focal point of a minus lens, which, because it is formed in front of the lens, can only be stipulated to exist.

image jump: Apparent shift in an object's position when viewed through a prism (eg, as vision is moved from one segment of a multifocal lens to another due to the prismatic effect of the segment edges).

immune response: A collective term used to describe the body's response to an antigen.

immune system: In combination, those tissues, structures, and mechanisms that help the body fight off infection.

immunity: The state of being unaffected by a specific antigen due to the presence of antibodies that recognize and destroy it.

immunocompromised (im-yoo-no-KOM-pruh-mized): Having an immune system that is depressed, weak, or damaged and thus unable to satisfactorily ward off infection.

impairment: A physical or mental condition or disorder that renders a person disabled; *compare* disability.

implant: General term for man-made material designed for surgical insertion into the human body; *see also* filtering implant, intraocular lens, orbital implant.

incident light: Ray of light that enters a medium; *see also* reflection, refraction (definition 1).

incise: General medical term meaning to surgically cut into a tissue (versus remove tissue); *compare* excise.

incision: General medical term referring to surgically cutting into tissue or to the cut itself; *compare* excision.

inclusion bodies or **inclusions:** General medical term for foreign particles seen within cells or tissues where they do not belong; in ophthalmic usage, often referring to particles of an unknown nature seen in the cornea.

inclusion conjunctivitis: *See* conjunctivitis.

incomitant (strabismus) (in-KAHM-uh-tent): *See* strabismus.

incongruous (in-KAHN-groo-us): General term indicating dissimilarity in form.

incongruous field defect (in-KAHN-groo-us): Visual field defects in both eyes that do not match each other; *compare* homonymous field defect.

incycloduction/intorsion (in-sy-kloh-DUK-shun): Inward rotation (ie, toward the midline of the face) of the eye around the visual axis, generally seen when the head is tilted; *compare* excycloduction/extorsion.

indentation tonometer: *See* tonometer.

index of refraction (IR): A comparison between the speed of light traveling through air versus the speed of light as it moves through an optical medium (eg, a lens); the mathematical formula is: speed of light in air/speed of light in material = refractive index; a more dense material causes light to pass more slowly through it, and thus has a high refractive index and a higher refracting ability; denser lens materials with a high index of refraction can be fashioned into high-power lenses that are relatively thin.

indirect illumination: In slit lamp biomicroscopy, method of viewing an ocular structure by reflected light in which the slit lamp light is directed onto some ocular structure other than the one to be viewed; *see also* retroillumination; *compare* direct illumination.

indirect lens: A hand-held lens used during indirect ophthalmoscopy.

indirect ophthalmoscopy: Process of viewing the inside of the eye through instrumentation consisting of a light source and lens/prism viewer worn on the examiner's head and a loose lens held in front of the patient's eye; called indirect because the image is seen upside-down and reversed; because the examiner uses both eyes, however, the image is three-dimensional; *compare* direct ophthalmoscopy.

indocyanine green (ICG) (in-doh-SY-uh-nine): Dye used in ophthalmology to image the choroid.

indocyanine green (ICG) angiography: Imaging technique in which ICG dye is injected into the arterial system; the dye remains inside the blood vessels, revealing the larger choroidal vessels.

induced: 1. In ophthalmic surgical usage, usually referring to a condition that is a result (often unwanted) of surgery, such as induced astigmatism following cataract surgery; *also called* consecutive; 2. in optics, the prismatic effect that occurs when the optical centers of a lens do not coincide with the patient's optical axis; *see* prism (definition 2).

infantile: General medical term describing a feature or process (eg, glaucoma or cataract) that occurs during the first 2 years of life; *compare* congenital, juvenile, senile.

infection: General medical term for invasion of the body/tissue by microorganisms; illness may or may not result.

inferior oblique (IO) muscle: Extraocular muscle lying underneath the eye around the equator of the globe and supplied by CN III (oculomotor nerve); responsible for elevating, abducting, and extorting the eye.

inferior rectus (IR) muscle: Extraocular muscle lying underneath the eye and supplied by CN III (oculomotor nerve); responsible for adducting, depressing, and extorting the eye.

infiltrates (IN-fil-trayts): Small particles that appear in tissue that is normally free of such particles; **corneal i.** whitish, cloudy particles in the cornea, often associated with infection or contact lens wear; **sterile i.** infiltrates, usually of the cornea, that are not associated with infection.

infiltrative keratitis (in-fil-trayt-iv kehr-uh-TY-tis): *See* keratitis.

infinity: In optics, imaginary point at distance from which rays of light travel in parallel paths; in clinical settings, 20 feet or more is considered to be infinity (thus, the numerator 20 for distance acuity measured using the Snellen's test chart).

informed consent: Process of explaining a treatment or procedure to the patient prior to its implementation, including risks and benefits such that the patient can sign a legal form stating that he or she understands the information presented; no surgery should ever be performed without prior informed consent by the patient or the patient's guardian.

infraduction (in-frah-DUK-shun): *Another term for* depression.

infraorbital (in-frah-OR-bit-al): At the bottom of or beneath the bony eye socket.

infusion: The act of introducing fluid into a closed anatomic structure, usually during surgery, or the fluid itself; *see also* irrigation.

injection: 1. The act of introducing fluid into tissue through a needle; 2. condition in which tissue is red, swollen, and engorged with dilated blood vessels; most often in ophthalmic usage referring to conjunctival injection.

inner granular or molecular layer (of retina): Cell layer within the retina composed primarily of nerve synapses and containing the amacrine cells, located between the ganglion cell layer and the inner nuclear layer; *see also* retina.

inner nuclear layer (of retina): Cell layer within the retina composed primarily of bipolar cells and containing the capillaries that supply blood to the retina; located between the inner and outer molecular layers; *see also* retina.

insertion: General medical term referring to: 1. location where a muscle attaches to bone or organ; 2. act of placing an object into the body (eg, a intraocular lens implant into the posterior chamber).

in situ (in SY-too): Latin term meaning "in place," denoting that an organ or tissue is in its normal and proper location.

inter-blink interval (IBI): Measurement of the time between blinks.

intercept: In retinoscopy, that part of the light that falls outside the subject's pupil (ie, on the face or phoropter); *compare* reflex (definition 3).

interferometer (in-ter-fuh-ROM-eh-ter): Instrument that measures visual acuity by using a laser to project a target onto the retina, bypassing the ocular media (and any opacities therein); the target is a grating, which is adjustable to decrease in size and spacing; the results indicate what the patient's probable vision would be if any media opacities were removed; *see also* potential acuity meter.

intermediate uveitis: *See* uveitis.

intermittent: Not present at all times; in ophthalmology, often referring to strabismus; *see also* definitions for esotropia, exotropia, strabismus.

internal limiting membrane (of the retina) (ILM): Innermost layer of the retina, in direct contact with the posterior hyaloid; *see also* retina.

internal rectus muscle: *Another term for* medial rectus muscle.

internal strabismus: *Another term for* esotropia.

International Code of Diseases (ICD): A system of designating conditions, disorders, injuries, and illnesses by number for statistical, regulatory, and other purposes.

interpupillary distance (IPD): *Another term for* pupillary distance.

interval of Sturm: *Another term for* Sturm's interval.

intort: To induce motion of an eye so that the "north pole" (ie, 12:00 position) of the globe tilts inward toward the other eye (ie, clockwise in the right eye and counterclockwise in the left); *compare* extort.

intracameral (in-tra-KAM-er-al): General medical term describing an entity located or occurring within a chamber; in ophthalmic usage, either within the anterior or posterior chamber.

intracameral anesthesia (in-truh-KAM-er-uhl): Anesthetic agent injected into the anterior chamber of the eye, usually during cataract surgery.

intracapsular cataract extraction (ICCE): General term for surgical techniques in which cataract extraction is accomplished either by grasping the lens (within its intact capsule) with forceps or cryoextraction; ICCE has been almost completely abandoned (except in economically underdeveloped areas of the world) in favor of extracapsular procedures; *see also* cataract extraction; *compare* extracapsular cataract extraction.

intracapsular ligament: Connective tissue joining the extraocular muscles to the globe.

intracorneal: Within the cornea.

intracorneal implant: *Another term for* intrastromal corneal ring.

intracranial pressure (ICP): Pressure inside the cranium (skull) governed by the formation and drainage of cerebrospinal fluid.

intraocular (in-trah-AHK-yuh-ler): General anatomic term for structure, entity, or process appearing or occurring within the eye.

intraocular lens (IOL) (in-trah-AHK-yuh-ler): Artificial lens surgically implanted into the eye to correct a refractive error, especially after cataract extraction; the age of contemporary IOLs is considered to have begun in 1949 with the first implantation of an IOL made of polymethylmethacrylate; contemporary IOLs are manufactured in many designs from a variety of materials, but all have in common a central focusing portion (the optic) and supporting structures (the haptics); *also called* pseudophakos; **acrylic IOL** foldable IOL manufactured from a polymer containing acrylic materials; **accommodating IOL** specially designed IOL that can be positioned so that the ciliary muscle will move it, changing the lens's effective power and providing both distance and near vision; *also called* pseudoaccommodative IOL; **anterior chamber IOL/ lens (A/C IOL or ACL)** IOL designed to be implanted in front of the iris, either after cataract extraction to correct aphakia or with the crystalline lens still in place to correct a refractive error; *compare* posterior chamber IOL; **C-loop IOL** IOL whose haptics are shaped like the letter C; **disk IOL** IOL with one circular haptic, designed to be implanted in the lens capsule to achieve centration; **foldable IOL** lens implant that can be folded, by virtue of either lens design or choice of soft lens material, and inserted into the eye through a small incision; *also called* soft IOL; **hydrogel IOL** foldable IOL manufactured from a polymer based upon the hydroxyethylmethacrylate (HEMA) molecule; **iris fixation IOL** largely obsolete anterior chamber IOL that was kept in place by attachment to the iris; **J-loop IOL** IOL with haptics shaped like the letter J; **phakic IOL** lens implanted to improve visual acuity while the natural crystalline lens remains in place; **piggyback**

IOLs two IOLs implanted in the same eye in order to provide higher refractive correction than is possible with a single IOL; **plate-haptic IOL** IOL designed with flat, more or less solid plates instead of "arms" for haptics; **posterior chamber IOL/lens (P/C IOL** or **PCL)** IOL designed to be implanted behind the iris, in either the lens capsule ("in the bag") or in the ciliary sulcus; *compare* anterior chamber IOL; **pseudoaccommodative IOL** *another term for* accommodating IOL; **secondary IOL (2° IOL)** IOL implanted in a separate procedure some time after the crystalline lens has been removed; **silicone IOL** foldable IOL manufactured from a polymer based upon the silicone molecule; **soft IOL** *another term for* foldable IOL.

intraocular lens exchange (in-trah-AHK-yuh-ler): Surgical procedure to remove one IOL and replace it with another, either to replace a damaged or dislocated IOL or to insert the appropriate power lens if the first lens failed to correct vision sufficiently.

intraocular pressure (IOP) (in-trah-AHK-yuh-ler): Pressure within the eye caused by the dynamics of the formation and drainage of aqueous humor; measured like atmospheric pressure as the height of a column of mercury that the pressure can support, thus the unit of measure is millimeters of mercury (mm Hg); *see also* glaucoma, hypotony, ocular hypertension, tonometry.

intraorbital (in-truh-OHR-bit-uhl): Within the bony eye socket.

intraorbital implant (in-truh-OHR-bit-uhl): Device, usually composed of a bone-like substance, implanted in the orbit after the eye is removed due to disease; often designed to accept a prosthetic eye.

intrascleral nerve loops (in-tra-SKLAYR-uhl): *Another term for* loops of Axenfeld.

intrastromal (in-tra-STROH-mal): General medical term for location within the main substance of a tissue; in ophthalmic usage, referring to the corneal stroma.

intrastromal corneal ring (in-tra-STROH-mal): Device, shaped like a lens, ring, or portion of a ring, implanted within the cornea to correct a refractive error; *also called* intracorneal implant.

intravitreal (in-tra-VIT-ree-uhl): Located within the vitreous humor.

intumescent cataract (in-too-MES-ent): *See* cataract.

invisible bifocal/trifocal: *Another term for* progressive addition lens.

ipsilateral (ip-suh-LAT-er-ul): Anatomic term meaning on the same side; *compare* bilateral, contralateral, unilateral.

irid-: Root word meaning iris.

iridectomy (ir-i-DEK-tuh-mee): Surgical procedure to remove iris tissue to facilitate the flow of aqueous humor and thus lower or prevent a rise in intraocular pressure; *compare* iridotomy; **peripheral i. (PI)** removal of a small wedge of iris tissue near its edge (ie, away from the pupil); **sector** or **total i.** iridectomy in which a portion of the iris from the edge of the pupil to the outer edge of the iris is removed (resulting in a keyhole pupil).

iridemia (ir-uh-DEE-mee-uh): Bleeding from the iris.

irides (IR-i-deez): Plural of iris.

iridocorneal angle (IR-ih-doh-KOHR-nee-uhl): *See* angle (definition 2).

iridocorneal endothelial syndrome (IR-ih-doh-KOHR-nee-uhl): Condition in which corneal and iris endothelial cells proliferate, causing adhesions between the iris and cornea as well as blocking the iridocorneal angle, resulting in intraocular pressure rise.

iridocyclitis (ir-id-oh-sy-KLY-tis): Inflammation of the iris and ciliary body; type of anterior uveitis; *see also* uveitis.

iridodialysis (ir-id-oh-dy-AL-uh-sis): Detachment of the root of the iris from the ciliary body.

iridodonesis (ir-id-oh-duh-NEE-sis): Abnormal antero-posterior movement ("flopping") of the iris, most often seen in aphakia or other situations in which the crystalline lens is displaced.

iridoplasty (ir-id-oh-PLAS-tee): Procedure using the argon laser to open the anterior chamber angle to lower IOP in angle closure glaucoma; *compare* iridectomy, iridotomy.

iridoplegia (ir-id-oh-PLEE-jee-uh): Partial or total paralysis of the iris.

iridotomy (ir-i-DOT-uh-mee): Surgical procedure to create an opening in the iris to provide a drainage point for aqueous and prevent build-up of intraocular pressure; *see also* laser iridotomy; *compare* iridectomy.

iris: Mobile, vascular, ring-shaped structure that lies behind the cornea and in front of the crystalline lens; its movements control the size of the pupil and, thus, the amount of light passing through to the retina; attached at its outer edge to the ciliary body and covered with a (usually) highly pigmented epithelial layer; the pupillary zone of the iris contains the iris sphincter (sphincter pupillae), which constricts the pupil, and the ciliary zone contains the outer dilator muscle (dilator pupillae), which dilates the pupil; the collarette is the border between the sphincter and dilator; the iris divides the anterior and posterior chambers of the eye, although surgical procedures involving the lens and ciliary body, both of which lie behind the iris, are described as anterior segment surgery; plural: irides.

iris-block glaucoma: *See* glaucoma.

iris bombé (bahm-BAY): "Ballooning" of the iris outward into the anterior chamber caused by a build-up of fluid behind the iris; *see also* pupillary block.

iris coloboma: *See* coloboma.

iris crypts: Normally occurring furrows in the front surface of the iris.

iris dilator: Peripheral circular muscle of the iris that widens (dilates) the pupil; *compare* iris sphincter.

iris freckle: *Another term for* iris nevus.

iris hooks: Surgical instruments used to catch the edge of the iris in order to pull and hold open the pupil during surgery.

iris nevus: Small benign area, either smooth or slightly elevated, of excess pigment on the iris; *also called* iris freckle.

iris plateau: *See* plateau iris.

iris prolapse: Protrusion of part of the iris through a wound or surgical incision.

iris root: Area of the iris where it inserts into the ciliary body.

iris sphincter: Circular muscle within the iris surrounding the pupil and responsible for constriction of the pupil; *compare* iris dilator.

iritis (i-RY-tis): Inflammation of the iris characterized by pain, photophobia, and redness; type of anterior uveitis; *see also* uveitis.

iron lines: Brown to black lines in the cornea caused by iron deposits.

irregular astigmatism: *See* astigmatism.

irrigation: General surgical term for washing a surface or cavity with fluid; *see also* infusion.

irrigation and aspiration (I&A, IA, or I/A): Surgical instrument and technique for removing intraocular tissue by simultaneously injecting fluid (ie, irrigation) and applying suction (ie, aspiration).

ischemia (is-KEE-mee-uh): General medical term denoting a lack of blood due to blockage of the blood supply; in ophthalmology, frequently referring to retinal ischemia.

ischemic optic neuropathy (ION) (is-KEE-mik): Damage to the optic nerve because of obstructed blood flow, usually resulting in sudden blindness with a poor prognosis for recovery; **anterior ION** damage is located in the area of the optic nerve that is most proximal to the globe.

iseikonia (i-suh-KOH-nee-uh): Normal condition in which each eye receives an image of similar size; *compare* aniseikonia.

Ishihara's test or **Ishihara color plates (ish-ee-HAR-ah):** Screening test for red/green color deficiency using pseudoisochromatic plates.

Island of Traquair or **island of vision (TRAH-kwahr):** Analogy that likens the visual field to an island with corresponding topography (eg, the macula is the highest point, the blind spot is a bottomless pit, and the outermost isopter is the shoreline).

isochromatic (i-soh-kruh-MAT-ic): Uniformity of color, either between two or more objects or between different parts of the same object (as in an iris that is of uniform color); *compare* anisochromatic, heterochromic.

isocoria (i-so-KOR-ee-uh): Normal condition in which the pupils of the two eyes are the same size; *compare* anisocoria.

isometropia (i-soh-mi-TROH-pee-uh): State in which both eyes have basically the same refractive power; *compare* anisometropia.

isopter (I-sop-ter): General term for line on a chart or map connecting similar numerical values; in ophthalmic usage, lines on a visual field test chart connecting the border of an area that responds to the same test object.

J-loop lens: *See* intraocular lens.

jack-in-the-box phenomenon: Distortion seen in high plus lenses in which the prismatic effect of the lenses creates a scotoma, thus an object may seem to suddenly appear and disappear as the wearer moves his or her head, causing the image to move in and out of the scotoma.

Jackson cross cylinder: *See* cross cylinder.

Jaeger acuity (J) (YAY-ger): Measurement of visual acuity at near distances (reading acuity) based upon standard sizes of printed block letters, recorded as J1, J2, etc.

Jaeger test (YAY-ger): A near vision test using targets (numbers, letters, E's, etc) of decreasing size and held at near, usually 14 inches.

jaw-winking phenomenon/syndrome: *Another term for* Marcus Gunn syndrome.

Jones I test: Test for nasolacrimal obstruction; fluorescein dye is instilled into one eye; the system is open if there is dye in the nasal passages after 5 minutes; *also called* primary dye test.

Jones II test: Test for nasolacrimal obstruction after a failed Jones I test; sterile saline is introduced into a dilated puncta; the system is open if the saline drains into the patient's throat; *also called* secondary dye test.

joule (J) (jool): Measurement unit of laser energy.

just noticeable difference (JND): In refractometry, the least amount of change in power for a patient to first distinguish any variation in visual acuity from that of the starting point (the patient's current correction).

juvenile: Describing a feature or process (eg, cataract or glaucoma) appearing or occurring in late childhood; *compare* congenital, infantile, senile.

K-reading: Radius of corneal curvature as measured during keratometry and expressed in millimeters (Europe) or diopters (United States).

kappa angle: *See* angle kappa.

Kaposi's sarcoma: *See* sarcoma.

Karickhoff lens (kah-RIK-of): *See* goniolens.

karyotype (KAR-ee-uh-typ): In genetics, an arranged picture of an individual's chromosome pairs, generated from tissue samples and using photomicrography; *also called* gene map.

Kelman phacoemulsification (KEL-mun): *See entry under* phacoemulsification.

kerat-, -o-: Root word literally meaning horn; usually referring to the cornea but also describing other "hard" tissues such as fingernails.

keratectasia (kayr-uh-tek-TAY-zhee-uh): Outward bulging of the cornea that occurs when corneal tissue is thinned or weakened; *also called* corneal ectasia.

keratectomy (kayr-uh-TEK-tuh-mee): General term for surgical removal of corneal tissue, usually performed as part of a corneal graft procedure; *see also* keratoplasty; excimer laser surgery is described as photorefractive keratectomy because wide areas of corneal tissue are removed.

keratic precipitates (KPs) (keh-RAT-ik): Small white or yellow bodies composed of inflammatory cells that adhere to the corneal endothelium, usually in the lower portion of the anterior chamber, seen in cases of iritis and iridocyclitis; **granulomatous** or **mutton-fat k.p.** large keratic precipitates resulting from long-standing inflammatory conditions; **punctate k.p.** small keratic precipitates.

keratitis (kayr-uh-TY-tis): General term for inflammation of the cornea; *see also* keratopathy; *Acanthamoeba* **k.** inflammation of the cornea resulting from an infection with the *Acanthamoeba* organism, almost always associated with contact lens wear; **annular k.** inflammation and appearance of deposits around the periphery of the cornea; **bacterial k.** corneal inflammation caused by a nonviral infection; **band k.** *see* keratopathy; **dendriform** or **dendritic k.** branched lesion appearing on the cornea in herpes virus infections; **diffuse lamellar k. (DLK)** uncommon immune/inflammatory response in refractive surgery in which leukocytes emerge between the flap and the corneal tissue beneath; *also called* Sands of Sahara syndrome; **disciform k.** disk-shaped edema deep in corneal tissue, often as a result of previous viral infection or inflammation; **epithelial punctate k.** *another term for* superficial punctate k.; **exposure k.** condition of corneal dryness, usually resulting from deficiency of tear fluid and/or incomplete closure of the eyelids especially during sleep; **filamentary k.** appearance of filaments attached to the corneal epithelium, can be a result of many conditions such as dry eye, infection, corneal abrasion, etc; **Herpes** or **herpetic k.** herpes virus infection leading to inflammation and lesions that may progress to ulcers; **infiltrative k.** corneal inflammation associated with whitish, cloudy particles, often indicating an infection or sometimes as a result of contact lens wear; **interstitial k.** keratitis involving deposits in the deeper tissues, resulting in corneal haze; usually associated with syphilis; **lattice k.** *another term for* lattice dystrophy; *see entry under* corneal dystrophy; **punctate k.** condition in which infiltrates form in tiny points on the corneal endothelium, usually associated with viral infection; **superficial punctate k. (SPK)** condition in which elevated opacities (which stain when fluorescein is used) form in small points on the surface of the corneal epithelium, usually centrally; *also called* epithelial punctate k.; **viral k.** corneal inflammation caused by a viral infection.

keratitis sicca (kayr-uh-TY-tis SIK-uh): *See* keratoconjunctivitis sicca.

keratocanthoma (kehr-uh-toh-kan-THOH-muh): Elevated lesion of the lids usually caused by sun exposure; sometimes confused with squamous cell carcinoma because both have a pigmented, cratered center.

keratocentesis (kayr-uh-toh-sen-TEE-sus): Surgical puncture of the cornea into the anterior chamber in order to remove aqueous humor for evaluation or to lower intraocular pressure; *also called* AC tap, paracentesis (general term).

keratoconjunctivitis (kayr-uh-toh-kun-junk-tuh-VY-tis): Inflammation of the tissues of the cornea and conjunctiva simultaneously; **atopic k.** keratoconjunctivitis associated with unusual sensitivity to allergens; **epidemic k. (EKC)** viral conjunctivitis that is highly contagious; duration is up to 3 weeks to 4 weeks; **phlyctenular k.** inflammation of the cornea and conjunctiva associated with the appearance of small blisters on both tissues; *see also* phlyctenule; **vernal k.** allergic disorder beginning in prepubescence featuring itching and stringy discharge; *also called* spring catarrh, seasonal conjunctivitis, warm weather conjunctivitis.

keratoconjunctivitis sicca (KCS) (kayr-uh-toh-kun-juk-tuh-VY-tis SIK-uh): Condition in which there is dryness, redness, and itching of the cornea and conjunctiva, often associated with chronic insufficient tear production; *see also* dry eye syndrome.

keratoconus (KC) (kayr-uh-toh-KOH-nus): Progressive malformation of the cornea such that it is thin and cone-like in shape rather than rounded; causes painless visual distortion (due to astigmatism) and loss; *also called* ectatic corneal dystrophy.

keratoglobus (kayr-uh-toh-GLO-bus): Malformation of the cornea such that it enlarges and protrudes in a globe-like shape, often with associated myopia and astigmatism.

keratomalacia (kayr-uh-toh-muh-LAY-shuh): Progressive degeneration of the cornea as a result of vitamin A deficiency.

keratome: Surgical instrument used to cut the cornea, either to create an incision into the eye for cataract surgery or to slice across the cornea to create a button for transplantation or flap for refractive surgery; *see also* keratomileusis, keratoplasty.

keratometer (kayr-uh-TOM-eh-ter): Any of several types of instruments used to measure the curvature of the cornea; the term usually refers to an instrument that measures the central 1.5 mm of the cornea, as long as the meridians of curvature are 90 degrees from each other; used in fitting contact lenses and in intraocular lens selection; *see also* corneal topography.

keratometry (kayr-uh-TOM-eh-tree): Measurement of corneal radius of curvature using a keratometer; *see also* K reading, keratometer.

keratomileusis (kayr-uh-toh-muh-LOO-sis): Any of several refractive surgical procedures in which a keratome is used to remove and/or reshape corneal tissue to correct a refractive error; *also called* corneal lathing; **automated lamellar k. (ALK)** *see entry under* keratoplasty; **Barraquer's k.** procedure no longer in use in which corneal tissue was removed, frozen, reshaped, thawed, and replaced on the eye; **hyperopic k.** keratomileusis performed to correct farsightedness; **laser epithelial k. (LASEK)** keratomileusis in which the corneal epithelium is loosened and pushed away from the central cornea, excimer laser ablation is applied, then the epithelium is replaced; **laser in-situ k. (LASIK)** keratomileusis in which a keratome is used to remove an outer layer of corneal tissue, a laser is used to reshape the exposed corneal tissue, and then the outer layer of corneal tissue is replaced (this technique is usually written and spoken as its abbreviation: LASIK); **myopic k.** keratomileusis performed to correct nearsightedness.

keratopathy (kayr-uh-TOP-uh-thee): General term for unhealthy condition of the cornea; *see also* keratitis; **band k.** condition, usually resulting from some underlying ocular or systemic disease, marked by calcium deposits in Bowman's layer that, as the name implies, appear across the cornea in narrow bands; *also called* ribbon k.; **bullous k.** degenerative condition of the cornea in which the epithelial cells form small blisters (ie, bullae) that eventually burst; usually the result of some previous ocular disease; **pseudophakic bullous k.** degenerative condition of the cornea resulting from improper intraocular lens implantation in which the endothelial cells form bullae; **ribbon k.** *another term for* band k.

keratophakia (kayr-uh-toh-FAY-kee-uh): Refractive surgical procedure in which a thin slice of cornea is removed then replaced over a suitably shaped piece of donor cornea (called a lenticle).

keratopigmentation (KAYR-uh-toh-pig-men-TAY-shun): Cosmetic procedure in which pigmentation is impregnated into corneal tissue to camouflage a cornea scar or to create the illusion of an iris in aniridia; *also called* corneal tattooing.

keratoplasty (KAYR-uh-toh-plas-tee): General term for corneal grafting procedure (commonly called a corneal transplant or corneal graft) in which a patient's cornea is removed with a keratome and replaced with donor tissue (as is commonly done in cases of corneal disease) or after being reshaped (as is done in some refractive surgical procedures); **automated lamellar k. (ALK or AK)** procedure in which a keratome is used first to remove an outer layer of corneal tissue and then to remove an inner layer of tissue; the outer layer of tissue is then replaced on the eye; the shape of the removed inner layer determines the change in the eye's refractive state; **full-thickness k.** *another term for* penetrating k.; l**amellar k. (LK or LKP)** or **partial penetrating k.** surgical procedure to treat corneal opacity by removing the layer of corneal tissue in the area of the opacity and replacing it with a clear corneal graft; **penetrating k. (PKP)** surgical procedure to treat corneal opacity in which the entire depth of a section of cornea is removed and replaced by a graft; *also called* full-thickness k.; **refractive k.** general term for keratoplasty performed to correct a refractive error.

keratoprosthesis (kayr-uh-toh-pros-THEE-sis): Artificial device used to replace the cornea either permanently in an attempt to restore sight (rarely used and rarely successful) or temporarily to facilitate some other operative procedure prior to replacing the cornea with a graft.

keratorefractive surgery (kayr-uh-toh-ree-FRAK-tiv): *See* refractive surgery.

keratoscopy (kayr-uh-TOS-kuh-pee): Technique for measuring the shape of the cornea by projecting evenly spaced, concentric circles of light (ie, keratometric mires) onto it; irregularities in the shape of the circles or the width of the space between them show deviations from a perfectly spherical shape; *see also* photokeratoscope, Placido's disk.

keratotomy (kayr-uh-TOT-uh-mee): Surgical procedure in which incisions are made into the cornea; usually referring to refractive surgical procedures in which incisions are carefully placed in the cornea so that the natural healing response and structural changes that ensue will reshape the cornea and correct any refractive errors present; **arcuate** or **astigmatic k. (AK)** keratotomy consisting of curved incisions (with the arc centered on the optical axis) performed to correct astigmatism; **radial k. (RK)** refractive surgical procedure in which corneal incisions are placed radially, like the spokes of a wheel (leaving a central optical zone free of incisions), in order to flatten the cornea and correct nearsightedness; the degree of flattening depends upon the depth (about 90% of the corneal thickness) and number (typically from 4 to 8) of incisions.

keyhole pupil: Condition in which the pupil resembles a keyhole following a sector iridectomy.

kinetic perimetry: *See* perimetry.

Koeppe lens (KEH-pee): *See* goniolens.

Krimsky measurement/test (KRIM-skee): Method of measuring a tropia in which the examiner uses prisms to move a light reflex in the patient's pupils until the reflexes are both centered; *see also* Hirschberg test.

Krukenberg's spindles (KROO-ken-burgz): Small, round deposits of pigment on the corneal endothelium arranged in a central, vertical pattern; often associated with iritis, diabetes, and pigmentary glaucoma; *also called* spindle cells.

Krupin implant, shunt, or **valve (KROO-pin):** Device implanted to control intraocular pressure by allowing aqueous fluid to flow from the anterior chamber into a filtering bleb.

laceration: General medical term denoting tissue damage by tearing.

lacri-: Combining form meaning tears; *see also* dacry-.

lacrimal apparatus: Collective term for the system that produces tears and drains them from the eye; it includes the lacrimal gland and accessory lacrimal glands (which produce tear fluid), the puncta (openings inside each upper and lower eyelid through which tear fluid drains), the lacrimal ducts or canaliculi (tubules that lead to the nasolacrimal sac), the nasolacrimal sac (which holds the overflow of tears), and the nasolacrimal duct (through which tears then drain into the nasal passages).

lacrimal bone: One of the bones of the orbit.

lacrimal caruncle (KAR-uhng-kul): Small mound of conjunctival tissue in the medial canthus.

lacrimal intubation: Surgical procedure in which a tube is implanted through the punctum, canaliculus, and nasolacrimal duct and into the nasal passage in order to restore tear drainage.

lacrimal lens: A reference to the refracting power of the tear film, generally as related to contact lens wear.

lacrimal probing: Surgical procedure in which a flexible probe is passed through the lacrimal duct in order to clear a blockage.

lacrimal sac: *See* nasolacrimal sac.

lacrimation (lak-ruh-MAY-shuhn): Flow of tears.

lactoferrin (lak-tuh-FER-in): Protein produced by the lacrimal gland and found in tear fluid.

lactoferrin test (lak-tuh-FER-in): Test in which a filter paper is placed on the eye to absorb tear fluid, then on a reactive plate that indicates the amount of lactoferrin present in the tears; in dry eye syndrome, lactoferrin levels are lower than normal.

lagophthalmos (lag-op-THAL-muhs): Incomplete closure of eyelids that may result in exposure keratitis.

lambda angle (LAM-duh): *See entry under* angle.

lamellar (luh-MEL-ur): Adjective describing a structure or process occurring in layers; partial-depth corneal transplants (as opposed to penetrating keratoplasty) are often described as lamellar grafts.

lamellar graft/keratoplasty (luh-MEL-ur KEHR-uh-toh-plas-tee): Surgical procedure in which only the damaged layers of the cornea are removed and replaced with donor tissue; *see also* keratoplasty.

lamina cribrosa (LAM-in-uh krib-ROH-suh): Mesh-like area of sclera at the back of the eye through which retinal ganglion cells and blood vessels pass; *also called* cribriform plate, scleral foramen.

laminar flow: Feature of the early venous phase of fluorescein angiography where the dye seems to coat the outside edges of the veins; *see also* fluorescein angiography.

Landolt's broken ring test: Vision test in which the optotypes are broken circles; the patient must identify the orientation of the breaks; *also called* Landolt's ring test.

Lanothony desaturated D-15 panel: *Another term for* desaturated 15 panel.

lase: To emit coherent light.

LASEK (laser epithelial keratomileusis): *See* keratomileusis.

laser: Acronym for light amplification by stimulated emission of radiation, a process invented in the early 1960s to produce coherent light; there are many types of lasers with diverse medical applications, all of which are based upon the fact that specific wavelengths of light are absorbed by specific tissues or compounds within tissues, with various consequent reactions; *see* Appendix 12; **argon fluoride (ArFl) l.** type of excimer laser that utilizes argon and fluorine; **argon l.** laser in which the light source is argon gas excited by electricity, producing laser energy in the blue-green part of the electromagnetic spectrum, which is absorbed by the red pigments of vascular tissue; action is via photocoagulation; current ophthalmic applications include treatment of diabetic retinopathy and macular degeneration, as well as trabeculoplasty and iridotomy; **carbon dioxide (CO_2) l.** laser in which the light source is carbon dioxide gas, producing laser energy at a fundamental wavelength of 10,600 nm; works via photovaporization; ophthalmic applications include removal of tumors from the orbit and cosmetic resurfacing of skin around the eyes; **diode l.** photocoagulating laser in which light is produced by electrical excitation of a solid-state semiconductor; used to treat retinal vascular disease; **dye l. (tunable dye l.)** photocoagulating laser in which a source of lased light is directed through a liquid dye that controls the wavelength of the energy that finally exits the laser; used in retinal vascular disease and glaucoma; **erbium:yttrium-aluminum-garnet (Er:YAG) l.** laser in which an Er:YAG crystal is excited by electricity and induced to emit laser light; ophthalmic applications include cosmetic procedures of the skin around the eyes; **excimer l.** photoablating laser in which the light source is an electrically excited dimer (a gas with two component elements, such as argon and fluoride); used to reshape the cornea by the process of photoablation; **helium-neon (HeNe) l.** laser producing light of a visible wavelength used as an aiming beam for ophthalmic surgical lasers that operate at invisible wavelengths; **holmium:YAG l.** laser that uses infrared wavelength; used to treat hyperopia via laser thermal keratoplasty; **l. interferometer** *see* interferometer; **krypton l.** photocoagulating laser used to treat the deeper choroid; **mode-locked l.** type of Q-switched laser that employs a dye; **neodymium:yttrium-aluminum-garnet (Nd: YAG) l.** laser in which an Nd:YAG crystal is excited by electricity and induced to emit laser light of infrared wavelength; the principal ophthalmic application of the Nd:YAG laser is posterior capsulotomy, although there are applications in vitreous and glaucoma surgery; **Q-switched l.** general term for photodisrupting lasers that concentrate energy into short pulses by employing filters to prevent light from exiting the laser until a certain threshold of energy is achieved; used for "fine cutting" as in iridotomy, breaking adhesions, etc; **ruby l.** original laser using an electric arc to produce light that is made coherent by a rod composed of synthetic ruby crystal; **YAG l.** *see* Nd:YAG l.

laser epithelial keratomileusis (LASEK): *See* keratomileusis.

laser in-situ keratomileusis (LASIK) (in sy-too): *See* keratomileusis.

laser iridotomy (ir-i-DOT-uh-mee): Creation of a hole in the iris using a laser; performed to enhance the flow of aqueous humor, thus maintaining normal intraocular pressure in eyes suffering from or predisposed to angle-closure glaucoma.

laser reversal of presbyopia (LARP or LRP): Laser is applied to the sclera in the area of the ciliary body in order to create more tension on the zonules; *compare* surgical reversal of presbyopia (SRP).

laser thermal keratoplasty (LTK) (KAYR-uh-toh-plastee): Refractive surgical procedure to correct hyperopia by applying infrared wavelength laser light to the peripheral cornea; usually referring to a proprietary treatment employing the holmium:YAG laser; *also called* holmium laser thermokeratoplasty; *compare* conductive keratoplasty.

laser trabeculoplasty (trah-BEK-yoo-loh-plas-tee): Destruction of small areas of the trabecular meshwork using a laser; performed to open the trabecular meshwork and lower intraocular pressure in eyes with glaucoma by improving aqueous outflow.

LASIK (laser in-situ keratomileusis): *See* keratomileusis.

late phase: Final segment (around 6 to 7 minutes following injection) of fluorescein angiography where the dye is leaving the retinal vasculature; generally only a faint glow of the choroidal and the area around the optic nerve remain; *see also* fluorescein angiography.

latent: General term describing a condition that is not immediately evident, such as a phoria or latent hyperopia; *compare* manifest.

lateral: General anatomic term describing a structure or process appearing or occurring at the side, away from the midline; in ophthalmic usage, referring to the side of the eye nearest the temple; *see also* temporal; *compare* medial, nasal.

lateral angle or **canthus (CAN-thus):** Area where the upper and lower eyelids join at the side of the face nearest the temple; *also called* temporal canthus; *compare* medial canthus.

lateral geniculate body (juh-NIK-yuh-lit): Area of the midbrain that receives visual impulses from the nerve fibers of the optic tract; *see also* visual pathway.

lateral rectus (LR) muscle: Extraocular muscle lying along the side of the eye near the temple, supplied by CN VI (abducens nerve) and responsible for abducting the eye; *also called* external rectus muscle.

lattice degeneration (of the retina): Condition in which the retinal tissues thin and blood vessels harden (leading to the "lattice" appearance), with break-up of the internal limiting membrane and adhesion of the vitreous to the retina; although most eyes with lattice degeneration do not progress to retinal detachment, about one third of eyes with retinal detachments have lattice degeneration as the underlying cause.

lattice dystrophy (of the cornea): *See* corneal dystrophy.

lazy eye: Colloquial term for amblyopia; laypeople sometimes misapply the term to strabismus (ie, an eye that is lazy and thus turns or drifts).

legal blindness: *See* blindness.

lens: General term for a transparent object (with two polished surfaces, at least one of them curved) that bends light rays from their original path, either to bring them together to a focus or spread them apart; *compare* prism; *see also* type of lens (Bagolini l., bifocal l., contact l., intraocular l., etc); **crystalline l.** reference to the natural lens of the eye.

lens blank: Unfinished spectacle or contact lens that has not yet been ground or fabricated to its final refractive power.

lens capsule: Thin, transparent, membranous envelope encasing the crystalline lens and to which the zonules are attached.

lens clock: Instrument used to measure the base curve of a spectacle lens; *also called* Geneva lens measure.

lens epithelium: The one-cell-thick layer of epithelial cells that covers the crystalline lens of the eye; when left in the lens capsule after cataract extraction, these cells can proliferate to form Elschnig's pearls.

lens glide: Surgical instrument used to support and guide an intraocular lens as it is being implanted into the eye.

lens loop: Surgical instrument consisting of a handle with a small loop at the end, usually notched with small "teeth," that is used to remove the crystalline lens during extracapsular cataract extraction; sometimes simply called a loop.

lens nucleus: *See* nucleus.

lens vault: *Another term for* apical clearance (definition 1).

lensectomy (len-ZEK-tuh-mee): Surgical procedure in which the crystalline lens is removed.

lenslet (LENZ-let): Small lens; *see also* Shack-Hartmann array.

lensmeter/lensometer (LENZ-mee-ter/lenz-AH-muh-ter): Instrument used to measure (or neutralize) the various components of curvature, and thus the refractive properties (ie, the "prescription") of an artificial lens.

lensometry (lenz-AH-muh-tree): The act of reading a lens prescription using a lensmeter/lensometer.

lenticle (LEN-tik-ul): Small "button" of donor corneal tissue used in refractive keratoplasty; *see also* keratophakia.

lenticular (len-TIK-yoo-ler): General term meaning of or like a lens, commonly referring to the natural crystalline lens of the eye; also used to describe "carrier" lenses for spectacle and contact lenses of high power.

lenticular astigmatism (len-TIK-yoo-ler): *See* astigmatism.

lenticular cataract (len-TIK-yoo-ler): Opacity of the crystalline lens; *see also* cataract.

lenticule (LEN-tuh-kyool): Alternate spelling for lenticle.

Leudde exophthalmometer (lood ex-op-thal-MAH-muh-ter): A clear ruler that is placed on the temporal bony orbit and used to measure ocular protrusion.

leukocoria (loo-koh-KOR-ee-uh): Literally, "white pupil," in which a dense white reflex is seen behind the pupil; associated with childhood retinoblastoma and retrolental fibroplasia.

leukocyte (LOO-kuh-syt): *Another term for* white blood cell.

leukoma (loo-KOH-muh): Dense white opacity of the cornea.

levator complex (leh-VAY-ter): Two-part muscle that lifts the upper eyelid, made up of the levator muscle and Müller's muscle.

levator muscle (luh-VEY-ter): Striated muscle portion of the levator complex that lifts the upper eyelid; more properly called the levator palpebrae superioris; *see also* Müller's muscle.

lid: Either of two flaps of skin that cover the eye during blinking; *see also* combining forms beginning with blephar-, palpebr-, and tars-; **l. eversion** flipping the lid inside out (eg, checking for a foreign body).

lid lag: Delay in downward motion of upper eyelid when the eye looks downward; *see also* von Graefe's sign.

lid lift: *Another term for* blepharoplasty.

lid retraction: Opening of the upper and/or lower lids wider than normal, resulting in excessive exposure of sclera; *see also* Dalrymple's sign.

lid speculum: Instrument used to hold the eyelids open.

light: Portion of the electromagnetic spectrum visible to the human eye.

light adaptation: *See* adaptation.

light/lightning flashes: *Another term for* flashes.

light peak: In electro-oculography, the response with the greatest width during the light-adapted phase of testing; *compare* dark trough; *see also* Arden ratio.

light perception (LP) vision: Very low visual acuity in which the subject can perceive only the presence or absence of light and is unable to see objects; *see also* count-finger vision, hand-motion vision; *compare* light projection, no light perception.

light projection (LP w/proj) vision: Low visual acuity in which the subject cannot see objects but can perceive not only the presence of light (ie, light perception), but also the direction from which it is shining; *see also* count-finger vision, hand-motion vision, visual acuity; *compare* light perception, no light perception.

limbal (LIM-bul): General medical term meaning near the line along which two structures meet; in ophthalmic usage, usually referring to the circular border between the cornea and sclera.

limbal conjunctiva (LIM-bul): *See* conjunctiva.

limbus (LIM-bus): General anatomic term for the line along which two structures meet; most commonly in ophthalmic usage, the circular border between the cornea and sclera; *also called* corneoscleral junction.

limiting membranes (of retina): *See* retina.

line of sight: *Another term for* visual axis; *see* axis.

line(s) of visual acuity: Reference to Snellen's visual acuity measurement in which the notation for distance visual acuity ranges from very low (20/400) to "normal" (20/20) and corresponds to lines of letters of diminishing size on the test chart; for example, a change from 20/30 to 20/40 visual acuity would be described as a "one-line loss," a change from 20/30 to 20/60 would be a "three-line loss," etc.

lipid: Substance composed of fat or oil and not soluble in water.

lipid layer: Outer layer of the tear film consisting of oily secretions (meibum) produced in the meibomian glands; *see also* tear film.

lissamine green (LIHS-uh-meen): Corneal dye that stains dry, dead, and deteriorated epithelial cells; used in diagnosing dry eye.

location: Part of the patient history where the patient identifies where a problem is occurring (eg, behind the eye, right upper lid, etc); *see also* history.

locus (LOH-kuhs): In genetics, a specific place on a chromosome occupied by a gene.

loop: 1. *Another term for* haptic; 2. *another term for* lens loop.

loops of Axenfeld: Branches off the long ciliary nerve that appear as tiny, dark spots on the inferior limbal sclera (usually nasally); *also called* intrascleral nerve loops.

loupe: Low-power magnifying device for viewing objects at very close range; usually referring to two loupes attached to a spectacle frame, employed by professionals performing close work on small objects (eg, jeweler's loupes) or by low-vision patients; before the operating microscope came into wide use, the patient's eye would be viewed during surgery through loupes worn by the surgeon.

low-pressure or **low-tension glaucoma:** *See* glaucoma.

low vision (LV): Visual impairment that cannot be remedied with corrective lenses or surgical intervention, usually describing a condition in which bilateral retinal pathology (eg, macular degeneration) renders an individual unable to perform normal daily functions; low vision is not synonymous with legal blindness; low vision has no objective definition because people have such widely varying needs for near versus distance vision or the ability to discern colors or fine detail.

low vision aids: General term for devices designed to help low-vision patients perform their daily tasks; *see* bioptics, loupe, magnifier, telescope, and typoscope.

lower-order aberration: *See* aberration.

LR6(SO4)3: Mnemonic for extraocular muscle innervation: lateral rectus innervated by CN VI, superior oblique by CN IV, and the other four by CN III.

lubricant: Substance designed to moisturize.

lumen (LOO-mun): 1. General term for the hollow area inside a duct or tube (eg, the lumen of the lacrimal duct); 2. in optics, the standard unit of the amount of light flowing through a solid angle (ie, a space shaped like a cone); 1 lumen (1 lm) is defined as the flux of light through 1 steradian emitted by a light source with 1 candela intensity.

luxation: General medical term meaning dislocation; in ophthalmology, often referring to displacement of the crystalline lens or an implant.

lymph (limf): Plasma-like fluid of the body containing mostly white and some red blood cells that is part of the immune system; found in lymph nodes and tissue spaces and carried by lymph capillaries and vessels; lymph eventually drains into the venous system.

lymph node (gland) (limf): Structure where lymph is filtered; of specific interest in ophthalmology is the preauricular node just in front of the ear, as it contains lymph from the conjunctiva and eyelids.

lymphocyte (LIM-fuh-syt): Inflammatory white blood cell that is formed in the lymph tissues and associated with chronic inflammation; **B-l.** lymphocyte that forms in the bone marrow; **T-l.** lymphocyte that forms in the thymus gland.

lyse (lahys): General medical term referring to the destruction of a cell by disrupting the cell membrane.

lysis (LY-sis): To destroy a cell by disrupting its cell membrane.

lysozyme (LY-so-zime): Natural enzyme found in tears that kills bacteria and viruses by lysis.

MacKay-Marg tonometer: *See* tonometer.

macrophage (MAK-ruh-fahj): A monocyte that has left the blood stream and can engulf bacteria and other antigens as part of the immune response; *also called* phagocyte.

macrophthalmia, -os (mac-rop-THAL-mee-uh): Condition in which the eyeball is abnormally large; *also called* megalophthalmia, megophthalmia; *see also* buphthalmos; *compare* microphthalmia.

macropia, -sia (meh-KROP-see-uh): Visual defect in which objects appear larger than they really are; *also called* megalopia; *compare* micropia.

macula (MAK-yu-luh): General anatomic term derived from the Latin for spot or stain; most commonly in ophthalmic usage, the small yellowish area of the retina where cone cells are most densely packed (more properly called the macula lutea); it is usually just below and temporal to the optic disk; the center of the macula is slightly depressed and known as the fovea, which in turn has a pit at its center called the foveola; *also called* macula lutea, retina, yellow spot; **corneal m.** area of cloudiness or white opacity on the cornea; **false m.** area of the retina that has an anomalous retinal correspondence with the macula of the fixating eye; *see* anomalous retinal correspondence.

macula lutea (MAK-yu-luh LOO-tee-uh): *Another term for* macula, referring to the macula's yellow hue (from Latin *lutea,* meaning yellow).

macular degeneration (MD) (MAK-yu-lar): General term for conditions in which the macular tissue breaks down, resulting in a loss of central vision; the visual loss is generally irreversible, although vitamin therapy, laser treatment, and surgical therapies are employed to slow its progression; **age-related m.d. (ARMD)** macular degeneration resulting from age-related changes in the small blood vessels, nerve cells, pigment epithelium, and other tissues in the macula; *also called* senile m.d.; **dry m.d.** relatively mild form of macular degeneration that is not accompanied by the formation of retinal exudates; *compare* wet m.d.; **senile m.d. (SMD)** *another term for* age-related m.d.; **wet m.d.** more severe form of macular degeneration that is accompanied by the formation of retinal exudates as a result of new, abnormal blood vessel growth (choroidal neovascularization); *compare* dry m.d.

macular ERG (MAK-yu-lar): *See* electroretinography.

macular hole (MAK-yu-lar): A small, well-defined opening in the macula through the entire thickness of the retina, possibly as a result of the vitreous body pulling on its attachments in the area of the macula.

macular photostress test (MPT) (MAK-yu-lar): Test to evaluate the macula's ability to recover after exposure to a bright light; useful in assessing macular disease; *also called* photostress test.

macular pucker (MAK-yu-lar): *See* epiretinal membrane.

macular sparing (MAK-yu-lar): Condition in which the central vision remains functional although the rest of the field exhibits extensive damage; seen in lesions affecting the optic radiations or the occipital lobe of the brain.

macular splitting (MAK-yu-lar): Condition in which the left or right side of the visual field, including the central field, is divided (ie, half of the field, specifically including the central field, remains).

maculopathy (mak-yu-LOP-uh-thee): General term for disorders of the macula.

madarosis (mad-uh-ROH-sis): Loss of lashes due to destruction of the follicles (as by disease), or congenital absence of lash and brow hairs.

Maddox rod: A red lens composed of cylinders; a point source of light viewed through the Maddox rod appears as a red streak of light; used in measuring muscle deviations, especially phorias.

magnetic resonance imaging (MRI): Use of radio waves (created by a strong magnetic field) to create an image of the body's interior; best used to view soft tissues; in ophthalmology, used to evaluate conditions involving swelling, tumors, and nerves; *compare* computerized tomography.

magnification: In optics, making an image appear larger; *compare* minification.

magnifier: In ophthalmic usage, a device used by low-vision patients to enlarge objects for better viewing, usually to facilitate reading and writing; **hand-held m.** magnifier consisting of a high-power plus lens that is held by the user; **projection m.** magnifier that projects an enlarged image of the object to be viewed onto a screen; **stand m.** magnifier consisting of a high-power plus lens that is mounted on a stand, leaving the user's hands free.

magnify: To visually enlarge, generally by the use of plus spherical lenses; *compare* minify.

malar bone: *Another term for* zygomatic (cheek) bone.

malignant: Generally used to describe a growth or condition that is uncontrolled, especially if invasive and ultimately life-threatening; *compare* benign.

malignant glaucoma: *See* glaucoma.

malignant melanoma: *Another term for* melanoma.

malignant myopia: *Another term for* degenerative myopia; *see entry under* myopia.

malingering (muh-LING-ger-ing): Situation in which the patient purposely gives false information (usually to make the vision, etc, appear worse than it is) during subjective testing in order to gain something (financial reimbursement, a pair of glasses, sympathy, etc); includes memorizing the eye chart to make vision seem better than it is (to get driver's license, a job, etc).

manifest: General term describing a condition that is evident, such as a tropia or manifest hyperopia; *compare* latent.

manifest refraction (MR): 1. Determining the refractive error at distance so that the eye does not accommodate, but without using drugs that actually prevent accommodation; 2. the refractive error measured in this manner.

manual vitrectomy: *See entry under* vitrectomy.

map-dot-fingerprint dystrophy (MDF): *See* corneal dystrophy.

Marcus Gunn pupil (MG): Impairment of the normal response of the affected pupil to bright light when stimulated by the light; verified by the swinging flashlight test, in which the examiner shines a light first into one eye, then into the other, then again into the first, comparing the response of the two pupils; Marcus Gunn pupil usually appears as a constriction of both pupils when the unaffected eye is illuminated, followed by an apparent dilation of both pupils when the affected eye is illuminated; the defect is sometimes manifest by the affected pupil constricting less to a direct light stimulus than does the unaffected pupil when presented with the same stimulus; *also called* afferent pupillary defect, Gunn's pupil, relative afferent pupillary defect; **reverse M.G.p.** situation in which the pupil of the affected eye is fixed; during the swinging flashlight test, the unaffected pupil will dilate when the light is shown into the affected pupil; when the light is swung to the unaffected pupil, that pupil will constrict very rapidly.

Marcus Gunn syndrome: Abnormal regeneration of the oculomotor branch of the trigeminal nerve that causes the eyelid to close when the mouth is opened; *also called* jaw-winking phenomenon/syndrome.

Marfan syndrome (MAR-fan): Genetic disorder that may be associated with subluxation of the crystalline lens; affected individual often has long, spindly limbs and digits.

mast cell: Inflammatory white blood cell (present in various tissues including those of the eye) that plays a role in the release of histamine and other substances involved in allergy; *also called* basophil; **m.c. stabilizer** in ophthalmic usage, a topical drug that acts to prevent mast cells from releasing histamines, and thus prevent or diminish the severity of ocular allergies.

maxillary bone: One of the bones of the orbit.

medial: General anatomic term describing a structure or process appearing or occurring in the middle; in ophthalmic usage, referring to the area of the eye nearest the nose; *see also* nasal; *compare* lateral, temporal.

medial angle/canthus: Area where the upper and lower eyelids join at the side of the face nearest the nose; *also called* nasal canthus; *compare* lateral canthus.

medial rectus (MR) muscle: Extraocular muscle lying along the side of the eye near the nose, supplied by CN III (oculomotor nerve) and responsible for adducting the eye; *also called* internal rectus muscle.

medium, -ia: 1. In optical usage, transparent object(s) or substance(s) through which light travels; the fact that light travels at different speeds in different substances accounts for the different degrees to which light is bent (refracted) by various media; *see also* index of refraction; **ocular m.** or **refracting m.** tissues in the eye through which light is transmitted: the cornea, aqueous humor, lens, and vitreous humor; sometimes includes the tear film; 2. in microbiology, a substance formulated for the culturing of microorganisms in the lab; *also called* culture medium, growth medium.

megalocornea (meg-uh-loh-KOHR-nee-uh): Abnormally large, otherwise normal, cornea due to an X-linked recessive gene.

megalophthalmia, -os (meg-uh-loh-op-THAL-mee-uh): *Another term for* macrophthalmia.

megalopia, -sia (meg-uh-LOH-pee-uh): *Another term for* macropia.

megophthalmia, -os: *Another term for* macrophthalmia.

meibomian cyst (my-BOH-mee-uhn): Inflammation of the eyelid that results in the collection of fluid within the meibomian gland; may develop into a chalazion; *see also* chalazion, hordeolum.

meibomian glands (my-BOH-mee-uhn): Glands located within the eyelids that produce oil; their secretions form the outer layer of the tear film; *also called* tarsal glands.

meibomianitis or **meibomitis (my-BOH-mee-uh-ny-tis):** Inflammation of the meibomian glands.

meibum (my-bum): The oily secretions of the meibomian glands that make up the lipid layer of the tear film.

melanin: Dark pigment present in the skin, hair, and retina.

melanoma: Generally referring to a pigmented, aggressive form of cancer that usually metastasizes; *also called* malignant melanoma; *compare* basal cell carcinoma, squamous cell carcinoma.

melting: *See* corneal melting.

membrane: General medical term for a thin tissue layer that acts as a "skin" or covering, lining, or connection between tissues, either as part of normal anatomy or a disease process; *see also* specific entry (Bruch's m., choroidal neovascular m., hyaloid m., etc); **anterior basal m.** *another term for* Bowman's capsule; **basement m.** general medical term for the thin membrane that lies underneath the epithelium of certain tissues; in ophthalmic practice, often referring to the basement membrane of the choroid or corneal epithelium.

membranectomy: Surgical removal of a membrane; in ophthalmic usage, usually referring to removal of retinal membranes.

meniscus (muh-NIS-kus): Curved, crescent-shaped surface; in ophthalmology, often referring to the surface of a concavoconvex or convexoconcave lens or to the curved surface of the tear film pooled at the lower lid.

meniscus lens (muh-NIS-kus): *Another term for* convexoconcave or concavoconvex lens.

meridian: Geometric term for a line passing through the poles (two points diametrically opposite) of a sphere; in ophthalmic usage: 1. standard reference lines used to describe positions on the eyeball; 2. used to describe the positions of the greatest and least curvature, generally on the cornea or a contact lens; 3. used to describe the plane of a cylindrical lens where the power lies; *compare* cylinder axis *under* axis.

meshwork: *See* trabecular meshwork.

mesopia (mez-OH-pee-uh): Vision under conditions of partial lighting, such as dimly lit rooms or outdoors at sunset and sunrise; *compare* photopia, scotopia.

mesopic ERG (mez-AH-pic): *See* electroretinography.

metamorphopsia (met-uh-mohr-FAHP-see-uh): Distorted vision, often associated with macular conditions.

methylcellulose (mehth-uhl-SELL-yoo-lohs): Organic compound that is a component of some artificial tears and viscoelastic substances.

microbiology: The study of microorganisms.

microorganism: Any very tiny living organism that cannot be seen without a microscope; may be single- or multi-celled; includes bacteria, protozoans, viruses, and some fungi.

microphakia (my-kroh-FAY-kee-uh): Abnormally small crystalline lens.

microphthalmia, -os (my-kroh-op-THAL-mee-uh): Abnormally small eye; *also called* nanophthalmia; *compare* macrophthalmia.

micropia, -sia (my-KROH-pee-uh): Visual defect in which objects appear smaller than they really are; *compare* macropia.

microsaccades (MY-kroh-seh-KAYDZ): Extremely fine involuntary movements of the eye that occur while the eye is fixated on an object; *see also* saccades.

microscope: Optical instrument that uses lenses to magnify objects; **biomicroscope** *another term for* slit lamp m.; **operating m.** microscope used by the ophthalmic surgeon to obtain an enlarged view of the eye; it is typically outfitted with a bright light and often has multiple eyepieces for use by other personnel or attachment of a camera; **slit lamp m.** *see* slit lamp.

microstrabismus: *See* strabismus.

minification: In optics, making an image appear smaller; *compare* magnification.

minify: To decrease the apparent size of an object, usually with minus spherical lenses; *compare* magnify.

mini-stroke: *Another term for* transient ischemic attack.

minus: 1. Property of an optical system such that it causes rays of light to diverge (eg, a biconcave lens); 2. in spoken ophthalmic usage, synonym for myopia (eg, a "minus 2 diopter patient").

minus cylinder: 1. Cylindrical lens that diverges light rays; *see also* cylinder; *compare* plus cylinder; 2. lens prescription written using minus cylinder power.

minus lens: Lens that causes incoming rays of light to diverge (*see* concave lens, cylinder [definition 2]); *also called* divergent lens; in common ophthalmic usage, the power of the minus sphere lens needed to correct nearsightedness is often used to describe the degree of myopia (thus, a "high minus" or "minus six" patient); *compare* plus lens.

miosis (my-OH-sis): Constriction of one or both pupils in response to stimulation by bright light, to accommodation, or to certain drugs or disease processes; *compare* mydriasis.

miotic (my-OT-ik): 1. State in which one or both pupils are constricted (generally meaning 2 mm or smaller); 2. any process or agent that constricts the pupils (as in a miotic drug).

mire: General term for a reference line of standard shape on a measuring device (eg, lensometer, keratometer, etc).

Mittendorf's dot (MIT-in-dorfs): Small opacity sometimes found on the posterior surface of the mature lens, indicating the former attachment site of the hyaloid artery; *see also* hyaloid artery.

mixed astigmatism: *See* astigmatism.

mixed nerve: Nerve that has both sensory (afferent) and motor (efferent) components; *see* motor nerve, sensory nerve.

Miyake photography or **view (mee-YAH-kee):** Method for viewing the anterior segment of a cadaver eye from the rear by dissecting the front part of the eye and fixing it to a clear plate behind which the camera is located.

model eye: *Another term for* schematic eye (definition 1).

modulation transfer function: Laboratory method for determining the light-transmitting characteristics of an optical system by analyzing light of known wave form after it passes through the system.

Moll (glands of): Modified sweat glands in the eyelid margin.

molluscum contagiosum (meh-LUS-kum KUN-tay-jee-OH-sum): Small, benign, wart-like skin lesions caused by a virus and thus contagious.

monochromatic (mon-oh-kroh-MAT-ik): Characterized by a single color, as in an image of only one hue or light of a single wavelength (eg, laser light).

monochromatism (mon-oh-KROH-muh-tiz-uhm): Very rare condition in which only one of the three visual pigments is present, usually cyanolabe and thus termed blue cone m.; *compare* achromatism, dichromatism, trichromatism.

monocular: Literally, "one eyed"; used alone to describe a patient with one functional eye or combined with another term to describe an ocular condition involving only one eye, as in monocular vision (ie, seeing with only one eye), monocular diplopia (ie, double image in one eye), etc; *see also* unilateral (as in one eye), uniocular; *compare* binocular.

monocyte (MON-oh-syt): Large white blood cell formed in bone marrow; called a macrophage if found outside the blood stream.

monovision: Situation in which one eye sees at near and the other at distance, usually artificially created for the presbyope using either contact lenses or intraocular lens implants.

morgagnian cataract (mohr-GAHN-yun): *See* cataract.

motility: Referring to movement; in ophthalmology, the study of extraocular muscles and their role in ocular alignment; *see also* strabismus.

motor fusion: *See* fusion.

motor nerve: Efferent nerve that carries an impulse (response to sensory input) from the brain to muscle tissue or glands; *compare* mixed nerve, sensory nerve.

mucin: Protein that is the primary component of mucus; in the eye, goblet cells in the conjunctiva produce the mucin that is found in tear fluid.

mucous: Adjective referring to membranes, glands, or other tissues that produce mucus.

mucus: A viscous substance produced by certain glands for lubrication and protection of tissues.

Müller's cells (MYOO-lerz): Retinal cells located in the inner nuclear layer with fibers extending to the internal and external limiting membranes; Müller's cells serve as part of the structural meshwork of the retina and supply nutrients and other metabolic materials to retinal nerve cells.

Müller's muscle (MYOO-lerz): Smooth muscle portion of the levator complex that opens the upper lid; *also called* superior tarsal muscle; *see also* levator muscle.

multifocal lens: Artificial lens that is designed to provide more than one, and usually more than two, focal points; several multifocal systems have been developed for spectacle, intraocular, and contact lenses; *see also* aspheric lens, bifocal lens, diffractive multifocal lens.

multiple vision: *Another term for* polyopia.

mutation: In genetics, a permanent change in the structure of a gene that is capable of being passed on to progeny.

mutton-fat precipitates: *See* keratic precipitates.

myasthenia gravis (MG) (my-uhs-THEE-nee-uh GRAV-is): Chronic systemic disease characterized by muscle weakness; in the eye, ptosis and diplopia are typical.

mydriasis (mi-DRY-uh-sis): Widening of one or both pupils, usually as a response to reduced light but also to certain drugs or disease processes; *see also* dilation; *compare* miosis.

mydriatic (mid-ree-AT-ik): Condition or agent that dilates the pupils, as in a mydriatic drug.

mydriatic provocative test: Use of a topical mydriatic ("dilating drop") to ascertain if this will cause angle closure; *see also* dark room provocative test, provocative test.

myelin (MY-uh-lin): Fatty sheath that covers some nerve cell axons.

myope: Individual with myopia; *compare* hyperope.

myopia: Refractive error in which the eye focuses rays of light so that the focal point is in front of the retina, with the result that distant objects are not clearly seen; *also called* nearsightedness; *compare* hyperopia; **axial m.**

nearsightedness attributable to the length of the eye (ie, the eye is too long for images to be focused on the retina); *compare* refractive m.; **degenerative m.** nearsightedness attributable to severe, ongoing structural changes in the eye, eventually resulting in permanent damage to the retina; *also called* malignant m.; **high m.** nonspecific term for extreme myopia beyond what is found in most of the population, usually referring to myopia of 6 D or greater; **index m.** nearsightedness resulting from a crystalline lens of more plus power than normal (eg, in cataract progression); **lenticular m.** nearsightedness attributable to excessive (plus) power of the crystalline lens; **low m.** nonspecific term for small amount of myopia, usually referring to myopia of –2 D or less; **malignant m.** *another term for* degenerative m.; **moderate m.** nonspecific term referring to an amount of myopia that causes significant but not extreme visual impairment, usually referring to myopia between –2 D and –6 D; **night m.** difficulty seeing at a distance in dim light, occurring because the dilated pupil reduces the depth of field; **progressive m.** nearsightedness that continues to worsen; **pseudomyopia** temporary nearsightedness associated with drugs or systemic disorders (such as diabetes) that resolves when the underlying cause is removed; **refractive m.** nearsightedness that is attributable to the refractive power of the eye (ie, the refractive power of the cornea and lens is too great and brings incoming rays of light to focus in front of the retina); *compare* axial m.; **school m.** nearsightedness that seems to arise from prolonged use of near vision for reading during the school year.

myopic: Adjective referring to myopia or nearsightedness; *compare* hyperopic.

myopic keratomileusis: *See* keratomileusis.

myotonic pupil (mahy-uh-TON-ik): *Another term for* Adie's pupil; *also called* pupillotonia, tonic pupil.

nanophthalmia, -os (nan-op-THAL-mee-uh): *Another term for* microphthalmia.

narrow angle: *Another term for* shallow angle.

narrow-angle glaucoma (NAG): *See* closed-angle glaucoma *under* glaucoma.

nasal: General anatomic directional term meaning toward the nose; *see also* medial; *compare* lateral, temporal.

nasal bone: Either of two bones lying between the orbits and forming the bridge of the nose.

nasal canthus: *Another term for* medial canthus.

nasal step: Visual field defect in which a two-part defect "steps" from nasal to temporal with a normal field in between; corresponds to damage of nerve fibers near the central portion of the retina's nasal side; most often associated with glaucoma.

nasolacrimal duct (NLD) (nay-zoh-LAK-ruh-mul): Canal through which tear fluid drains from the nasolacrimal sac into the nasal passages; *see also* lacrimal apparatus.

nasolacrimal probing (nay-zoh-LAK-ruh-mul): Procedure to open an obstructed nasolacrimal passage; a thin wire is passed through the canaliculus and into the nasolacrimal sac and duct.

nasolacrimal sac (nay-zoh-LAK-ruh-mul): Internal sac adjacent to the eye that holds tears that have drained off the eye; *also called* dacryocyst, lacrimal sac, tear sac; *see also* lacrimal apparatus.

Nd:YAG laser: Neodymium:yttrium-aluminum-garnet; *see entry under* laser.

near acuity: *Another term for* near vision.

near point of accommodation (NPA): Distance from the eye to the nearest point clearly visible when accommodation is at its maximum.

near point of convergence (NPC): Nearest point where the eyes can maintain binocular vision by pulling together; the greatest degree of convergence that the eyes can attain.

near vision: Measurement of acuity for close-up tasks, generally tested at 14 inches using a standard reading card; *compare* distance vision; *also called* near acuity, reading vision; *see also* vision.

nearsighted/nearsightedness: *Another term for* myopia.

necrosis (neh-KRO-sus): General term referring to abnormal death of cells or tissue (eg, as part of a disease process or injury).

neoplasm: Abnormal growth of cells that form a tumor or new tissue; may be benign or malignant.

neovascular glaucoma: *See* glaucoma.

neovascularization (nee-oh-vas-cu-lar-eh-ZAY-shun): Abnormal growth of blood vessels caused by some disorder or disease state, most often seen in diabetic retinopathy; these new vessels are generally weak and prone to leakage and bleeding; **corneal n.** abnormal blood vessel growth into the cornea, usually associated with contact lens wear; **retinal n.** abnormal blood vessel growth into the retina, usually associated with diabetes and hypertension.

nerve fiber bundle defect: Visual field defect caused by damage to the nerve fiber layer; *see* nerve fiber layer; characteristically these monocular defects include nasal step and scotomas in the central field.

nerve fiber layer (NFL): Retinal nerve fibers (actually, axons of the ganglion cell layer) that come together at the optic nerve head; their unique pattern of distribution plays a key role in the appearance of visual field defects, most notably in glaucoma; *see also* retina.

neuritis (nuhr-I-tiss): General medical term referring to inflammatory condition of nerves in the peripheral nervous system.

neuroblastoma (nuhr-o-blass-TOH-muh): Malignant orbital tumor of childhood.

neuron (NOO-ron): A nerve cell consisting of the cell body from which radiate short, branched extensions (dendrites) and long, myelin-encased process (axon).

neuro-ophthalmology: Medical subspecialty concerned with the nervous system's involvement with the eye, both sensory and motor; includes ocular movements, pupillary responses, and the structures of the brain involved in vision.

neuropathy (nuhr-OP-ah-thee): General medical term meaning a disorder (usually noninflammatory) affecting nerves in the peripheral nervous system.

neurotransmitter (NURH-o-TRANZ-mit-uhr): Biochemical that crosses the synapse (gap) between nerve cells, attaches to specific receptor sites, and thus carries messages from the brain; *see* acetylcholine, epinephrine, norepinephrine.

neutrality: In retinoscopy, the point where the pupillary reflex seems to "wink" on and off, rather than displaying against or with motion; *compare* "against" motion (definition 1), "with" motion (definition 1).

neutralize/neutralization: 1. In optics, the act of determining the power of an unknown lens; *see also* lensometry; 2. in retinoscopy, the act of determining the refractive state of the eye by adjusting lenses before the eye until the pupil is uniformly illuminated by the retinoscope; 3. the act of correcting a refractive error with lenses or strabismus with prisms.

neutrophil (NOO-truh-fil): Mature, inflammatory white blood cell that engulfs bacteria and releases enzymes as a response to infection or injury; *also called* polymorphonucleocyte (PMN).

nevus (NEE-vuhs): A nonmalignant lesion on the skin or other tissue; may or may not be pigmented and/or raised and/or smooth; in the eye, it is more frequently found on the lids, conjunctiva, iris, and choroid but can appear on other tissues/structures as well; plural: nevi.

nictitation (nic-tih-TAY-shun): Blinking, especially in animals that have a thin, translucent membrane (ie, nictitating membrane) instead of fleshy eyelids.

night blindness: *Another term for* nyctalopia.

night vision: *Another term for* scotopia.

no light perception (NLP) vision: Total blindness; *see also* count-finger vision, hand-motion vision, visual acuity; compare light perception vision, light projection vision.

nocturnal amblyopia (nahk-TERN-uhl am-blee-OH-pee-uh): *Another term for* nyctalopia.

nodal point: *Another term for* optical center.

nominal power (of a lens): The algebraic sum of the front and back surface powers of a lens; *compare* effective power.

nomogram (NOM-uh-gram): A mathematical formula or graph used to calculate necessary action for a specific outcome; ocular procedures using nomograms include contact lens fitting, intraocular lens selection, refractive surgery methods (ie, how many incisions, how deep, and where to place them; size of pupillary zone; how much tissue to remove; etc); such a formula or graph allows each practitioner or surgeon to enter numbers specific to his or her own methods, experience, and other data that will enable the best results.

nonaccommodative esotropia: *See* esotropia.

nonconcomitant (strabismus) (non-con-KAHM-eh-tent): *See* strabismus.

noncontact tonometer (NCT): Another term for air-puff tonometer, *see entry under* tonometer.

nondominant eye: The eye that is subjectively less preferred for use by an individual, much the way one hand is less preferred than the other; *compare* dominant eye.

nonproliferative: General medical term meaning an entity or condition that does not spread; *compare* proliferative.

nonproliferative retinopathy: Retinal abnormality/pathology that does not spread, especially in diabetic retinopathy; *compare* proliferative retinopathy.

nonsteroidal anti-inflammatory drug (NSAID): A drug used to reduce inflammation that does not contain steroids, thus avoiding the undesirable side effects of steroids; *compare* corticosteroid.

noradrenaline (nohr-ah-DREN-uh-lin): *Another term for* norepinephrine.

norepinephrine (nohr-ep-uh-NEF-rin): One of two biochemicals that conducts messages for the sympathetic nervous system (the other is epinephrine); *also called* noradrenaline; *see also* epinephrine; *compare* acetylcholine.

normal retinal correspondence (NRC): *Another term for* harmonious retinal correspondence.

Nu value (NOO): *Another term for* Abbe value.

nuclear adhesions: Small areas where the nucleus and cortex of the crystalline lens normally are attached.

nuclear cataract/sclerosis: *See* cataract.

nuclear layer (of the retina): One of two layers of retinal nerve tissue; the outer nuclear (or bacillary) layer consists of the rod and cone cells, and the inner layer consists of the amacrine and bipolar cells, as well as the capillaries that carry blood through the retina; *see also* retina.

nucleus: General term for a central structure; in ophthalmic usage, most commonly referring to the nucleus of the crystalline lens.

null point: In congenital nystagmus, the head/eye position where ocular movement is either neutralized or maximally reduced.

nyctalope (NIK-ta-lohp): Individual with nyctalopia.

nyctalopia (nik-ti-LOH-pee-uh): Visual defect in which vision is greatly reduced in low light conditions, most often as a result of retinal pigment insufficiency; commonly called night blindness; *also called* nocturnal amblyopia.

nystagmus (ny-STAG-muhs): Rapid, rhythmic, involuntary eye movements; nystagmus is classified according to the direction of motion (horizontal is the most common) and the stimuli that cause it to occur; *see* Appendix 6; **amaurotic n.** nystagmus of a blind eye; **caloric n.** nonpathological vestibular nystagmus that results when the semicircular canals of the inner ear are stimulated by irrigating the ear with warm or cold fluid; *also called* labyrinthine n.; **congenital n.** nystagmus present from birth; **conjugate n.** nystagmus in which the eyes move in the same direction and with the same rhythm; **disconjugate n.** nystagmus in which the eyes exhibit different directions or rhythms; **dissociated n.** nystagmus in which the amplitude of the movements are not the same in both eyes; **endpoint n.** nonpathological nystagmus that sometimes occurs when the eyes are turned as far in one direction as possible; **fixation n.** nystagmus that occurs as the eyes attempt to maintain prolonged fixation; **induced n.** nonpathological nystagmus caused by an outside source, including drugs; other types include caloric n., optokinetic n., and rotational n.; **jerk n.** *another term for* rhythmic n.; **labyrinthine n.** *another term for* caloric n.; **latent n.** nystagmus that either appears or increases when one eye is covered; **optokinetic n. (OKN)** nonpathological, rapid movements of the eyes as they move to fixate on rhythmic, repeating stimuli; *also called* railroad n.; **pendular n.** nystagmus in which the eye's movement in one direction is equal to the movement in the other; **physiologic n.** nonpathological nystagmus that can be evoked in the normal person; **railroad n.** *another term for* optokinetic n.; **rhythmic n.** pattern of eye movement that is slower in one direction followed by a more rapid movement back to the original position; *also called* jerk n.; **rotatory n.** nystagmus in which the eyes revolve around the visual axis; **vestibular n.** nonpathological vestibular nystagmus that results when the semicircular canals of the inner ear are stimulated.

object of regard: *Another term for* fixation object.

objective: 1. Method of testing that does not require input from the patient (eg, retinoscopy, Krimsky measurement, slit lamp exam); *compare* subjective; 2. *another term for* objective lens.

objective lens: In optical systems, especially telescopes and microscopes, the lens nearest to the object being viewed; *compare* ocular (definition 2).

obligatory suppression: Constant mental "blocking out" of the image from one eye in order to prevent double vision, whether the eye is deviated or not; *compare* facultative suppression.

oblique astigmatism: *See* astigmatism.

oblique muscles: *See* inferior oblique muscle, superior oblique muscle.

O'Brien block: Injection of anesthetic agents to achieve akinesia (prevention of movement) of the eyelids.

occipital cortex (ok-SIP-i-tl): The outer part of the occipital lobe.

occipital lobe (ok-SIP-i-tl): That area of the brain, specifically the cerebrum, that is responsible for vision; located at the back of the brain.

occluder: Opaque instrument, lens, or patch used to cover one eye during ophthalmic testing.

occlusion: General term for blockage or closing; 1. in surgery the blockage of the aspiration port of an irrigation and aspiration probe; 2. in most common ophthalmic usage, covering an eye, typically during a vision examination; **o. therapy** treatment for amblyopia that involves patching the strong eye in order to force the weak eye to work.

occupational bifocal or **segment:** Multifocal lens with a near segment at the top instead of or in addition to the bottom, designed to provide close vision overhead.

Occupational Safety and Health Administration (OSHA): Governmental agency that establishes and enforces standards regarding the safety and health of employees; in part, these standards are designed to reduce/eliminate risks associated with exposure to harmful pathogens (such as hepatitis and human immunodeficiency virus [HIV]).

ocul-: Combining form meaning eye.

ocular: 1. General anatomic adjective meaning of or related to the eye (eg, ocular testing, ocular surgery, etc); 2. eyepiece of a microscope or other optical instrument; *compare* objective lens.

ocular adnexa: *See* adnexa.

ocular albinism (AL-buh-niz-um): X-linked recessive genetic disorder in which skin and pigment in the affected male is normal, but ocular pigment is deficient and the macula is underdeveloped, reducing visual acuity.

ocular angle: *Another term for* canthus.

ocular blood flow pneumotonometer (OBFT): *See entry under* tonometer.

ocular histoplasmosis: *Another term for* presumed ocular histoplasmosis syndrome.

ocular history: That part of the patient's history that is specifically eye related; *see also* history.

ocular hypertension (OHT): High intraocular pressure (IOP); IOP of 20 to 22 millimeters of mercury (mm Hg) is generally considered the border between "normal" IOP and ocular hypertension in otherwise healthy eyes; ocular hypertension is not the same as glaucoma because glaucoma only exists if there is some indication of damage; *see also* glaucoma suspect, intraocular pressure.

ocular media: Tissues in the eye through which light is transmitted: the cornea, aqueous humor, lens, and vitreous humor; *also called* refractive media.

ocular motility: General term for the processes by which the eyes move in a controlled, coordinated fashion, or the study of the function and disorders of alignment and movement of the eyes.

ocular pemphigoid (PEM-fih-goyd): *See* pemphigoid.

ocular prosthesis: Artificial cosmetic device resembling the eye that is placed in the socket after surgical removal of the eye (correct clinical term for "glass eye"); *compare* orbital implant.

ocular torticollis (tohr-tih-KAHL-uhs): Abnormal head posture assumed to improve vision; commonly due to extraocular muscle imbalance (usually congenital paralysis of the vertically-acting muscles), uncorrected astigmatism, other uncorrected refractive error, or nystagmus; posture may be chin up, chin down, head tilt, or head turn; *see also* head tilt, head turn.

ocularist: Individual trained to make and fit ocular prostheses.

oculi uterque (AHK-yuh-lie YOO-tuh-kwah): Latin phrase meaning either or both eyes, abbreviation for which (OU) is commonly used in ophthalmic speech and literature.

oculogyration (ok-yuh-loh-ji-RAY-shun): Circular motion or rotation of the eyes.

oculogyric crisis (ahk-yuh-loh-JY-rik): Condition in which the eyes involuntarily turn upwards; seen in Parkinson's disease.

oculomotor: General term referring to eye movement and the muscle and nerve systems that initiate and control it.

oculomotor nerve: The third cranial nerve (CN III) that innervates the extraocular muscles except the superior oblique and lateral rectus.

oculomotor nerve palsy: Paralysis of the oculomotor nerve (CN III) associated with dilated pupil, ptosis, double vision, and inability to elevate and adduct the eye; if the pupil is spared, the most likely causes are diabetes or hypertension; *also called* third nerve palsy.

oculopathy (ok-yuh-LOP-athy): General term for abnormal/unhealthy condition of the eye.

oculoplastics (ok-yuh-loh-PLAS-tiks): Surgical specialty concerned with reconstructive and cosmetic surgery of the orbit, eyelids, and ocular adnexa.

oculopupillary reflex (OK-yuh-loh-PYOO-pil-ayr-ee): Dilation of the pupils when the surface of the eyeball or eyelids is touched or irritated.

oculus dexter (OK-yuh-lus DEK-ster): Latin phrase meaning right eye, abbreviation for which (OD) is commonly used in ophthalmic speech and literature.

oculus sinister (OK-yuh-lus SIN-uh-ster): Latin phrase meaning left eye, abbreviation for which (OS) is commonly used in ophthalmic speech and literature.

oedipism (ED-uh-piz-um): Self-mutilation involving the eye; named for legendary Greek character Oedipus, who blinded himself.

off-label (use): Using a drug or substance as a treatment other than the recommended and common use.

onchocerciasis (on-koh-ser-KY-uh-sis): Condition in which a small parasitic worm infests the skin, connective tissues, and eyes of its host, causing optic atrophy and optic neuritis; a significant cause of blindness in areas of the world where clean water is not always available; *also known as* river blindness; *see also* filariasis.

oncology: The study and treatment of malignancies; **ocular o.** oncology as it relates to ocular lesions.

onset: In history taking, the patient's report of when symptoms began.

-op-, -opt-: Combining form meaning see or sight.

open angle: Subjective description meaning that the angle between the iris and cornea is wide enough to allow easy passage of aqueous and is not in danger of occlusion.

open-angle glaucoma: *See* glaucoma.

open-sky: General term for surgical procedures (usually vitrectomy) in which the whole cornea is removed to give the surgeon access to the internal structures of the eye; this very traumatic approach has been abandoned in most contemporary ophthalmic surgery.

operating microscope: *See* microscope.

operculated retinal hole or **tear (oh-PER-kyoo-lay-tid):** Retinal hole in which a piece of retinal tissue (operculum) is separated around its entire circumference (or nearly so) and pulled away from the surrounding retina by its attachment to the hyaloid membrane.

operculum (oh-PER-hyuh-luhm): A flap of torn retinal tissue that is partially or totally detached; *see also* operculated retinal hole.

ophthalm-: Combining form meaning eye.

ophthalmalgia (op-thal-MAL-gee-uh): Eye pain.

ophthalmia (op-THAL-mee-uh): General term for inflammation of the eye; *see also* sympathetic ophthalmia.

ophthalmia neonatorum (op-THAL-mee-uh nee-oh-nuh-TOHR-um): In general terms, any conjunctivitis in the newborn, more often referring to that caused by gonococcal organisms; also called neonatal conjunctivitis.

ophthalmic: Related to or involving the eye (eg, ophthalmic surgery or ophthalmic disease).

ophthalmic artery: Main vessel bringing blood into the eye and orbit, entering the optic foramen, and dividing into vessels that enter the retina, lacrimal apparatus, extraocular muscles, etc.

ophthalmic medical personnel (OMP): Person trained to assist an ophthalmologist; three certification levels and several subspecialties are available; *see* Appendix 23.

ophthalmic migraine: Visual aura often described as a scintillating scotoma that closes in and then recedes, lasting about 10 to 20 minutes; may be followed by headache; *also called* optic migraine.

ophthalmic nerve: A branch of the trigeminal nerve (CN V), which in part supplies sensation to the globe, eyelids, face, and forehead.

ophthalmitis (op-thal-MY-tis): General term for inflammation of the eye.

ophthalmodynamometry (ODM) (op-THAL-moh-DY-nuh-MAHM-uh-tree): Technique for measuring blood pressure in the central retinal artery by applying pressure to the sclera until the artery can be seen (via ophthalmoscopy) to stop pulsating.

ophthalmologist: Medical doctor (MD degree from an accredited medical school) specializing in care of the eye, including correction of refractive errors, diagnosis, and both pharmacological and surgical treatments.

ophthalmometer (op-thuh-MOM-eh-ter): General term for any instrument that measures the state of the eye; most commonly in ophthalmic usage referring to a keratometer.

ophthalmopathy (op-thal-MAH-puh-thee): General term for disease of the eye.

ophthalmoplegia (op-thal-mo-PLEE-jee-uh): Paralysis of the eye.

ophthalmoscope: Instrument for viewing the inside of the eye; **binocular o.** ophthalmoscope that allows the examiner to use both eyes when viewing a subject's eye, thereby obtaining a three-dimensional image; *see also* direct ophthalmoscopy, indirect ophthalmoscopy.

ophthalmoscopy: Using an ophthalmoscope to examine the eye's interior; *see also* direct ophthalmoscopy, indirect ophthalmoscopy.

opsoclonia (op-soh-KLO-nee-uh): Involuntary, arrhythmic, rapid movements of the eyes, usually resulting from injury or insult to the brain.

optic: 1. Related to or involving vision or the eye (eg, optic nerve); 2. an element of an optical system (eg, a lens or prism); 3. the central focusing portion of an intraocular lens; *see also* haptic.

optic atrophy: Degeneration of nerve fibers in the optic disk, described in its two major manifestations as primary and secondary optic atrophy.

optic canal: *Another term for* optic foramen.

optic chiasm (KY-az-um): Point at which the two optic nerves meet; the nasal nerve fibers from each eye cross here, while the temporal fibers continue on the same side; the impulses from the right and left sides of the retina of each eye are directed to the geniculate body and the occipital lobe in such a way that the right brain receives and fuses the right sides of the two retinal images and the left brain receives the left sides; *also called* chiasm, optic nerve decussation.

optic cup: *See* cup.

optic disk: Roughly circular area at the back of the eye where nerve fibers converge to form the optic nerve, creating a "blind spot" where images are not perceived; *also called* optic nerve head, optic papilla; *see also* blind spot, retina.

optic foramen (fuh-RAY-mun): Opening in the ethmoid bone of the orbit (eye socket) through which the optic nerve passes; *also called* optic canal.

optic migraine: *Another term for* ophthalmic migraine.

optic nerve (ON): Cranial nerve number two (CN II); the bundle of retinal nerve fibers that exits each eye; the optic nerves meet at the optic chiasm.

optic nerve decussation (dee-kuh-SAY-shun): *Another term for* optic chiasm.

optic nerve head: *Another term for* optic disk.

optic neuritis (nurh-I-tis): Inflammatory disorder of the optic nerve, often accompanied by pain, decreased vision, and central field defect; *compare* optic neuropathy.

optic neuropathy: General term referring to a noninflammatory disorder of the optic nerve; *compare* optic neuritis.

optic papilla: *Another term for* optic disk.

optic radiations: "Fan" of afferent neurons as they leave the lateral geniculate body and travel to the occipital lobe of the brain; *see also* visual pathway.

optic tract: Visual nerve fibers that run from the chiasm to the lateral geniculate body; *see also* visual pathway.

optical: Related to or involving a system through which light is transmitted.

optical axis: *See* axis.

optical center (OC): Point of a lens through which a ray of light may pass without being bent (ie, refracted); *also called* the nodal point of a lens; the OC of a lens is generally aligned with the patient's optical axis (line of sight).

optical coherence tomography (OCT) (koh-HEER-ens tuh-MAH-gruh-fee): High-resolution imaging technique that uses backscattering of light to evaluate the retina and its layers (including thickness measurements).

optical cross: A way of visualizing the power of a lens in each meridian, based on the fact that the meridians of power in a spherocylindrical lens are perpendicular to each other.

optical zone (OZ): Area of a lens or ocular tissue through which the eye sees; used in describing corrective spectacle, contact, or intraocular lenses to designate the optically functioning part of the lens from structural or other parts; in corneal refractive surgery, the portion of the cornea that is intended to provide the refractive correction.

optician: Individual trained to make vision-correcting lenses and to dispense and adjust eyewear.

optics: Study of the nature and behavior of light; **geometric o.** that branch of optics that deals with the properties of light (eg, wavelength, color, lasers, etc); **physical o.** the behavior of light as it passes through media, on which optical instruments, lenses, and prisms are based; for important optical principles, *see* electromagnetic spectrum, focus, lens, light, prism, reflection, refraction.

optometrist: Doctor of optometry (OD degree from an accredited school of optometry) trained in the diagnosis and treatment of refractive errors and medical conditions of the eye, with some training in general medical principles; most are authorized (depending on their state's optometric practice laws) to use some prescription pharmaceuticals in diagnosis and treatment of ocular conditions; with very few highly controversial exceptions, no state authorizes optometrists to perform any type of surgery, including laser surgery.

optotype: General term for standardized image used in visual acuity tests (derived from Snellen's term for the letters on his original chart).

ora serrata (OHR-uh ser-RAT-uh): Irregular anterior border of the retina where it attaches to the choroid, located adjacent to the pars plana of the ciliary body and approximately 8 mm posterior to the corneoscleral limbus; *see also* retina.

orb: In ophthalmic usage, *another term for* globe.

orbicularis oculi muscle (ohr-BIK-yoo-layr-uhs AWK-yuh-lie): Muscle that controls blinking and closure of the eyelids; it encircles the eye with fibers in the upper and lower lids.

orbit: Either of two spherical hollows in the skull that protect and provide attachments for the eyes, extraocular muscles, and surrounding tissues; commonly known as the eye socket, the orbit consists of the ethmoid, frontal, lacrimal, maxillary, palatine, sphenoid, and zygomatic bones.

orbital cellulitis: Inflammation of the subcutaneous tissues around the orbit.

orbital crest: Area of the skull just above the orbit at the level of the eyebrow.

orbital decompression: Surgical procedure to increase the volume of the orbit by removing bone from its wall and thus relieve pressure on the eye, usually in treatment of an ocular tumor.

orbital fissure: One of two openings (superior [*also called* sphenoid fissure] and inferior) in each orbit through which blood vessels and nerves pass.

orbital implant: Biologically inert device implanted in the orbit and under the conjunctiva after enucleation in order to maintain the volume of the orbit; *also called* enucleation implant; *compare* ocular prosthesis.

orbital septum: Tissue that lies between the rim of the orbit and the tarsal plate; as a barrier tissue, it prevents infections of the eyelid from passing back into the orbit.

orbitopathy (or-buh-TOP-o-thee): General term referring to disorder/abnormality of the orbit (versus the globe).

orthokeratology (ortho-K) (or-thoh-kayr-uh-TOL-uh-jee): Treatment of refractive error by prescribing rigid contact lenses designed to gradually reshape the cornea.

orthophoria (or-thoh-FOR-ee-uh): Normal state in which the eyes remain properly oriented even if one or the other is occluded; *see also* phoria.

orthoptics (ohr-THOP-tiks): System for nonsurgical correction of strabismus and other defects of ocular motility; *see also* vision therapy/training.

orthoptist (or-THAHP-tist): Person trained and certified in evaluation and treatment of ocular motility and binocularity disorders, including amblyopia.

oscillating vision: *Another term for* oscillopsia.

oscillopsia (ahs-uh-LAP-see-uh): State in which objects appear to move back and forth; *also called* oscillating vision.

OSHA: *See* Occupational Safety and Health Administration.

osmotic (oz-MAH-tik): General chemical term for a process or agent that influences the flow of liquids across a membrane; in ophthalmic usage, osmotics are used topically or systemically to draw water out of the eye, thus reducing intraocular pressure.

osteopath (OSS-tee-o-path): *Another term for* Doctor of Osteopathy; *see* osteopathy.

osteopathy (oss-tee-OP-a-thee): Philosophy of medicine based on the interrelationship of bones, organs, nerves, and muscles; treatments can include alignment and nutrition as well as medication and surgery; graduates have the designation of Doctor of Osteopathy (DO) and may specialize in ophthalmology.

outer granular or outer granular layer (of retina): Cell layer within the retina where the synapses of the outer and inner nuclear layers meet; *see also* retina.

outer limiting membrane (of retina): *Another term for* external limiting membrane (of retina).

outer nuclear layer (of retina): Cell layer within the retina composed primarily of bipolar cells and containing the rod and cone cell bodies, located between the inner and outer molecular layers; *see also* retina.

outflow facility: The ease with which aqueous humor drains from the anterior chamber into Schlemm's canal; in glaucoma, the outflow facility is inadequate for the amount of aqueous produced; *also called* facility of outflow.

overcorrection: Excessive correction of refractive error, making a nearsighted eye farsighted or a farsighted eye nearsighted, usually referring to a refractive surgical procedure or intraocular lens implantation that missed its intended target; *compare* undercorrection.

over-refraction: Technique of determining the amount of corrective power needed in addition to the corrective lenses currently in place; determined by using an autorefractor, trial lenses, or phoropter to perform refractometry while the patient wears eyeglasses or contact lenses.

overwear syndrome (OWS): Painful corneal erosions caused by excessive wearing of contact lenses; lack of tear flow leads to hypoxia to the point of corneal decompensation.

oxygen deprivation: *Another term for* hypoxia.

P

pachymetry (pak-im-uh-tree): Measurement of the thickness of the cornea using light or ultrasound; the instrument used to make the measurement is a pachymeter.

palatine bone (pal-uh-tahyn): One of the bones of the orbit.

palinopsia (pal-uh-NAP-see-uh): Persistent afterimage.

pallor (PAL-er): General term for abnormal whiteness (paleness) of tissue; in ophthalmic usage, change in color of the optic disk from yellow to white, indicative of retinal damage (as in glaucoma).

palpebra (PAL-pee-brah): Proper medical term for the eyelid; plural: palpebrae; **inferior p.** lower eyelid; **superior p.** upper eyelid.

palpebral (pal-PEE-brahl): Referring to the eyelids.

palpebral conjunctiva: Mucosal tissue lining the inner surface of the eyelids; *see also* conjunctiva; *compare* bulbar conjunctiva.

palpebral fissure: The gap between the upper and lower eyelids.

palpate (PAL-pait): General medical term meaning to evaluate by touch.

palsy: *Another term for* paralysis; for palsies affecting the eye, *see* entry for specific disorder (eg, Bell's palsy, etc).

PAM: Acronym for potential acuity meter; *see* potential acuity meter.

pannus (PAN-uhs): In ophthalmic usage, condition in which blood vessels grow into the cornea, which then becomes fibrous and loses its transparency; may be classified according to type as allergic, glaucomatous, etc.

panophthalmitis (pan-OP-thahl-my-tus): Wide-spread inflammation of the tissues of the eye.

panretinal photocoagulation: Laser surgical procedure in which laser energy is applied across wide areas of the retina in an attempt to stop the progression of retinopathy.

pantoscopic tilt (PAN-tuh-SKAH-pik): Fit of spectacles so that the bottom of the frame front is angled closer to the cheeks; ideal is between 4 degrees and 18 degrees; *compare* retroscopic tilt.

Panum's fusion area or **fusional space (PAN-umz):** Area in front of and behind the horopter where fusion occurs, making stereopsis possible; *see also* horopter.

papilla: In ophthalmic usage, small elevated area of palpebral conjunctiva with central blood vessels, present in conjunctival infection or allergy; plural: papillae; **lacrimal p.** slightly elevated area on the edge of the eyelid, near the nose, where the punctum is located; **optic p.** *another term for* optic disk.

papillary conjunctivitis: *See* giant papillary conjunctivitis *under* conjunctivitis.

papilledema (PAP-eh-luh-DEE-mah): Noninflammatory swelling of the optic disk with engorgement of blood vessels, usually as a result of increased intracranial pressure; *also called* choked disk.

papillitis (pap-uh-LY-tis): Inflammation of the optic nerve head; type of posterior uveitis; *see also* uveitis.

papilloma (pap-uh-LOH-mah): Benign epithelial lesion commonly seen on the eyelids and occasionally on the conjunctiva.

papillomacular bundle (pap-uh-loh-MAK-yoo-ler): Dense, oval bundle of retinal nerve ganglion cell fibers extending from the macula into the central optic nerve.

paracentesis (payr-uh-sen-TEE-sis): General medical term for a surgical technique that involves puncturing a cavity in order to remove fluid; in ophthalmic usage, an incision into the anterior chamber of the eye; *see* keratocentesis.

paracentral scotoma: *See* scotoma.

paradoxical: General term describing a sign or symptom, such as visual field loss or diplopia, that has a peculiar feature or is of uncertain cause.

parakinesia (payr-uh-kuh-NEE-zee-uh): In ophthalmic usage, general term for abnormal motor function of the muscles of the eye.

parallax: Optical phenomenon in which an object shifts in the field of view when the observer changes position; nearer objects appear to shift opposite to the direction of the observer's head while distant objects seem to move in the same direction; **binocular p.** a shift in the relative position of objects when the observer views first with one eye alone and then with the other eye alone.

paralysis: General term meaning immobile or lack of sensation; *also called* palsy.

paraoptometric: Personnel trained to assist an optometrist; three certification levels are available; *see* Appendix 23.

parasite: Organism that requires a host organism in order to live and/or reproduce.

parasympathetic nervous system (payr-uh-sim-pah-THET-ik): Division of the autonomic nervous system that encourages digestion and maintains energy reserves; in the eye, this system causes pupil miosis and accommodation; *see also* acetylcholine; *compare* sympathetic nervous system.

parasympatholytic   (payr-uh-sim-path-o-KIT-ik): Substance that blocks the parasympathetic system, thus causing a sympathetic response; *also called* cholinergic-blocking; cyclopentolate (a cycloplegic) is an example; *compare* sympatholytic.

parasympathomimetic (payr-uh-sim-path-o-my-MET-ik): Substance that causes a parasympathetic-like response in the autonomic nervous system; pilocarpine (a miotic) is an example; *compare* sympathomimetic.

parophthalmia (payr-op-THAHL-mee-uh): Inflammation of the tissues surrounding the eye.

pars: General anatomic term meaning part.

pars plana (pahrz PLAY-nah): Commonly used term for the outermost ring of the ciliary body; also called pars plana corporis ciliaris, pars plana ciliaris; vitrectomy is sometimes carried out through an incision at the level of the pars plana.

pars planitis (parhz plah-NY-tis): *Another term for* intermediate uveitis; *see entry under* uveitis.

pars plicata (parhz plih-KAH-tuh): The innermost ring of the ciliary body consisting of the ciliary processes.

particle: *Another term for* photon.

passive forced duction test: *Another term for* forced duction test.

past medical history: That part of the patient history where the patient relates previous disorders, procedures, treatments, etc; *see also* history.

patching: 1. Treating amblyopia by occluding the eye with better acuity to force the weaker eye to improve; 2. covering an eye with a protective or therapeutic bandage.

patent: General term meaning open (eg, a patent iridotomy).

patent blue: Stain used as a visualization aid during anterior and posterior segment surgery.

pathway: *See* pathway of light, visual pathway.

pathway of light: The route light travels through the eye; order is as follows: tear film, cornea, aqueous, pupil, lens, vitreous, and retina.

pathogenesis (path-o-JEN-uh-sis): General medical term denoting the origin and course of a disease.

patient history: *See* history.

pattern ERG: *See* electroretinography.

pattern VER: *See* visual evoked response.

peak delay: In electroretinography, the time between stimulus presentation and the peak of the b-wave; *see also* b-wave.

peaked pupil: Abnormal pupil shape where the pupillary margin is drawn, often described by using clock designations (eg, pupil peaked at 10:00); may be the result of injury, surgery, congenital abnormality, or pathology; *also called* ectopic pupil.

pedigree: In genetics, tracing the expression of a specific, inherited trait through a family tree.

pemphigoid (PEM-fi-goyd): In ophthalmic usage, a condition in which the conjunctiva blisters, leading to dryness of the eye and adhesion to the eyelids.

penetrating keratoplasty (PKP): Surgical procedure in which the entire cornea is removed and replaced with donated tissue, popularly known as corneal transplantation; *compare* lamellar graft/keratoplasty; *see also* keratoplasty.

penalization: Method of treating amblyopia by fogging the eye with the better vision, forcing use of the weaker eye; **chemical/cycloplegic p.** use of atropine in the stronger eye to blur vision; **optical p.** use of increased plus or a filter in the spectacle lens of the stronger eye.

perfluorocarbon (per-FLOHR-oh-kar-bun): Class of heavy gases, such as perfluoropropane (C3F8), used in retinal detachment repair; *see also* gas-fluid exchange.

perforation: Piercing of a tissue or structure, usually as a result of trauma or a complication of surgery.

peribulbar (payr-ee-BUHL-bahr): Term describing the area around the eye; *compare* retrobulbar.

peribulbar anesthesia: Anesthesia administered in several injections around the periphery of the eyeball; *compare* retrobulbar anesthesia.

perimeter: In ophthalmic usage, an instrument used to perform perimetry (visual field testing).

perimetry: Technique of visual field testing that determines the boundaries of the field of view by presenting test targets (most often points of light) to the test subject, who fixates upon the middle of a blank screen and reports when the target becomes visible in the periphery; **automated p.** or **computerized p.** perimetry in which a computer assists in selecting and recording the position of targets and provides a printout of the test results; **Goldmann p.** perimetry in which a machine controlled by an examiner is used to map out the visual field (versus automated, where a computer performs this function); results are recorded manually; **kinetic p.** perimetry in which the target moves from the periphery of the visual field toward the central fixation point until the subject reports that it is visible; **manual p.** perimetry that is controlled by an examiner (eg, Goldmann p., tangent screen); **static p.** perimetry in which the target is a stationary point of light that gradually increases in brightness until the subject reports that it is visible.

periocular (payr-ee-OC-u-lur): General term meaning around the eye.

periodic strabismus: *See* strabismus.

periorbital (pehr-ee-ORB-it-uhl): Near the eye or the bony eye socket.

peripheral cataract: *See* cataract.

peripheral iridectomy: *See* iridectomy.

peripheral uveitis: *Another term for* intermediate uveitis; *see entry under* uveitis.

peripheral vision: Perception of objects in the outer areas of the field of view; *also called* side vision; *see also* visual field.

peritectomy/peritomy (payr-uh-TEK-tuh-mee/payr-RIHT-uh-mee): In ophthalmic usage, an incision into the conjunctiva at the limbus.

persistence of vision: *See* afterimage.

petechia (peh-TEE-kee-uh): General medical term referring to tiny hemorrhages on the surface of the skin (eg, the eyelids) or mucous membrane (eg, the conjunctiva).

pH: Measure of the acidity or alkalinity of a substance; a pH of 7 is neutral, below 7 denotes acidity, and over 7 denotes alkalinity.

phaco- or **phako-:** Combining form meaning lens, usually referring to the natural crystalline lens of the eye but also applicable to artificial lenses; note that in British usage, phako- is the only acceptable combining form.

phaco (FEY-koh): *See* phacoemulsification.

phacoablation (fay-koh-uh-BLAY-shun): A still-experimental surgical technique of cataract removal by which lens tissue is vaporized by the action of a laser.

phacoanaphylaxis (fay-koh-an-uh-fuh-LAK-sis): Condition in which leakage of proteins from the crystalline lens leads to inflammation within the eye.

phacodonesis (fay-koh-duh-NEE-sis): Movement of the crystalline lens, usually as a result of broken zonules.

phacoemulsification/phacofragmentation (phaco) (fay-koh-ee-muhl-suh-fi-KAY-shun): Surgical technique for cataract extraction using a probe that vibrates at ultrasonic frequency (approximately 40,000 cycles per second) and emulsifies the lens nucleus so that it may be aspirated from the eye through a small incision; **endocapsular p.** technique in which the emulsification of the nucleus is carried out within the area usually enclosed by the lens capsule, which is opened to allow access to the crystalline lens (*compare* Kelman p.); **endolenticular p.** technique in which the emulsification of the nucleus is carried out entirely within the lens capsule and with the lens nucleus remaining in its natural position within the cortex; **extracapsular p.** technique in which the anterior lens capsule is opened and the nucleus is emulsified through this hole;

intercapsular p. technique in which the emulsification of the nucleus is carried out through a small slit in the lens capsule; **Kelman p.** original phacoemulsification procedure described by the inventor of phaco, Dr. Charles Kelman, in which the lens nucleus is maneuvered into the anterior chamber and then emulsified; **one-handed p.** general term for techniques of phacoemulsification in which only one instrument (the phaco probe) is used during emulsification of the nucleus; **two-handed p.** general term for techniques in which a second instrument is used by the surgeon to maneuver the lens as it is being emulsified by the phaco probe.

phacolytic glaucoma (fay-koh-LIT-ik): *See* glaucoma.

phacomatoses (fay-koh-mah-TOH-sis): A collective term for a group of inherited diseases distinguished by the presence of tumors in various tissues (eg, neurofibromatosis, etc); alternate spelling: phakomatoses.

phagocyte (FAG-uh-syt): *Another term for* macrophage.

phakic (FAY-kik): Adjective describing an eye in which the natural crystalline lens is present; *compare* aphakic, pseudophakic.

phakic lens implant: Intraocular lens placed inside the eye as a means of correcting a refractive error, without removing the crystalline lens.

phako-: *See* phaco-.

phase: 1. Property of wave energy such that the "peaks" and "troughs" of many individual waves can coincide with each other or cancel each other; waves with peaks and troughs that coincide are said to be in phase; *see also* coherent light; 2. referring to a stage of fluorescein angiography; *see* fluorescein angiography.

phenotype (FEE-noh-typ): The visible expression of dominant genes, including the effect of environmental interaction (ie, the inherited genetic characteristics exhibited in an individual).

phlyctenular keratoconjunctivitis (flik-TEN-yuh-ler): *See* keratoconjunctivitis.

phlyctenule (flik-TEN-yool): Small, fluid-filled blisters that can lead to ulcerations on the conjunctiva; corneal involvement can occur; linked to a hypersensitivity to bacterial products; *see also* phlyctenular keratoconjunctivitis *under* keratoconjunctivitis.

phoria (FOHR-ee-uh): General term for misalignment of the eyes present only when fusion is disrupted (eg, by occluding one eye); it is a latent deviation, usually held in check by fusion; *also called* heterophoria; *see also* esophoria, exophoria, hyperphoria, hypophoria, orthophoria; *compare* tropia; *see also* strabismus; **horizontal p.** phoria in the horizontal plane; **vertical p.** phoria in the vertical plane.

phoropter (FOHR-op-ter): Instrument fitted with a number of different types of lenses that are rotated into place in front of a test subject's eyes to determine the amount of vision correction necessary; formerly a brand name of one such instrument (commonly called a refractor) but now used generically.

phosphene (FOS-feen): Sensation of seeing a light when the visual cortex or retina is stimulated nonvisually; *see also* entopic phenomenon; **pressure p.** phosphene that appears when mechanical pressure is applied to the eye.

photo-: Combining word meaning light.

photoablation (foh-toh-ay-BLAY-shun): In ophthalmology, use of laser energy (ie, short wavelength ultraviolet light as in the excimer laser) to cause tissue to decompose at the chemical level; *also called* photodecomposition.

photocoagulation (fo-toh-co-ag-yoo-LAY-shun): In ophthalmic usage, application of laser light that is absorbed by the pigmented tissues of the eye and converted into heat energy; used to seal blood vessels and for trabeculoplasty; **panretinal p. (PRP)** treatment in which laser is applied to a large area of the retina, as in diabetic retinopathy; *see also* laser.

photodecomposition (fo-toh-de-comp-o-ZISH-uhn): *Another term for* photoablation.

photodisruption (fo-toh-dis-RUP-shun): In ophthalmology, use of laser energy (ie, high-energy such as nd: YAG) that causes tissue damage at the atomic level.

photodynamic therapy (PDT): Use of low-intensity light (usually from a laser) and photosensitive agents to ablate tissue in a very localized area; in ophthalmology, used to treat ocular tumors, neovascularization, and refractory glaucoma.

photo-evaporation: *Another term for* photovaporization.

photokeratoscope (foh-toh-KAYR-uh-tuh-skohp): Photographic instrument for evaluating corneal surface using a reflected image/rings.

photon: Smallest unit of light energy; *also called* particle, quantum.

photophobia (foh-toh-FOH-bee-uh): Excessive sensitivity of the eyes to light.

photopia (foh-TOH-pee-uh): Daylight vision in which the rod cells of the retina are suppressed and the cones are the primary light perceiving cells; *compare* mesopia, scotopia.

photopic ERG (foh-TAHP-ik): *See* electroretinography.

photopic vision (foh-TAHP-ik): Light-adapted vision; *see also* photopia; *compare* scotopic vision.

photopsia (foh-TAHP-see-uh): Appearance of flashes of light in the field of view attributable to some defect of the retina or optic tract.

photoreceptors: The cells in the retina that transmit nerve impulses when stimulated by light (ie, rod cells and cone cells); *also called* sensory receptors.

photorefractive keratectomy (PRK) (foh-toh-ree-FRAK-tiv kayr-uh-TEK-tuh-mee): Application of the excimer laser to remove corneal tissue in order to change the surface curvature of the eye and thus correct refractive errors.

photostress test: *Another term for* macular photostress test.

phototherapeutic keratectomy (PTK) (foh-toh-thayr-uh-PYOO-tik kayr-uh-TEK-tuh-mee): Application of the excimer laser to remove corneal tissue in order to treat pathology rather than to change any refractive error of the eye.

phototoxicity: Property of bright light such that it damages the retina upon prolonged exposure.

photovaporization: In ophthalmology, use of laser energy (ie, long wavelength infrared) to evaporate the water out of a tissue; used to remove lesions and cauterize; *also called* photo-evaporation.

phthisis (TY-sis): General term for gradual loss of the bulk and structure of a bodily organ; in ophthalmic usage, most commonly referring to phthisis bulbi.

phthisis bulbi (TY-sis BUHL-by): Condition in which a blind eye shrivels, sometimes necessitating surgical removal.

physical optics: Segment of optics that deals with theories of light and the electromagnetic spectrum; *compare* geometric optics, physiological optics.

physiologic astigmatism: *See* astigmatism.

physiologic blind spot or **scotoma:** *Another term for* blind spot; *see also* scotoma.

physiological optics: Science of light as it reacts specifically with the eye; *compare* geometric optics, physical optics.

pie-on-the-floor: *Another term for* inferior quadrantanopsia; *see entry under* quadrantanopsia.

pie-in-the-sky: *Another term for* superior quadrantanopsia; *see entry under* quadrantanopsia.

piggyback: In ophthalmology, placing two lenses on top of each other, as in piggyback intraocular lenses (*see* intraocular lens) or piggyback contact lenses (in which case a rigid lens is worn over a soft lens).

pigment epithelium (PE): *Another term for* retinal pigment epithelium.

pigmentary dispersion syndrome: Condition in which iris pigment is scattered and appears as small deposits on other anterior segment structures but no glaucoma occurs; *compare* pigmentary glaucoma *under* glaucoma.

pigmentary glaucoma: *See* glaucoma.

pincushion distortion: Bowed-in distortion of images that results from the steep curvature of spectacle lenses used to correct high farsightedness (ie, strong plus lenses); *compare* barrel distortion.

pinguecula (ping-GWEK-yuh-luh): Abnormal, benign growth of yellowish membrane at the junction of the sclera and cornea.

pingueculitis (ping-GWEK-yuh-LY-tis): Inflamed pinguecula; *see* pinguecula.

pinhole (PH): Opaque disk or lens with one or more tiny holes; looking through a pinhole reduces the amount of scattered light, improving any vision decrease due to refractive errors; reduced vision due to pathology is not improved, making pinhole vision an important diagnostic test.

pink eye: Common term for conjunctivitis.

placebo (pluh-SEE-boh): A treatment (usually oral medication) with no medicinal value, given for psychological reasons (ie, to gratify the patient) or testing purposes (as a control).

Placido's disk (pluh-SEE-dohz): Disk with concentric circles used to evaluate corneal curvature; *see also* keratoscopy.

plano lens (PLAY-noh): Lens that has no refracting power; rays of light passing through such a lens (which has no curvature of either surface) continue on their straight-line paths; also, a lens may have one convex or concave surface in combination with one plano surface, in which case it is called planoconvex or planoconcave, respectively.

plaque: 1. Small discriminant area on the surface of a tissue, organ, etc; 2. patch of cholesterol or other material clinging to the inner surface of a blood vessel; **Hollenhorst p.'s** embolus of cholesterol lodged in the retinal arterioles and causing occlusion; they are sparkly and orange-yellow.

plateau iris: Congenital condition in which the depth of the anterior chamber is normal, but the angle is narrow because iris insertion is abnormally high; dilation causes the iris to bunch up and block the angle, precipitating angle closure glaucoma.

platysmal reflex (pluh-TIZ-muhl): Constriction of the pupil in response to manipulation of the platysma, a muscle that runs from the neck into the area of the lower jaw.

pleoptics (plee-AHP-tiks): Optical treatment for eccentric fixation.

plica (PLY-kuh): General anatomic term for a fold of tissue.

plica ciliaris (PLY-kuh sil-ee-AYR-us): The small folds of tissue in the ciliary body.

plica lacrimalis (PLY-kuh lak-ruh-MAY-luhs): Fold of skin that acts as the valve of the tear gland.

plica semilunaris (PLY-kuh sem-ee-loo-NAYR-uhs): Half-moon-shaped fold of tissue formed where the nasal portion of the bulbar conjunctiva joins muscle tissue.

plus: 1. Property of an optical system such that it causes rays of light to converge (eg, a convex lens); 2. in spoken ophthalmic usage, synonym for hyperopia (eg, a "plus 2 diopter patient").

plus cylinder: 1. Cylindrical lens that converges light rays; *see also* cylinder; *compare* minus cylinder; 2. lens prescription written using plus cylinder power.

plus lens: Lens that causes rays of light to converge (*see* convex lens, cylinder [definition 1]); in common ophthalmic usage, the power of the plus sphere lens used to correct farsightedness is often used to describe the degree of hyperopia (thus, a "high plus" or "plus six" patient); *also called* convergent lens; *compare* minus lens.

pneumatic retinopexy (noo-MAT-ik): *See* retinopexy.

pneumotonometer (noo-moh-tuh-NAHM-eh-tur): *See entry under* tonometer.

polar cataract: *See* cataract.

polarized light: Light that has been altered so that the normally random planes of its transverse wave motions (ie, the plane in which the theoretical "peaks" and "troughs" lie) are aligned along the same pole; polarizing filters are used in various optical instruments and also in some types of sunglasses.

poliosis (poh-lee-OH-sis): General term meaning lack of hair pigment (ie, graying), which may include the eyelashes.

poly: Shortened term for polymorphonucleocyte.

polycarbonate: Lightweight, shatter-resistant polymer used as a spectacle lens material.

polycoria (pahl-ee-KOHR-ee-uh): Condition in which there is more than one pupillary opening in the iris.

polymegethism (pahl-ee-MEG-uh-thiz-uhm): In ophthalmic usage, condition in which corneal endothelial cells become irregular in size and shape; note that this spelling is based on authorities' citation of Greek poly ("many") being joined with megethos ("size") rather than megalos ("large").

polymethylmethacrylate (PMMA) (pahl-ee-METH-el-meth-ACK-ruh-layt): Acrylic polymer used in the manufacture of contact lenses ("hard lenses") and intraocular lenses.

polymorphonucleocyte (PMN) (pahl-ee-MOHR-foh-NOO-klee-oh-site): *Another term for* neutrophil; *also called* "poly."

polyopia, -sia, -y (pahl-ee-OH-pee-uh): General term for visual defect in which one object appears as multiple images; *see also* diplopia, triplopia.

polypropylene (pahl-ee-PROH-puh-leen): Flexible polymer used in the manufacture of sutures and some intraocular lens haptics.

polytrichosis (pahl-ee-trik-OH-sus): Abnormal increase in the number of eyelashes.

popping: *See* eye popping.

posterior capsulotomy: *See* capsulotomy.

posterior chamber (PC): Portion of the eye behind the iris and in front of the crystalline lens-zonule apparatus and ciliary body; it is part of the anterior segment and aqueous is formed here; not to be confused with posterior segment; *compare* anterior chamber.

posterior chamber intraocular lens: *See* intraocular lens.

posterior hyaloid membrane: *See* hyaloid membrane.

posterior pole (of the eye): Imaginary point at the rear surface of the sclera directly opposite the anterior pole of the eye; *compare* anterior pole (of the eye).

posterior pole (of the lens): Point at the very back and center of the crystalline lens; *compare* anterior pole (of the lens).

posterior segment (of the eye): General term describing the structures of the eye lying behind the lens-zonule apparatus and ciliary body; ophthalmic surgery is roughly divided into the categories of anterior segment (cornea, glaucoma, and cataract procedures) and posterior segment (retina and vitreous procedures); not to be confused with posterior chamber; *compare* anterior segment (of the eye).

posterior staphyloma: *See* staphyloma.

posterior subcapsular cataract (PSC): *See* cataract.

posterior synechia (PS): *See* synechia.

posterior toric: Method of stabilizing toric contact lenses by incorporating the toric optics into the posterior surface of the lens, theoretically achieving a shape complementary to that of the cornea, helping to prevent rotation and maintaining the orientation of the lens to correct astigmatism in the proper axis; *also called* back surface toric; *compare* dynamic stabilization, prism ballast, truncation.

posterior uveitis: *See entry under* uveitis.

posterior vitreous detachment (PVD): Separation of all or part of the vitreous body from its normal attachment to the retina and optic nerve, usually following syneresis (ie, degenerative shrinking of the vitreous) but sometimes as a result of trauma; symptoms include flashes and floaters; posterior vitreous detachment sometimes causes retinal breaks, as the anterior vitreous is firmly attached to the peripheral retina; often simply called vitreous detachment.

potential acuity: Visual acuity that theoretically could be attained in an eye if all correctable defects (usually referring to opacities of normally clear refractive ocular media) were corrected.

potential acuity meter (PAM): Device that measures potential acuity by projecting an eye chart through any ocular opacities in the ocular media and directly onto the retina; *see also* interferometer.

preauricular node (pree-au-RIC-u-lur): Lymph node lying just anterior to the ear, which can swell in infections of the eye, notably those of viral origin.

precorneal tear film: *Another term for* tear film.

pre-chiasmal: Occurring before the retinal nerve fibers reach the chiasm; pre-chiasmal lesions cause visual field defects in the affected eye only; *see also* chiasm.

preferential looking technique (PLT): Visual acuity test used with infants and small children; patient is presented with a set of side-by-side cards, one blank and the other with an acuity-graded figure (a grid, picture, etc), and the response is noted. The figure cards are reduced in detail until there is no particular response to either card.

Prentice's law/rule: Optical formula defining the amount that a ray of light deviates (measured in prism diopters, Δ) from its original straight path when passing through a point at a given distance (measured in centimeters, cm) from the center of a lens of a given power (measured in diopters, D), expressed as Δ = D × cm.

preocular tear film: *Another term for* tear film.

preretinal: Located in the area between the posterior face of the vitreous and retina.

preretinal membrane: Condition in which a membrane forms between the retina and the vitreous humor in the region of the macula.

presbyope (PREZ-bee-ohp): Individual with presbyopia.

presbyopia (prez-bee-OH-pee-uh): Naturally occurring process of aging whereby changes in ocular tissues result in loss of accommodation and thus near vision, usually first noticeable soon after age 40; these changes are generally considered to be due to increasing rigidity of the crystalline lens and decreasing tone of the ciliary muscle.

press-on lens/prism: Flexible plastic lens that can be cut to fit a spectacle lens and applied without adhesive; *see also* Fresnel lens/prism.

pressure: *See* intraocular pressure.

presumed ocular histoplasmosis syndrome (POHS) (his-toh-plaz-MO-sus): Benign infection caused by the *Histoplasma* fungus; characterized by minute, roundish lesions with pigmented borders in the retina, commonly called histo spots; usually referred to as "presumed" based on the presence of these lesions alone; *also called* ocular histoplasmosis; *see also* histoplasmosis.

primary: Occurring initially (ie, before a secondary condition, procedure, etc, but not necessarily causing it); *compare* secondary (definition 1); for entities described as primary, look up entry under main word, such as primary glaucoma *see* glaucoma, etc.

primary deviation: Measurement of a paralytic strabismic deviation in which the normal eye fixates and the fellow eye (with the muscle paralysis) is allowed to deviate; *compare* secondary deviation.

primary dye test: *Another term for* Jones I test.

primary gaze/position: *See* gaze.

Prince rule: Ruler marked off in inches and/or centimeters, along with dioptric values used to evaluate accommodation; *see also* near point of accommodation *under* accommodation.

principal axis: *Another term for* optical axis, *see entry under* axis.

prism: 1. General term for a transparent object having at least two flat surfaces at an angle to each other (most commonly a triangle in cross section, the top of which is the apex and the bottom of which is the base) that bends light rays from their original trajectory but in parallel paths; *compare* lens; a prism bends light toward its base, thus when viewed through a prism, an object appears to move toward the prism's apex; prisms are used to measure and/or correct various types of strabismus; **base-down, base-in, base-out,** and **base-up p.** description of the orientation of prisms in front of the eye when measuring strabismus or vergences, or when prescribing in a spectacle lens; 2. any component of an optical system that functions as a prism (eg, a concave spectacle lens is thicker around the edges than in the center, bending light more in the periphery of the lens); **induced p.** prismatic effect that occurs when the visual axis of the patient is not aligned with the optical center of a lens.

prism angle: Angle at which the two refracting surfaces of a prism meet.

prism apex: Line formed by the junction of the refracting surfaces of a prism (the top of the triangle).

prism ballast: Method of stabilizing toric contact lenses by thickening the bottom with prism, thereby making the bottom of the lens heavier and/or the top of the lens less resistant to the mechanical action of the lids during blinking, which helps prevent rotation and maintain the orientation of the lens to correct astigmatism in the proper axis; *compare* dynamic stabilization, posterior toric, truncation.

prism bar: Device in which prisms of increasing power are attached together and arranged in a row so that they can be easily moved in front of the eye; **horizontal p.b.** prism bar in which the bases of the prisms are aligned; used for measuring horizontal strabismus; **vertical p.b.** prism bar in which the prisms are arranged apex-to-base-to-apex; used for measuring vertical strabismus.

prism base: Flat, thick surface of a prism opposite the apex.

prism and alternate cover test (PACT): *See entry under* cover test.

prism diopter (Δ, PD): Measure of the refracting power of a prism or the prismatic effect of a lens; 1 prism diopter displaces a ray of light 1 centimeter from its original path at a point 1 meter from the prism; *see also* diopter, Prentice's law/rule.

prism and cover test: *Another term for* prism and alternate cover test; *see entry under* cover test.

privacy: Generally referring to the patient's right to confidentiality; **p. act** *see* Health Insurance Portability and Accountability Act.

probing (nasolacrimal): *See* nasolacrimal probing.

progressive addition lens (PAL): Spectacle lens in which the refractive power increases from the center toward the lower periphery to provide a range of correction from far to near; used in the correction of presbyopia to avoid visible lines on the lens (as seen with traditional bifocal or trifocal lenses); *also called* invisible bifocal/trifocal, no-lines, progressive adds, progressives).

progressive myopia: *See* myopia.

progressive power lens (PPL): *Another term for* progressive addition lens.

projection: In ophthalmic usage, process by which objects are mentally connected (via the image on the retina) to various points in space; **anomalous p.** mental connection of an image to a point in space by processes other than those that occur in normal, healthy visual systems; *see also* anomalous retinal correspondence; **erroneous p.** visual defect in which objects are referred to points in space to which they do not actually correspond (ie, the objects seem to be "in the wrong place"); **light p.** *see* light projection vision.

projector: Instrument used to display optotypes for visual acuity and targets for other tests, usually to simulate a 20-foot distance.

prolapse: General term for shifting of an anatomic structure out of its normal position and through another structure; *see also* iris prolapse.

proliferative: General medical term meaning an entity or condition that spreads or grows; *compare* nonproliferative.

proliferative diabetic retinopathy (PDR): *See* diabetic retinopathy.

proliferative retinopathy: Retinal abnormality/pathology that spreads, especially as applies to neovascularization and fibrosis in diabetic retinopathy; *compare* nonproliferative retinopathy.

proliferative vitreoretinopathy (PVR): *See* retinopathy.

proptosis (prop-TOH-sis): *Another term for* exophthalmia.

prostaglandin analogue (PGA) (prahs-tuh-GLAN-din ANN-eh-log): Class of drugs for reducing intraocular pressure by increasing outflow (eg, latanoprost, travoprost).

prosthesis (prahs-THEE-sus): General medical term referring to an artificial body part; in ophthalmology, referring to a cosmetic, artificial eye.

protan (PROH-tan): Color vision defect involving the red color mechanism and linked to the X chromosome; *see* protanomaly, protanopia.

protanomaly (proh-tuh-NAHM-uh-lee): Partial impairment of the red color mechanism, resulting in red/green confusion with red appearing duller than normal.

protanopia, -opsia (proh-tuh-NOH-pee-uh): Severe or total lack of the red color mechanism; reds appear black and gray, the orange-yellow-greens all look yellow, blue/green is grayish, and blue looks the same as purple.

protozoa: Single-celled animals such as amoebae; of concern in ophthalmology are those that cause ocular infections; *see also Acanthamoeba*, toxoplasmosis; singular: protozoan.

provocative test: General term for test in which the examiner attempts to elicit an abnormal response to a stimulus; an example in ophthalmology is provoking high intraocular pressure (eg, when glaucoma is suspected); *see also* dark room provocative test, mydriatic provocative test.

pseudo- (SOO-doh): Prefix meaning false (eg, pseudostrabismus, where the eyes appear crossed to the observer but on testing are found to be straight).

pseudoaccommodation: 1. Ability to see to some degree at both near and distance when true accommodation is impossible (either because of the onset of presbyopia or in some other circumstance); used to describe range of vision achieved (eg, when a monofocal intraocular lens is implanted in an eye with a low degree of astigmatism); 2. the change in effective power seen in an accommodating intraocular lens implant as the ciliary muscle moves the IOL; *see* accommodating IOL *under* IOL.

pseudoexfoliation syndrome: *Another term for* exfoliation syndrome.

pseudoisochromatic charts/plates (SOO-doh-ice-o-kroh-MAT-ik): Color vision test using dots of varying shades that make up numbers or patterns (eg, Ishihara plates, Hardy-Rand-Rittler plates); some figures are not visible or are misinterpreted if color vision is abnormal; *see also* Hardy-Rand-Rittler plates, Ishihara's test.

pseudomyopia (SOO-doh-my-OH-pee-uh): *See* myopia.

pseudophake: Eye in which there is an intraocular lens implant; *compare* aphake.

pseudophakia (SOO-doh-FAY-kee-uh): State in which an intraocular lens is present in the eye.

pseudophakic: Adjective describing an eye with an intraocular lens; *compare* aphakic, phakic.

pseudophakic bullous keratopathy (SOO-doh-FAY-kik BUHL-uhs): *See* keratopathy.

pseudophakos (soo-doh-FAY-kuhs): *Another term for* intraocular lens.

pseudopsia (soo-DAHP-see-uh): Visual hallucination.

pseudopterygium (soo-doh-tuh-RIJ-ee-um): *See* pterygium.

pseudoptosis (soo-doh-TOH-sis): *See* ptosis.

pseudostrabismus: The eyes appear crossed to the observer but on testing are found to be straight; this optical illusion may be due to epicanthal folds or a large kappa angle.

pseudotumor cerebri (soo-doh-TOO-mer SER-uh-bry): Increase in intracranial pressure (on the brain) that is not due to the presence of a tumor, resulting in ocular symptoms such as blurred and double vision, swelling of the optic nerve head (papilledema), and strabismus.

pseudo-von Graefe's sign (soo-doh-vahn-GRAY-feez): Failure of the upper eyelid to move downward when the eyeball is turned downward; occurs when nerve fibers serving the eyelid muscles have been damaged and do not heal properly; *compare* von Graefe's sign.

pterygium (tuh-RIJ-ee-uhm): Fully attached triangular membrane of fleshy tissue extending from a base in the conjunctiva of the canthus toward and possibly onto the cornea, sometimes arising from a pinguecula; usually caused by excessive exposure of the eye to irritation (eg, dust, wind, and direct sunlight); usually found nasally or temporally; removed surgically if it begins to impinge on the optic axis; **cicatricial p., pseudop., or scar p.** triangular adhesion of the conjunctiva to the cornea, resembling pterygium but attached only at its apex.

ptosis (TOH-sis): In ophthalmic usage, a drooping of the upper eyelid; *also called* blepharoptosis; **p. adiposa** ptosis caused by the deposit of fatty tissue in the upper eyelid; **apparent p.** the lid appears to be ptotic, but in actuality it is not (eg, in hypotropia the elevated eye is more covered by the upper lid, causing the optical illusion that the lid is lower); **false p.** *another term for* pseudoptosis; **guarding p.** tendency of the lid to droop when the eye has been injured in some way; **Horner's p.** ptosis accompanied by miosis and lack of sweating on one side of the face, caused by a nerve defect; *see also* Horner's syndrome; **levator p.** ptosis caused by a defect of the levator muscle; **mechanical p.** ptosis caused by a mass or scar tissue that prevents the lid from rising fully; **morning** or **waking p.** normal drooping of the upper eyelid noted upon waking from sleep; **neurogenic p.** ptosis caused by nerve palsy; **pseudop.** apparent drooping of the eyelid that is actually a result of an abnormally narrow fissure; *also called* false ptosis; **upside down p.** abnormal position in which the margin of the lower lid is higher than is typical, often associated with Horner's syndrome.

ptotic (TAHT-ik): General medical term (adjective) meaning drooping (eg, a ptotic eyelid).

puff tonometer: *Another term for* air-puff; *see entry under* tonometer.

pulsed phaco power: Phacoemulsification instrument setting in which ultrasound power is automatically switched on and off rapidly so that the needle is alternately vibrating and stationary; used to prevent heat build-up of the metal phaco tip; *see also* duty cycle.

puncta: Plural of punctum.

punctal occlusion: 1. Method for treating dry eye syndrome by blocking the outflow of tears through the puncta, either temporarily by inserting a punctal plug or permanently by laser cauterization; 2. method of keeping eye drops on the eye and out of systemic circulation by applying pressure to the nasal canthus (with the fingers) after medication has been instilled.

punctal plug: Device that is designed to be inserted into (and later removed from) the punctum in order to treat dry eye by blocking the outflow of tears.

punctate: Appearing as tiny dots (eg, punctate keratopathy).

punctum: In ophthalmic usage, one of the openings in the eyelids through which tear fluid drains off of the eye; there is one in the upper (ie, **superior p.**) and the lower (ie, **inferior p.**) of each lid, located 2 mm to 4 mm from the medial canthus; plural: puncta.

pupil (P): Normally circular opening in the center of the iris that controls the amount of light passing through the eye to the retina by opening (dilating) in dim light in a process called mydriasis and closing (constricting) in bright light in a process called miosis; for a number of unusual states and abnormal conditions of the pupil that are noteworthy, *see also* Adie's p., Argyll Robertson p., Behr's p., cat's eye p., keyhole p., Marcus Gunn p., miotic (definition 1); **ectopic p.** pupil with an eccentric position in the iris; **fixed p.** pupil in which there is no reaction to light or near; **peaked p.** pupil drawn to a point instead of being totally round, usually as a result of surgery or injury; **tonic p.** pupil in which the near reaction of miosis is stronger than the miosis caused by direct light; usually referring to Adie's p.

pupillary axis: *See* axis.

pupillary block: Condition in which the iris presses against the structures behind it, blocking the normal flow of aqueous humor into the anterior chamber and resulting in a build-up of intraocular pressure; *see also* iris bombé, pupillary block glaucoma *under* glaucoma.

pupillary dilator muscle: Iris muscle encircling the outer edge of the iris and extending into the ciliary body, responsible for dilating the pupil; *compare* pupillary sphincter muscle.

pupillary distance (PD): Measurement of the distance from one pupil's nasal edge to the temporal edge of the pupil of the fellow eye; the idea is to figure the distance between the eyes' visual axes; *also called* inter-pupillary distance (IPD).

pupillary margin: Heavily pigmented edge of the iris immediately surrounding the pupil.

pupillary muscle: *See* pupillary dilator muscle, pupillary sphincter muscle.

pupillary response: Any one of a number of responses of the pupil to a stimulus, usually referring to the reaction of pupil size to varying intensities of light (*see also* pupil), but also including **accommodative p.r.** constriction of the pupil in near vision; **consensual p.r.** normal state in which dilation or constriction of one pupil in response to a stimulus is accompanied by a similar response in the pupil of the fellow eye, even if the stimulus is only delivered to one eye; its absence is an indication of a disorder of the ocular nervous system; **direct p.r.** reaction of pupil size to varying intensities of light in that eye only; **oculosensory p.r.** or **oculopupillary reflex** dilation of the pupils when the surface of the eyeball or eyelids is touched or irritated.

pupillary sphincter muscle: Iris muscle encircling the pupil, responsible for constricting the pupil; *compare* pupillary dilator muscle.

pupillary zone: Area of the iris adjacent to the pupil.

pupillography (pyoo-pil-AH-grah-fee): Rarely-done photography of the undilated pupil using infrared lighting; may utilize video to record light responses.

pupillometer (pyoo-pil-AH-muh-ter): 1. Most commonly, *another term for* corneal reflection pupillometer used to measure interpupillary distance; 2. device used to measure pupil size by projecting a numeric scale onto the pupil.

pupillometry (pyoo-pil-AH-muh-tree): Measuring interpupillary distance or pupillary diameter using a pupillometer.

pupilloplasty (PYOO-pil-oh-PLAS-tee): General term for surgical procedure to alter the appearance or function of the pupil, usually referring to repair of a damaged pupil.

pupilloplegia (pyoo-pil-oh-PLEE-jee-uh): Paralysis of the pupil; *see also* fixed pupil *under* pupil.

pupillotonia (pyoo-pil-uh-TOH-nee-uh): *Another term for* Adie's pupil.

Purkinje entopic test (per-KIN-jee): *Another term for* entopic test.

Purkinje images (per-KIN-jee): Reflections from the anterior and posterior surfaces of the cornea and crystalline lens, useful in measuring strabismus as well as determining the curvature and relative position of these surfaces (eg, in ophthalmoscopy).

Purkinje shift (per-KIN-jee): Change in sensitivity of vision from daylight to dark in which the retina becomes more sensitive to the blue-green part of the electromagnetic spectrum; *see also* scotopia.

purulent (PYOOR-uh-luhnt): Producing or appearing like pus.

push plus: Refractometry technique in which the patient is given as much plus power (or the least amount of minus power) possible and still retain clear vision; especially important in patients who can accommodate.

Q-switched laser: *See* laser.

quadrafoil: *Another term for* tetrafoil.

quadrant: General term meaning four equal parts; in ophthalmic usage, usually referring to the visual field (ie, upper left, upper right, lower left, and lower right).

quadrantanopia, -opsia (kwah-dran-tuh-NOH-pee-uh or kwah-drah-tuh-NOHP-see-uh): Loss of one quarter of the visual field in one or both eyes; *also called* quadrant hemianopia; *compare* hemianopia; **crossed binasal q.** quadrantanopia of the lower nasal portion of one visual field and the upper nasal portion of the other visual field; **crossed bitemporal q.** quadrantanopia of the lower temporal portion of one visual field and the upper temporal portion of the other visual field; **heteronymous q.** quadrantanopia affecting different portions of the two visual fields (eg, the upper temporal region of one and the lower nasal region of the other visual field); **homonymous q.** quadrantanopia affecting similar portions of both visual fields (eg, the upper temporal regions of both visual fields); **inferior q.** visual field defect in one of the lower quadrants; defect occurs in the parietal lobe; *also called* "pie-on-the-floor"; **pie-in-the-sky q.** *another term for* superior quadrantanopia; **pie-on-the-floor q.** *another term for* inferior quadrantanopia; **superior q.** visual field defect in one of the upper quadrants and respecting the vertical; defect occurs in the temporal lobe; *also called* "pie-in-the-sky."

quadrantic defect (kwah-DRAN-tik): Visual field defect that occurs in one quadrant of one eye.

quantum: *Another term for* photon.

radial keratotomy (RK): *See entry under* keratotomy.

radiopaque (ray-dee-oh-PAYK): Object or material that does not allow X-rays to pass through and are thus rendered visible; alternate spelling radio-opaque.

radiuscope (RAY-dee-uh-skohp): Instrument for measuring the curvature of contact lenses.

radix (RAY-diks): General anatomic term for the "root" of a structure, as in the **optic nerve r.**, which joins the optic nerve to the geniculate body of the brain.

range of accommodation: *See* accommodation.

range of motion: In ophthalmology, diagnostic test in which the eyes are rotated to each of the cardinal positions in order to evaluate the action(s) of the extraocular muscles; *see also* gaze.

raphe (RAY-fee): General anatomic term for the junction line between two halves of a structure; **horizontal or retinal r.** horizontal line on the temporal side of the macula, dividing superior and inferior fibers of the retinal nerve fiber layer; from the raphe, the nerve fibers follow diverging paths to the optic disk.

reading vision: *Another term for* near vision.

recession: In ophthalmology, strabismus surgery in which a muscle is weakened by detaching then reattaching it behind its original insertion point.

recessive: In genetics, a gene whose expression is masked by a dominant gene at the same locus; if both loci contain recessive genes, then they will be expressed rather than masked; *see also* allele; *compare* dominant.

reciprocal innervation: *See* Sherrington's law.

recovery point: In ocular motility, the initial amount of prism that resolves prism-induced diplopia and restores fusion; *compare* break point (definition 2).

rectus muscle: *See* specific muscle (inferior r., lateral r., medial r., superior r.).

recurrent corneal erosion: *See* corneal erosion.

red blood cell (RBC): Blood cell that contains hemoglobin and thus carries oxygen; *also called* erythrocyte.

red-free filter: Filter that absorbs red light, rendering blood, blood vessels, and nerve fibers more easily observed; used in ophthalmoscopy and ophthalmic photography.

red-free photography: Photography of the eye using green ("red-free") light, so structures that appear red in white light instead appear black, thereby increasing contrast and enhancing images of blood vessels, inflammation, and hemorrhages.

red-green test: 1. *Another term for* duochrome test; 2. referring to color vision testing for red-green defects; 3. test to map strabismic deviations (**Lancaster r-g t.**).

red reflex: Reflection of light from the retina; appears as a bright red area through the pupil, due to the retina's blood supply and pigmentation; an opacity will cast a shadow or dull the reflex's brightness; *also called* retinal reflex.

reduced eye: *See* schematic eye (definition 2).

reflection: Property of light such that it bounces back from the surface of an object or from an interface between two substances with different indices of refraction; light rays striking the surface or interface are called incident and those bouncing back are called reflected.

reflex: 1. Muscle reaction to stimulation; **accommodative r.** the triad of focusing, convergence, and miosis that occurs with near vision; **oculopupillary r.** dilation of the pupils when the globe or lids are irritated; **pupillary r.** *see* pupillary reflex; 2. reflection of light, as in corneal reflex; *see also* red reflex; 3. in retinoscopy, that part of the light that reflects from the pupil; *compare* intercept.

reflex tearing: *See* tearing.

reflux: General medical term meaning to flow backward from the normal pathway.

refract: 1. To bend light by refraction; *see* refraction (definition 1); 2. to perform a refraction; *see* refraction (definition 2).

refraction: 1. Bending of light as it passes from one transparent media to the next such that light is bent from its normal straight-line course; *see* index of refraction; 2. in ophthalmic practice, the act of determining what power lens is needed to correct an ametropia, including the generation of a prescription for corrective lenses (which may be done only by a licensed professional); *see also* cycloplegic refraction, manifest refraction (definition 1), over-refraction; *compare* refractometry; 3. in ophthalmic speech and literature, the power of a lens needed to correct an ametropia is referred to as the refraction of a given individual, leading to informal descriptions such as "the (patient's) refraction was minus 2 diopters."

refractive amblyopia: *See* amblyopia.

refractive error: *Another term for* ametropia.

refractive index: *Another term for* index of refraction.

refractive keratoplasty (KAYR-uh-toh-plas-tee): Corneal surgery performed to correct refractive error; *see also* keratoplasty, refractive surgery.

refractive media: *Another term for* ocular media; *see also* medium (definition 1).

refractive surgery: Surgical procedure that has the correction of an ametropia as its primary objective; *see also* clear lensectomy, epikeratophakia, intrastromal corneal ring, keratomileusis, keratophakia, keratoplasty, keratotomy, laser, thermokeratoplasty.

refractometry (ree-frak-TAHM-uh-tree): Measuring the refractive error of a patient in order to yield information about that refractive error and without writing a prescription for corrective lenses; technical staff may legally perform refractometry but not refractions, as they do not have a license to prescribe; however, licensed personnel may use the refractometric measurement to generate a lens prescription; *compare* refraction (definition 2).

refractor: Instrument containing rotating lenses for the measurement of a patient's refractive error; commonly called a phoropter, although that term actually refers to a specific brand of refractor; **automated r. (AR)** computerized instrument that objectively measures a patient's refractive error (and often K readings and pupillary distance as well).

registration: In refractive surgery, process of locating diagnostic data and customized laser ablation patterns in relation to some physical or anatomic landmark on the eye so that the final treatment is centered and also rotated to the same axis in which the original diagnostic data were obtained.

regression: In refractive surgery, phenomenon in which the correction achieved in the immediate postoperative period drifts back toward the original refractive error.

regular astigmatism: *See* astigmatism.

relapse: General medical term meaning that the symptoms of a disorder (or the disorder itself) have increased or returned; *compare* remission.

relative afferent pupillary defect (RAPD): *Another term for* Marcus Gunn pupil.

remission: General medical term meaning that the symptoms of a disorder have decreased or ceased; *compare* relapse.

resection: In ophthalmology usage, strabismus surgery in which a muscle is strengthened by shortening and then reattaching it to its original insertion point.

respect the horizontal (meridian): *See* horizontal meridian.

respect the vertical (meridian): *See* vertical meridian.

reticle or **reticule:** Pattern of lines or grid, usually a standardized scale, inscribed in the eyepiece of optical instruments to allow the examiner to make quantitative observations of the subject.

retina: Transparent, light-sensitive structure lining the inside of the eye; lies between the vitreous body and the choroid; light striking the retina passes through the internal limiting membrane, the retinal nerve fiber layer, the ganglion cell layer, the inner molecular and inner nuclear layers (which, like the outer molecular and outer nuclear layers just beneath them are composed of nerve cells and synapses), the external limiting membrane, the bacillary layer (composed of the light-sensitive rod and cone cells), and finally the retinal pigment epithelium (which plays no part in visual sensation but has a key role in retinal nutrition), which is attached to the choroid; *see also* amacrine cells, bipolar cells, external limiting membrane, fovea, inner nuclear layer, internal limiting membrane, macula, nerve fiber layer, optic disk, ora serrata.

retinal accommodation: Accommodation triggered by the perception of an unfocused image (usually at near) on the retina.

retinal adaptation: Process whereby the retina adjusts to the level of light in the environment, becoming more or less sensitive to light under relatively dark and light conditions, respectively.

retinal apoplexy (AP-uh-plek-see): Condition in which the central retinal vein is blocked, leading to an impairment of the retina's blood supply and eventual damage.

retinal artery: *See* branch retinal artery, central retinal artery.

retinal branch vein occlusion: *See* branch retinal vein occlusion.

retinal central artery occlusion: *See* central retinal artery occlusion.

retinal central vein occlusion: *See* central retinal vein occlusion.

retinal correspondence: Property of vision such that a point on one retina becomes associated (in the brain) with a point on the retina of the fellow eye; if intact, it is known as normal retinal correspondence (NRC); *see* anomalous retinal correspondence, harmonious retinal correspondence.

retinal dehiscence (de-HISS-uns): *Another term for* retinal dialysis.

retinal detachment (RD): Condition in which the bacillary layer (rod and cone cells) of the retina is partially or completely separated from the pigment epithelial layer, resulting in a loss of vision in the area that is detached; *see also* giant retinal break, retinal tear; **rhegmatogenous r.d.** retinal detachment that begins as a break or tear in the retina, then vitreous seeps in between the layers; **serous r.d.** detachment in which the layers are forced apart by blood or plasma leaking from retinal blood vessels; **traction r.d.** detachment in which the retina is pulled away from the pigment epithelial layer (eg, as a complication of vitrectomy or due to the progression of diabetic retinopathy).

retinal dialysis: Retinal tear in the area of the ora serrata; *also called* retinal dehiscence.

retinal dysplasia (diss-PLAY-zee-uh): General term for abnormal development of retinal tissue.

retinal exudates (EKS-yoo-dayts): Light-colored bodies that appear on the retina in a number of retinal conditions, may be either hard exudates (well-defined, waxy, yellowish bodies that are truly the result of exudation [leakage of substances from retinal tissue]), or soft exudates (which are not exudates at all but rather small areas of the retinal nerve fiber layer that have lost their blood supply and become wispy white zones with no clear borders; *also called* cotton-wool spots); usually appearing in diabetic and other types of retinopathy.

retinal hole: *See* retinal tear, operculated retinal hole.

retinal ischemia (ih-SKEE-mee-uh): Condition in which the blood supply of the retina is cut off, resulting in tissue damage; *see also* branch retinal artery occlusion, branch retinal vein occlusion, central retinal vein occlusion, central retinal artery occlusion, retinal exudates.

retinal pigment epithelium (RPE): Dark, posterior-most layer of the retina providing attachment to the choroid as well as functioning in retinal nutrition; *also called* pigment epithelium; *see also* retina.

retinal recovery: *Another term for* retinal adaptation.

retinal reflex: *Another term for* red reflex.

retinal rivalry: Blurring of an area of the visual field when different, nonfusable images are presented to corresponding areas of the two retinae as first one image, then the other, is suppressed.

retinal tear: Opening in the retina caused by a pull from the hyaloid membrane, trauma, or surgical complication; *see also* giant retinal break, operculated retinal hold/tear, posterior vitreous detachment, retinal detachment.

retinal vasculitis (vas-kyuh-LAHY-tis): Inflammation of the retinal blood vessels; type of posterior uveitis; *see also* uveitis.

retinal vein: *See* branch retinal vein, central retinal vein.

retinitis (ret-in-I-tis): General term for inflammation of the retina, often associated with bacteria or fungi and characterized by loss of central vision and cells in the vitreous; type of posterior uveitis; *see also* uveitis; may be termed chorioretinitis if the choroid is also involved; **actinic r.** retinitis resulting from exposure to ultraviolet radiation; **cytomegalovirus (CMV) r.** opportunistic viral infection (belonging to the herpes group) of the retina in immunocompromised patients (such as those with AIDS); **exudative r.** retinitis marked by the appearance of retinal exudates; **purulent r.** retinitis caused by infection in the eye; **serous r.** inflammation of the retina characterized by swelling of the macula.

retinitis pigmentosa (RP) (ret-n-I-tis pig-men-TOH-sah): Inherited retinal dystrophy in which deposits of melanin pigment appear on the retina, accompanied by atrophy of retinal blood vessels and pallor of the optic disk, eventually leading to loss of vision.

retinoblastoma (ret-in-oh-bla-STOH-muh): Malignant tumor arising from the retinal cells of an embryo and developing in the first few years of life; its hallmark is leukocoria.

retinopathy (ret-in-AHP-uh-thee): General term for abnormal, noninflammatory condition of the retina, often associated with some systemic disorder; **cellophane r.** *another term for* cellophane maculopathy; **central serous r. (CSR)** sudden edema and swelling of the macula with leakage from blood vessels and central visual impairment and distortion, possibly leading to retinal detachment; **chloroquine r.** retinopathy resulting from use of the drug chloroquine; **circinate r.** retinopathy marked by the appearance of a circle of white patches around the macula, which can lead to retinal hemorrhaging; **diabetic r.** ocular effects of systemic diabetes mellitus characterized by retinal swelling, multiple small hemorrhages, retinal exudates, and growth of blood vessels into the retina, with progressive loss of vision if left untreated; **hypertensive r.** ocular effects of systemic hypertension, mainly affecting the retinal blood vessels; **proliferative (vitreo-) r.** neovascularization of the retina and vitreous in certain conditions involving the circulatory system, such as diabetes mellitus.

retinopathy of prematurity (ROP): Condition that affected premature infants in inappropriately high oxygen-enriched environments, occurring less frequently than in the past now that there is increased awareness of oxygen-related risks but still causing concern due to the numbers of premature infants; marked by neovascularization of the retina, which is followed by retinal hemorrhage, scarring and occasionally detachment, and growth of fibrous tissue into the vitreous humor; the possibility of serious ocular conditions such as glaucoma is increased following ROP (the advanced stage of which is called retrolental fibroplasia [RLF]).

retinopexy (RET-in-oh-PEK-see): Surgical procedure to repair a retinal detachment, most commonly through injection of air or heavy gas following vitrectomy (pneumatic retinopexy) or sometimes application of extreme cold to the external globe (ie, cryoretinopexy).

retinoschisis (RET-in-oh-SKEE-sis): Splitting of the tissue layers of the retina, usually in the periphery (so that central vision is unaffected) and infrequently leading to a detachment.

retinoscope (RET-in-uh-skohp): Hand-held instrument that projects a spot or streak of light that is reflected by the retina; the apparent motion and brightness of the reflected light when the instrument is moved allows the examiner to determine the refractive state of the eye (*see also* neutralization [definition 2]); it is an objective test in that it does not require patient responses.

retinoscopy (ret-in-AH-skuh-pee): Technique of objectively measuring a patient's refractive error using the retinoscope, usually refined via refractometry; *also called* skiascopy; **gross r.** the refractive measurement found with the retinoscope, including the power of the working lens; **net r.** the refractive measurement of the eye found with the retinoscope, minus the power of the working lens; this is the patient's actual refractive error.

retinosis (ret-in-OH-sis): General term for abnormal, noninflammatory condition of the retina.

retinotomy (ret-in-AHT-uh-mee): General term for surgical incision into the retina.

retraction syndrome: *Another term for* Duane's retraction syndrome.

retrobulbar (ret-roh-BUHL-bar): General term describing the area behind the eye; *compare* peribulbar.

retrobulbar anesthesia (ret-roh-BUHL-bar): Anesthesia administered by injection behind the eye; *compare* peribulbar anesthesia.

retrobulbar injection (ret-roh-BUHL-bar): Injection (usually anesthetic) directed behind the globe, into the muscle cone.

retroillumination: Method of viewing an ocular structure by light reflected from another structure (often the retina) lying behind the one to be viewed; usually referring to slit lamp biomicroscopy but can also describe a technique used with operating microscopes; *see also* indirect illumination.

retrolental (ret-roh-LEN-tul): Term describing the area behind the lens.

retrolental fibroplasia (RLF) (ret-roh-LEN-tul fy-broh-PLAY-zhah): The advanced stage of retinopathy of prematurity; *see* retinopathy of prematurity.

retroscopic tilt (ret-roh-SKAH-pik): Undesirable fit of spectacles where the top of the frame front is angled closer to the brow; *compare* pantoscopic tilt.

rhegmatogenous retinal detachment (reg-mah-TAH-jen-uhs): *See* retinal detachment.

rhodopsin (roh-DAHP-sin): Light-sensitive retinal pigment found in the rod cells; rhodopsin is synthesized in the dark, obliterated by light, and responsible for dark adaptation; *also called* visual purple; *see also* scotopia.

rigid gas-permeable (RGP) lens: *See* gas-permeable contact lens *under* contact lens.

ring scotoma: *Another term for* annular scotoma, *see entry under* scotoma.

Risley/Risley's prism: Two prisms mounted in a ring-like holder; prism power increases or decreases as the lenses are rotated by a thumbscrew; base may be oriented in any direction desired; *also called* rotary prism.

river blindness: *Another term for* onchocerciasis.

rod cells: One of two types of light-sensitive cells in the retina; often simply referred to as rods, they function primarily in peripheral and night vision; *compare* cone cells; *see also* rhodopsin, scotopia.

rod monochromatism (mon-oh-KROH-muh-tiz-uhm): *Another term for* achromatism.

rose bengal: Dye used in ophthalmic applications to stain the surface of the eye and detect damaged or dead conjunctival or corneal epithelial cells.

rotatory nystagmus: *See* nystagmus.

rotary prism: *Another term for* Risley prism.

Roth's spots: Infectious retinitis in which white areas appear in the optic disk surrounded by areas of hemorrhage.

rubeosis iridis (ru-bee-OH-sis IR-uh-diss): Abnormal growth of blood vessels into the iris in individuals with diabetes mellitus or following trauma.

rust ring: Localized corneal stain resulting from a metallic foreign body containing iron.

S

saccades (suh-KAYDZ): Rapid refixation movements of the eyes from one point of fixation to another in a series of jerky steps, or as an effort to maintain prolonged fixation; *also called* saccadic movement; *see also* microsaccades.

saccadic fixation (suh-KAD-ik): Rapid change of fixation from one point to another in the visual field.

saccadic movement (suh-KAD-ik): *Another term for* saccades.

Sands of Sahara syndrome: *Another term for* diffuse lamellar keratitis; *see entry under* keratitis.

sarcoma: A cancerous tumor derived from connective tissue.

scanning laser polarimetry: Measurement of the thickness of the retinal nerve fiber layer using polarized light; used to evaluate glaucoma.

scar pterygium: *Another term for* cicatricial pterygium; *see entry under* pterygium.

schematic eye: 1. Device used in training for retinoscopy; two telescoping cylinders are used to vary the length of the schematic eye (representing the axial length of a human eye) and auxiliary lenses are placed into the cells of the instrument to simulate astigmatism and other refractive errors; the examiner places trial lenses in front of the auxiliary lens while viewing the schematic eye though the retinoscope; *also called* model eye; 2. a theoretical eye composed of the average measurements and optical values of ocular structures; the values are used in mathematical computations, but not without inaccuracies; *also called* Gullstrand's schematic/reduced eye, reduced eye, schematic eye of Gullstrand; *see* Appendix 4.

Schiøtz tonometer (SHEE-ahtz): *See* indentation tonometer *under* tonometer.

Schirmer's test (SHER-merz): Test of tear production in which one end of a 5-x-25-mm strip of filter paper is placed into the cul-de-sac of the lower eyelid about 6 mm temporal to the punctum; the strips are left in place for a 5-minute test time; wetting of the paper at a rate of 2 mm to 3 mm per minute is considered normal; sometimes referred to as **S.t. number one**; **S.t. number two** same test as above, only the patient is given topical anesthetic prior to inserting the filter strips in order to eliminate tearing caused by irritation of the strips themselves.

Schlemm's canal (shlemz): Ring-shaped passage in the filtration angle through which aqueous humor drains into the bloodstream; *also called* canal of Schlemm, scleral canal.

Schwalbe's line (shuh-WAHL-beez): Border of Descemet's membrane, appearing on gonioscopy as a dark line at the edge of the cornea.

scintillating scotoma (SIN-tuh-lay-ting): *See* scotoma.

scissors motion: Confusing reflex in retinoscopy where aberration causes the reflex to break into two bands joined at one end.

sclera (SKLAYR-uh): Commonly called the "white" of the eye; the tough, fibrous tissue that makes up the major outer layer of the eye (lined inside by the choroid and retina); the optic nerve passes through it posteriorly at the lamina cribrosa, and anteriorly it joins with the clear cornea at the limbus; **blue s.** appearance of a thin sclera when pigment and blood from underlying tissue (the choroid) gives it a bluish tint.

scleral buckle (SB): Elastic band placed around the globe as part of a procedure to repair a retinal detachment; *also called* encircling band.

scleral buckling procedure: General term for surgical techniques to repair retinal detachment in which a device (such as a silicone band) is used to indent the sclera in the region of the detachment, bringing the pigment epithelium layer back into contact with the bacillary layer of the retina.

scleral canal: *Another term for* Schlemm's canal.

scleral conjunctiva: *See* conjunctiva.

scleral depression: While using the direct ophthalmoscope, a metal probe (scleral depressor) is used to indent the sclera, pushing more peripheral areas of the retina into the examiner's view.

scleral depressor: Short, curved, blunt probe inserted into the cul-de-sac and pushed against the sclera during scleral depression; *see* scleral depression.

scleral foramen (fuh-RAY-muhn): *Another term for* lamina cribrosa.

scleral lens: Large-diameter contact lens that covers the cornea and extends over the conjunctiva and onto the sclera; used in orthokeratology and treatment of certain conditions of the external ocular tissues; *compare* semiscleral lens; *see also* contact lens.

scleral rigidity: Elasticity of the sclera, which plays a role in measuring intraocular pressure; troublesome with indentation tonometry, where a low scleral rigidity (ie, tissues are more elastic) gives an incorrect lower reading and vice versa.

scleral shell: Cosmetic ocular prosthesis that is worn over a disfigured eye.

scleral show: Excessive exposure of the sclera due to abnormally wide opening of the eyelids.

scleral spacing procedure (SSP): Surgical treatment for presbyopia that uses scleral implants.

scleral spur: Band of scleral fibers in the anterior chamber, located between Schlemm's canal and the ciliary body, serving as part of the anchor tissue for the ciliary body and iris; *also called* corneoscleral spur.

scleral sulcus: Area where the tissues of the cornea insert into the similarly fibrous tissues of the sclera.

scleral trabeculae (SKLAY-ruhl truh-BEK-yuh-lee): *Another term for* trabecular meshwork.

sclerectasia, -asis (sklayr-ek-TAY-zee-uh): Stretching of the sclera caused by chronic elevated intraocular pressure in early life.

sclerectomy (sklayr-EK-tuh-mee): General term for surgical removal of scleral tissue.

scleritis (sklayr-I-tis): Inflammation of the sclera; **anterior s.** scleritis affecting the front, visible part of the sclera; **necrotizing s.** slowly progressive degeneration of the sclera to the point of perforation, often associated with rheumatoid arthritis; *also called* scleromalacia perforans; **posterior s.** scleritis affecting the back, nonvisible portion of the sclera and Tenon's capsule.

sclerocorneal (sklayr-oh-KOHR-nee-ul): Of or related to the sclera and cornea together.

scleromalacia (sklayr-oh-muh-LAY-shuh): Condition marked by the thinning and softening of the sclera.

scleromalacia perforans (sklayr-oh-muh-LAY-shuh PER-fer-uhns): *Another term for* necrotizing scleritis, *see entry under* scleritis.

scleronyxis (sklayr-oh-NIK-sis): Surgical procedure involving a puncturing of the sclera.

scleroplasty (SKLAYR-oh-plas-tee): General term for surgical procedure on the sclera.

sclerostomy (sklayr-AH-stuh-mee): General term for the surgical creation of an opening in the sclera, most commonly in an attempt to allow drainage of aqueous from the anterior chamber in the treatment of glaucoma.

sclerotic scatter: In slit lamp biomicroscopy, method of shining the light onto the corneal limbus from an angle, creating a bright ring around the cornea; this light is refracted throughout corneal tissue to provide a view of its structure, especially the general pattern of any opacities.

sclerotomy (sklayr-AH-tuh-mee): General term for an incision into the sclera.

scoto-: Combining word meaning dark.

scotoma (skuh-TOH-mah): Area within the borders of the visual field in which vision is impaired or absent, attributable to dysfunction of the retina or optic nerve; there is a natural scotoma where the optic nerve enters the eye, called the physiologic spot; plural: scotomata; *see also* hemianopia, quadrantanopia (both of which are contractions of the field rather than scotomata); **absolute s.** area within the visual field where there is no response to any stimuli (of that particular perimeter); **annular s.** ring-shaped scotoma, usually centered around the fixation point; *also called* ring s.; **arcuate s.** nerve fiber bundle defect that curves in an arc-like shape; *also called* comet s., scimitar s.; **Bjerrum's s.** scotoma extending from the physiologic blind spot (if it progresses it becomes an arcuate scotoma); **central s.** scotoma in the center of the visual field with corresponding impairment of macular function; **centrocecal s.** egg-shaped scotoma extending from the physiologic blind spot to the fixation point; **comet s.** *another term for* arcuate s.; **false s.** area of impairment in the visual field that is not attributable to dysfunction of the retina (eg, scotoma caused by a small undiagnosed cataract); **junction s.** scotoma arising from a defect in the optic chiasm (junction of the two optic nerves); **motile s.** type of false scotoma in which opaque material (eg, cells) floating through the vitreous results in the appearance of dark areas within the visual field that shift with the passing of time; **negative s.** scotoma that is dark and devoid of light perception; **paracentral s.** near-central scotoma attributable to an area of dysfunction close to the macula; **pericecal** or **peripapillary s.** scotoma occurring around the physiologic blind spot related to nerve fiber dysfunction near the disk; **peripheral s.** scotoma that is located well away from the fixation point; **physiologic s.** *another term for* blind spot; **positive s.** scotoma that is bright, often scintillating; **relative s.** area within an isopter where the retina does not respond to the target used to map the isopter; **ring s.** *another term for* annular s.; **scimitar s.** *another term for* arcuate s.; **scintillating s.** scotoma with a jagged outline surrounded by bright flashes, often reported to precede attacks of migraine; **Seidel's s.** arcuate defect that has extended from a Bjerrum's scotoma at the physiologic blind spot and curves around the central field.

scotopia (skuh-TOH-pee-uh): Night vision in which the rod cells of the retina are sensitized with the pigment rhodopsin in the process of dark (scotopic) adaptation; commonly called night vision; *compare* nyctalopia, photopia; *see also* mesopia, Purkinje shift.

scotopic adaptation: *Another term for* dark adaptation, *see* adaptation.

scotopic ERG (skuh-TAH-pik): *See* electroretinography.

scotopic vision (skuh-TAH-pik): Dark-adapted vision; *see* scotopia; *compare* photopic vision.

screen (tangent): *See* tangent screen.

screening: 1. Referring to preliminary testing, often to quickly detect gross defects or to rapidly obtain basic information; 2. use of specific tests or information to determine the population group falling into a specific category.

seasonal conjunctivitis: *See entry under* conjunctivitis.

sebaceous gland (suh-BAY-shus): Gland that produces sebum, a fatty oily exudate; in the eye these are the Zeiss and meibomian glands in lids and the caruncle in conjunctiva.

second cranial nerve (CN II): The optic nerve; *see* optic nerve.

second sight: Misnomer for the decrease in hyperopia (or increase in myopia) that accompanies cataract formation, allowing the patient to read without glasses; sometimes called the honeymoon stage of cataracts.

secondary: 1. General medical term for an event, procedure, or condition that occurs after a previous event, procedure, or condition (but not necessarily caused by it); *compare* primary; for entities described as secondary, look up entry under main word, such as secondary glaucoma *see* glaucoma; 2. general term for the second item in a group of related events, procedures, or conditions that is always described in the same order (eg, secondary astigmatism, secondary deviation, etc); *see definition under* main word.

secondary astigmatism: *See* astigmatism.

secondary deviation: The amount of deviation that occurs in paralytic strabismus when the eye that normally does not fixate is forced to do so; the secondary deviation is always larger than the primary deviation; *compare* primary deviation.

secondary dye test: *Another term for* Jones II test.

secondary membrane: *Another term for* capsule opacification.

sector iridectomy: *See* sector i. *under* iridectomy.

segment: 1. In general ophthalmology, referring to the anterior or posterior of the eye, with the crystalline lens being the dividing line; **anterior s.** front portion of the eye from (and including) the crystalline lens forward; comprised of both anterior and posterior chambers; **posterior s.** rear portion of the eye from behind the crystalline lens and back; 2. in opticianry, term used to describe the near vision optical element(s) placed into a portion of a corrective bifocal or trifocal lens; *see also* add (definition 2).

segment height: Millimeter measurement indicating the placement of any multifocal add(s) to a spectacle lens; measured from the deepest part of the eyewire.

Seidel's scotoma (SY-dellz): *See* scotoma.

Seidel's sign (SY-dellz): Leakage of aqueous humor from the anterior chamber onto the external surface of the eye made visible with the use of fluorescein dye.

semilunar fold: Flap of conjunctiva normally found in the medial canthus next to the caruncle.

semiscleral lens: Contact lens that covers the cornea and extends slightly past the limbus; modern soft lenses are of this type; *compare* scleral lens.

senile: General term meaning occurring in old age; *compare* congenital, infantile, juvenile.

senile cataract: *See* cataract.

senile ectropion: *Another term for* involutional ectropion, *see entry under* ectropion.

senile macular degeneration (SMD): *See* macular degeneration (age-related).

sensory fusion: *See* fusion.

sensory nerve: Afferent nerve that carries the sensation of touch, light, odor, taste, or sound to the brain; afferent nerves also carry input from visceral organs to the brain; *compare* mixed nerve, motor nerve.

sensory receptors: *Another term for* photoreceptors.

sensory retina: All layers of the retina involved in the perception of light (ie, all layers except the retinal pigment epithelium); *see also* retina.

separation difficulty: *Another term for* crowding phenomenon.

sequelae (suh-KWEL-ee): Unintended side effects of a surgery or medication (or other treatment); a condition arising as a result of another disorder.

seventh cranial nerve (CN VII): *Another term for* facial nerve.

seventh nerve palsy: *Another term for* Bell's palsy.

sex-linked (gene): A gene with a locus on the X or Y (sex) chromosome; *see also* X-linked gene, Y-linked gene.

Shack-Hartmann aberrometry: Aberrometry method in which a beam of light is shone into the eye, reflected from the retina, and collected by an array of small lenses (lenslets); the lenslets create a pattern that indicates any optical aberrations that have distorted the original wavefront of the light passing through the eye.

Shack-Hartmann array: Portion of an aberrometer using a group of small lenses (lenslets) to measure optical aberrations using Shack-Hartmann aberrometry.

shaken baby syndrome: Set of signs and symptoms classic of abusive shaking of a small child such that the head snaps back and forth; ocular findings include retinal hemorrhages and cotton-wool spots, especially near the macula.

shallow angle: Anatomical structure of the angle of the eye such that pupillary dilation may close the angle, causing a rise in intraocular pressure; *also called* narrow angle.

sheath syndrome: *Another term for* Brown's syndrome.

shell: *See* scleral shell.

Sherrington's law (of reciprocal innervation): General principle of physiology, also applicable to the extraocular muscles, that every stimulus inducing a muscle to contract is accompanied by an equal stimulus for the antagonistic muscle (ie, the one with the opposite effect) to relax.

shingles: Herpes zoster infection; in the eye, may produce a rash on the lids, scleritis, keratitis, iritis, or optic neuritis, or cause glaucoma.

side vision: *Another term for* visual field.

siderosis (sid-uh-ROH-sis): General term for condition in which deposits of iron appear in bodily tissues.

siderosis bulbi (sid-uh-ROH-sis BUHL-by): Siderosis within the eye.

siderosis conjunctivae (sid-uh-ROH-sis kahn-junk-TY-vee): Deposits of iron in the conjunctiva, usually from a foreign body.

sign: Objective finding associated with a disorder that can be perceived or detected by the examiner; *compare* symptom.

silicone contact lens: *See* soft contact lens *under* contact lens.

silicone IOL: *See* intraocular lens.

silicone oil: Heavy fluid used in surgery to repair retinal detachment; *see also* gas-fluid exchange.

sine-wave grating: The pattern of lines used as a target in contrast sensitivity testing.

sinistro-: Prefix describing processes or structures occurring or appearing toward the left; in ophthalmic usage, part of the phrase oculus sinister (OS), meaning the left eye; *compare* dextro-.

6/6 vision: Normal visual acuity as measured at a 6-m distance (ie, numerator is always 6); corresponds to 20/20 vision (a 20-ft test distance).

sixth cranial nerve (CN VI): *Another term for* abducens nerve.

sixth nerve palsy: Paralysis of the abducens nerve, prohibiting abduction; subject often adopts a head turn toward the affected side in order to reduce or eliminate diplopia.

Sjögren's syndrome (SHOH-grinz): Systemic disorder with symptoms including severe dry eye, dry mouth, and connective tissue disease (most commonly rheumatoid arthritis); *see also* arthro-ophthalmopathy.

skew deviation: *See* deviation.

skiascopy (skee-AH-skuh-pee): *Another term for* retinoscopy.

slab-off lens: Multifocal lens in which a portion of the lower near-vision segment is ground away (thus the term slab-off) in such a way as to shift the optical center of that segment closer to the optical center of the upper distance vision part of the lens; this is done to reduce the vertical imbalance (thus eliminating double vision and discomfort) present at near when there is a large difference in refractive error between the two eyes.

slit lamp: Microscope with a light source that projects a beam of light onto the eye, usually as a narrow vertical beam (thus, the term slit, but with other beam shapes possible), allowing an examiner to view ocular structures under varying magnifications and illuminations; *also called* biomicroscope.

slit lamp biomicroscopy: Examination of a patient using the slit lamp.

Sloan letters or **optotypes:** Eye chart or card using block capital letters C, D, H, K, N, O, R, S, V, and Z.

smear: Obtaining a sample of infected tissue or exudate to place onto a microscope slide for evaluation; the material placed on such a slide; the act of making such a slide.

snap back test: An assessment of lid elasticity in which the lower lid is gently pulled away from the globe then released; a lid with normal tone will quickly "snap" against the eye.

Snell's law: Optical formula defining the index of refraction of a substance as the sine of the angle of incidence divided by the sine of the angle of refraction.

Snellen acuity: Measurement of visual acuity based upon standard sizes of letters visible to the "normal" eye at specified distances using the Snellen chart.

Snellen chart: The traditional visual acuity test using letters as optotypes; the test type incorporated into Snellen's vision test target is the most commonly used eye chart in the United States; its standard testing distance of 20 feet gives us the familiar system of measuring distance visual acuity against a reference value of 20/20; *see also* visual acuity, visual acuity tests.

Snellen letters: Optotypes used on a Snellen chart; each letter subtends 5 minutes of arc.

soaking solution: Solution used to condition contact lenses for proper hydration and wetting.

socket: 1. *Another term for* orbit; 2. the pocket into which an ocular prosthesis is inserted.

Soemmering's ring (SOH-muh-rings): Ring-shaped collection of crystalline lens material left after cataract extraction, which sometimes opacifies.

soft contact lens (SCL): *See* contact lens.

soft exudates: *Another term for* cotton-wool spots; *see also* retinal exudates.

soft IOL: *Another term for* foldable IOL, *see entry under* intraocular lens (foldable).

solution: In pharmacology, a medication that completely dissolves in the vehicle; *compare* emulsion, suspension; *see* vehicle.

spasm: General term meaning sudden involuntary contraction of a muscle or set of muscles, usually accompanied by pain and/or dysfunction; *see also* tic; **accommodative s.** *see* accommodative spasm; **blepharospasm** *see* blepharospasm.

spasmus nutans (SPAZ-mus NOO-tanz): Combination of nystagmus (usually horizontal) and head nodding in infants; resolves itself during childhood.

spectacles: Eyeglasses; **aphakic s.** eyeglasses prescribed to correct vision after removal of a cataractous crystalline lens, usually requiring very thick plus lenses; **half-eye s.** small spectacles, often with a flat top, made to wear farther down on the nose than normal so that one may look through them when gazing down for near work and over them when looking straight ahead at a distance.

spectrum: *See* electromagnetic spectrum.

specular microscope: Instrument equipped with a video camera used to view and image the corneal endothelium; *also called* endothelial camera.

specular microscopy: Technique for viewing the corneal endothelium; used to assess the health of the cornea, particularly prior to intraocular surgery; *see also* endothelial cell count/density.

specular reflection: Slit lamp illumination technique for viewing the corneal epithelium and endothelium and crystalline lens surfaces; both light source and microscope are positioned 30 degrees to opposite sides.

speculum (SPEK-yoo-lum): General term for an instrument that facilitates the observation of some part of the body by holding open an orifice; in ophthalmic usage, a lid speculum (*also called* blepharostat) is a device placed between the upper and lower lids to hold them open.

sphenoid bone (SFEE-noyd): One of the bones of the orbit.

sphenoid fissure (SFEE-noyd): *Another term for* the superior orbital fissure, *see entry under* orbital fissure.

sphere (sph): 1. In optics, a lens that refracts all incoming light to a single focal point; 2. in refraction, the component of refractive error that can be corrected with a spherical lens (myopia or hyperopia); *compare* cylinder.

spherical aberration: In optics, the higher-order aberration that distorts an image by focusing too strongly in the center and around the entire periphery, with a ring of weak focus around the midperiphery (**positive s.a.**), or in a similar pattern with areas of strong and weak focus reversed (**negative s.a.**); often results in blurring of images, halo, and nighttime glare; *see also* aberration.

spherical equivalent (Deq or SE): 1. Representation of the refractive power of a toric lens defined as the spherical power plus one half the cylinder power; 2. similar calculation performed on the components of a spectacle prescription to describe the overall refractive error of an eye.

spherical lens: Lens that refracts all incoming light to a single focal point; *compare* aspheric, toric lens.

spherocylindrical lens: A lens combining spherical (for hyperopia or myopia) and astigmatic (cylindrical) correction; *see also* toric lens.

sphincter: General anatomic term for a circular muscle; in ophthalmic usage, referring to the pupillary sphincter; *see* pupillary sphincter muscle; *compare* pupillary dilator muscle.

sphincterotomy (sfink-ter-EK-toh-mee): In ophthalmic usage, an incision into the pupillary sphincter, usually performed when a small pupil makes intraocular surgery difficult.

spindle cells: *Another term for* Krukenberg's spindles.

spiral of Tillaux (teh-LOH): Configuration of the insertion-to-limbus distances of the extraocular muscles such that the distances decrease as you go around the limbus; on the right eye, beginning superiorly and moving counterclockwise, these measurements are superior oblique (7.7 mm), lateral rectus (7.0 mm), inferior rectus (6.5 mm), and medial rectus (5.5 mm).

spirillum (spy-RIL-um): Bacterium that is a spiral-shaped rod; plural: spirilla.

spot retinoscope: Retinoscope that projects a round light; *see also* retinoscope.

squamous cell carcinoma (skw-A-mus): Malignant skin lesion, most notably on sun-exposed areas of the face; this carcinoma begins as a superficial lesion, but may invade and metastasize into life-threatening cancer; *compare* basal cell carcinoma, melanoma.

squint: Largely out-of-date term for strabismus.

squint angle: *Another term for* angle of deviation.

stain: In general, dye used for diagnostic purposes; *see also* corneal staining; in microbiology, dyes used to render organisms visible on microscope slides or to identify organisms (eg, gram stain, Wright stain); *see* specific stain.

staining: *See* corneal staining.

standardized A-scan: Ultrasound used to differentiate tissue (eg, melanoma versus hemangioma); *also called* diagnostic A-scan.

staphyloma (STAF-uh-LOH-muh): Localized thinning of the sclera so that it bulges, often associated with high myopia; it appears dark because the choroid pushes into the bulging area; rarely referring to a thinned, bulging area of the cornea; **anterior s.** scleral staphyloma in the area of the ciliary body; **equatorial s.** scleral staphyloma occurring midway between the anterior and posterior poles of the eye, usually where the vortex veins exit the globe; **posterior s.** scleral staphyloma in the posterior segment, usually at the optic nerve head.

starburst: Subjective perception of bright lines emanating from a point source of light such as the sun or car headlights; may be caused by the natural optical system of an eye or appear as side effects of corrective lenses or eye surgery; *see also* glare, halo.

static perimetry: *See* perimetry.

statistically significant: The mathematical determination that a phenomenon probably did not occur by mere chance.

steamy cornea: *Another term for* corneal edema.

steep: In ophthalmic usage, describing the surface curvature of a lens or ocular medium that imparts the greatest refractive power; *compare* flat.

steep axis: In a toric lens or spherocylindrical ocular medium (usually the cornea), the most curved axis that hence has the most refracting power; the cylinder axis of astigmatism as measured on refractometry using plus cylinder is parallel to this steep axis (in minus cylinder it is perpendicular to it); *compare* flat axis.

steepening: In refractive surgery, increasing the curvature of the cornea to correct hyperopia; *compare* flattening.

stenopaic/stenopeic slit (sten-oh-PAY-ik): Opaque disk in which there is a single horizontal opening, used in refractometry to determine the axis of best vision in a patient with high or irregular astigmatism.

step: *See* nasal step.

stereopsis (ster-ee-OP-sis): Three-dimensional vision possible only when binocular vision and fusion are present; *see also* binocular vision and fusion; *compare* depth perception.

steroids: *Another term for* corticosteroids.

stigmatic lens: Lens that brings light from a point source into a point of focus.

stigmatoscopy (stig-muh-TAHS-kuh-pee): Technique for determining the refractive state of the eye by having the test subject view a pinpoint of light and report its appearance.

stimulus: In ophthalmology, any object or target used to elicit a response from any component(s) of the visual system.

strabismus (struh-BIZ-muhs): Misalignment of the visual axes of the eyes (ie, the eyes are not straight); *also called* cross-eyed; *see also* angle of deviation, primary deviation, secondary deviation; **absolute s.** strabismus present under all conditions and at all fixation distances; *also called* constant s.; **accommodative s.** strabismus (usually convergent) that occurs upon accommodation or attempted accommodation; *see also* esotropia; **alternating s.** strabismus in which either eye can maintain fixation (*also called* bilateral, binocular s.); **anatomic s.** strabismus resulting from malformation of the structure of the eye, ocular muscles, or orbit; **bilateral** or **binocular s.** other terms for alternating s.; **comitant** or **concomitant s.** strabismus in which the angle of deviation is the same for all directions of gaze regardless of which eye is fixating; *compare* incomitant s.; **constant s.** *another term for* absolute s.; **convergent s.** strabismus in which the deviation is inward/nasal/medial (*also called* esotropia, internal strabismus); **cyclic s.** strabismus that occurs and disappears at regular intervals of time; **divergent s.** strabismus in which the deviation is outward/temporal/lateral (*also called* exotropia, external strabismus); **dynamic s.** muscular imbalance that tends to make the eye deviate but is usually overcome in normal binocular vision; **external s.** *another term for* exotropia; **horizontal s.** strabismus in which the misalignment is to the left or right; *compare* vertical s.; **incomitant s.** paralytic strabismus in which the angle of deviation varies with the direction of gaze, fixating eye, or fixation distance; *also called* noncomitant, nonconcomitant s.; *compare* comitant s.; **intermittent s.** strabismus that is not present at all times; **internal s.** *another term for* esotropia; **kinetic s.** strabismus resulting from spasm of the extraocular muscles; **latent s.** misalignment of the eye that occurs only when one eye is deprived of fusional stimulus; *also called* phoria, suppressed s.; **manifest s.** strabismus that is not latent; *also called* tropia; **mechanical s.** strabismus resulting from some anatomic pull upon or displacement of the eye or extraocular muscles; **microstrabismus** strabismus of such a small degree that it is only noted upon close examination; **monolateral** or **monocular s.** *another term for* unilateral s.; **muscular s.** strabismus resulting from some imbalance of the extraocular muscles; **noncomitant** or **nonconcomitant s.** *another term for* incomitant s.; **nonparetic s.** strabismus not associated with muscle paralysis; *compare* paralytic s.; **paralytic** or **paretic s.** strabismus resulting from paralysis of one or more extraocular muscles; **periodic** or **relative s.** strabismus that occurs only at certain directions of gaze or fixation distances; **spasmodic** or **spastic s.** strabismus resulting from spasm of one or more extraocular muscles; **suppressed s.** *another term for* latent s.; **unilateral s.** strabismus in which one eye deviates while the fellow eye achieves normal fixation; *also called* monolateral or monocular s.; **vertical s.** strabismus in which the deviation is a turning up or down; *compare* horizontal s.

strabotomy (struh-BAHT-uh-mee): Surgical procedure to correct strabismus by cutting an extraocular muscle.

streak retinoscope: Retinoscope that projects a linear light reflex; *see also* retinoscopy.

striae (STREE-uh): General medical term for the appearance of lines or streaks in tissue; **corneal s.** fine, whitish lines in the corneal stroma resulting from edema;

retinal s. lines in the retina, usually originating from a visible point of pathology.

striate cortex (STRY-ayt): *Another term for* visual cortex.

stroma: General anatomic term for the main structural element of a tissue or organ; **corneal s.** central layer of fibrous corneal tissue lying between Bowman's and Descemet's membranes; **iris s.** connective tissue to which the sphincter muscles, nerves, and pigment of the iris adhere.

Sturm's interval: In astigmatism, the area between the point focus of the spherical component and the linear focus of the astigmatic component; light rays within this interval form a cone shape known as the conoid of Sturm; *also called* interval of Sturm.

sty/stye: *Another term for* external hordeolum; *see entry under* hordeolum.

subacute: Designation of a disorder as being somewhere between acute and chronic; *compare* acute, chronic.

subcapsular cataract: *See* cataract.

subchoroidal hemorrhage (sub-koh-ROYD-uhl): Bleeding between the retina and choroid, leading to retinal detachment if left untreated (*also called* suprachoroidal hemorrhage).

subconjunctival hemorrhage (SCH) (sub-kahn-junk-TY-vul): Bleeding between the conjunctiva and sclera, dramatic in appearance (initially a blood-red patch on the surface of the eye) but usually posing no threat to the eye or sight and resolving without treatment.

subcutaneous (sub-cu-TAY-nee-us): General medical term meaning under the skin.

subduction: General term for downward motion; in ophthalmic usage, downward movement of the eye.

subjective: Method of testing that relies on the patient's responses (eg, refractometry, Maddox rod, stereo testing); *compare* objective (definition 1).

subluxation: General term for dislocation, as in a subluxated lens.

subretinal neovascularization (SRNV) (nee-oh-vas-cu-lahr-i-ZAY-shun): Intrusion of abnormal blood vessels and scar tissue into the retinal layers when Bruch's membrane has been compromised; commonly seen in wet macular degeneration, but found in other disorders as well.

substantia propria corneae and **sclerae (sub-STAN-shuh PROH-pree-uh KOHR-nuh-ee and SKLAYR-ee):** Stroma of the cornea and sclera, respectively.

sulcus: General anatomic term describing a grooved or depressed area; *see also* ciliary sulcus, scleral sulcus.

sulfonamide (suhl-FON-uh-myd): Any sulfa-containing drug used as an antibacterial.

sulfur hexafluoride (SF6): Heavy gas used in surgery to repair retinal detachment.

sunburst dial: *Another term for* astigmatic clock.

sunglasses: Spectacles with lenses that are tinted to decrease the amount of light passing through them, thus increasing comfort in bright light; *see also* ultraviolet blocker.

sunrise and **sunset syndromes:** Dislocation of an intraocular lens upward or downward, respectively, behind the pupil.

super vision: 1. Theoretical visual acuity if the eye had perfect optics without any aberrations; also called supernormal vision; 2. visual acuity better than 20/20.

supercilium (soo-pur-SILL-ee-uhm): Proper term for the eyebrow.

superficial punctate keratitis (SPK): *See* keratitis.

superior oblique muscle (SO): Extraocular muscle lying across the top of the eye and supplied by CN IV (trochlear nerve) responsible for depressing, abducting, and intorting the eye.

superior oblique tendon sheath syndrome: *Another term for* Brown's syndrome.

superior rectus muscle (SR): Extraocular muscle lying across the top of the eye, supplied by CN III (oculomotor nerve), responsible for elevating, adducting, and intorting the eye.

superior tarsal muscle: *Another term for* Müller's muscle.

suppression: Action of the brain to ignore the image from one eye during binocular vision as a result of anisometropia, deviation, or other visual disturbance.

suprachoroid (soo-pruh-KOR-oid): The outer layer of the choroid and ciliary body consisting primarily of connective, avascular tissue.

suprachoroidal hemorrhage (soo-pruh-koh-ROYD-uhl): *Another term for* subchoroidal hemorrhage.

supraduction: In ophthalmic usage, upward turning of one eye; *also called* elevation, sursumduction; *compare* depression.

supraorbital: At the top of or above the bony eye socket.

suprathreshold: In visual field testing, the strategy of testing with a slightly brighter target than would normally be needed to obtain a response from a subject of given demographics; sometimes used as a screening strategy.

supraversion: In ophthalmic usage, upward turning of both eyes; *also called* sursumversion; *compare* deorsumversion.

surfactant: Soap element of some contact lens and other cleansers that binds with external debris and breaks its attachment to the lens surface.

surgical reversal of presbyopia (SRP): Four plastic segments are inserted into the sclera in the area of the ciliary body in order to create more tension on the zonules; *compare* laser reversal of presbyopia.

sursumduction: *Another term for* supraduction.

sursumversion: *Another term for* supraversion.

suspension: In pharmacology, a medication that does not dissolve but remains particulate matter in the vehicle; *compare* emulsion, solution; *see* vehicle.

swinging flashlight test: Pupil test in which the light source is moved rapidly from one eye to the other while evaluating pupillary reaction; *see also* Marcus Gunn pupil.

symblepharon (sim-BLEF-uh-ron): Condition in which the conjunctiva of the eyelid adheres to the bulbar conjunctiva.

sympathetic amaurosis: *See* amaurosis.

sympathetic nervous system: Division of the autonomic nervous system that diverts energy to the muscles for "fight or flight"; in the eye, this system causes pupil dilation; *see also* adrenergic, epinephrine; *compare* parasympathetic nervous system.

sympathetic ophthalmia (SO) (op-THAL-mee-uh): Condition in which trauma or intraocular foreign body leading to uveitis in one eye is followed by uveitis in the other uninjured eye a few weeks later; in some cases of trauma, a severely injured eye will be removed to prevent this complication; although rare, it causes a loss of sight in both eyes.

sympatholytic (sim-path-oh-LIT-ik): Substance that blocks the sympathetic system, thus causing a parasympathetic response; beta-blockers, used to treat glaucoma, are sympatholytic drugs; *compare* parasympatholytic.

sympathomimetic (sim-path-oh-my-MET-ik): Substance that causes a sympathetic-like response in the autonomic nervous system; phenylephrine (a mydriatic) is a sympathomimetic drug; *compare* parasympathomimetic.

symptom: Subjective indication or perception of a disorder as experienced and related by the patient; may or may not be objectively apparent to the examiner (eg, an examiner and patient can both see redness, but only the patient can feel pain); *compare* sign.

symptomatic: Having symptoms, especially those common to a particular disorder; *compare* asymptomatic; *see* symptom.

symptomatic tear film break-up time (SBUT): Test of tear function; the time between the subject's blink and becoming "aware" of the eye; normally should be within one second of the tear break-up time; *see also* break-up time.

synapse: A gap between the axon of one nerve cell and the dendrite of the next; impulses cross the synapse via neurotransmitters; *see also* axon, dendrite (definition 1), neurotransmitter.

syncanthus (sin-KAN-thuhs): Adhesion of the tissues of the eye to structures of the orbit.

synchysis (sin-KEE-sis): Condition in which the vitreous humor loses its normal consistency and liquefies; **s. scintillans** formation of sparkling crystals within the liquefied vitreous humor, related to ocular degenerative disease.

syncope (SING-koh-pee): Temporary loss of consciousness; *also called* faint.

syndrome: General medical term referring to specific combination of symptoms and signs typical of a given disorder; *see* specific syndrome (eg, Brown's syndrome, etc).

synechia (sin-IK-ee-uh *or* **sin-EEK-ee-uh):** General term for fibrous adhesion of organs or tissues; plural: synechiae; **anterior s.** adhesion of the iris to the cornea; *compare* posterior synechia; **posterior s. (PS)** adhesion of the iris to the lens; *compare* anterior synechia.

synechialysis (sin-eek-ee-uh-LY-sis): Surgical breaking of synechiae.

syneresis (sin-er-EE-sis): In ophthalmic usage, degenerative shrinking of the vitreous body as a result of aging, often resulting in vitreous detachment; *see also* posterior vitreous detachment.

synergist: Extraocular muscle (EOM) that assists another EOM in the same eye to accomplish a specific movement; **contralateral s.** *another term for* yoke muscle.

synoptophore (sin-AHP-tuh-for): Table-top instrument used in strabismus measuring, retinal correspondence testing, and orthoptic training.

systemic: General medical term meaning to affect the entire body.

taco test: Method of determining if a soft contact lens is inside out; center of the lens is gently pinched together between thumb and forefinger; if it curls up (like a taco), it is right side out; if the edges flare outward, it is inside out.

tamponade (tam-puh-NOD): Use of a plug as part of a surgical procedure; **gas t.** intraocular use of gas to push against a retinal tear as part of vitreoretinal surgery; **silicone oil t.** intraocular use of silicone oil to push against a retinal tear as part of vitreoretinal surgery.

tangent screen: A method of manual perimetry using a large black felt screen to find scotomata and map isopter borders in the central 30 degrees of the visual field; targets of varying sizes and colors are presented by the examiner, and the patient indicates when they are seen or not seen.

tangential illumination (tan-JEN-shul): In slit lamp biomicroscopy, method of viewing surfaces of ocular structures (especially their texture) by shining light at an oblique angle across the surface of the structure.

target: 1. *Another term for* fixation object/target; 2. the goal of treatment (eg, target intraocular pressure in glaucoma patient).

tarsal (TAHR-sul): Of or like the tarsus.

tarsal angle (TAHR-sul): *Another term for* canthus.

tarsal glands (TAHR-sul): *Another term for* meibomian glands.

tarsal muscle (TAHR-sul): One of the muscles that acts to open the eyelids, either upper (superior tarsal muscle, *also called* Müller's muscle) or lower (inferior tarsal muscle).

tarsal plate (TAHR-sul): *Another term for* tarsus.

tarsorrhaphy (tar-sohr-uh-fee): General term for surgical procedures in which the upper and lower eyelids are sutured together; *also called* blepharorrhaphy.

tarsus (TAHR-sus): "Plate" of connective tissue that serves as the underlying structure of the eyelids, either upper (superior tarsus) or lower (inferior tarsus); *also called* tarsal plate; plural: tarsi.

tear break-up time: *See* break-up time.

tear duct, gland, etc: *See* lacrimal apparatus.

tear film: The natural fluid covering of the surface of the eye, composed primarily of three strata: an inner layer of mucin (produced in the conjunctival goblet cells), a middle watery layer (produced in the lacrimal glands, which also produce various important tear proteins like lactoferrin), and an outer layer of oily lipid secretions (produced in the meibomian glands); contact lenses "ride" upon the tear film, which is constantly refreshed by the various glands mentioned above and continuously drains through the puncta and the nasolacrimal ducts into the nasal sinuses; *also called* precorneal tear film, preocular tear film.

tear sac: *Another term for* nasolacrimal sac.

tearing: Common term for lacrimation; **basal t.** lacrimation that occurs normally (ie, not due to some stimulus); is reduced in "dry eye"; **reflex t.** lacrimation resulting from strong stimulus (eg, odor, foreign body, wind, bright light, etc).

telecanthus (tel-uh-KAN-thus): A distance between the medial canthi of more than 30 mm.

telescope: 1. General term for an optical device consisting of an objective (either a convex lens or concave mirror) and an ocular (a concave or convex lens) to enlarge and focus the image of a distant object; **Galilean t.** telescope in which the objective is a convex lens and the ocular is a concave lens, producing an erect image; 2. low-vision aid that employs telescopic optics to magnify a relatively narrow field of view.

temple: In opticianry, part of the spectacle frame that attaches to the frame front, rests against the head, and usually extends over the ear; *see also* frame front; **t. length** frame measurement of the temple from where it joins the frame front (hinge) to the bend or tip (which depends on temple style).

temporal: General anatomic directional term meaning toward the side (ie, temple) of the head; *see also* lateral; *compare* medial, nasal.

temporal canthus (KAN-thus): *Another term for* lateral canthus.

tendon: General term meaning the fibrous tissue that attaches muscle to bone.

tenectomy (ten-EK-tuh-mee): Surgical procedure in which a tendon is cut and removed (not to be confused with tenonectomy).

Tenon's capsule, membrane, or **sac (TEE-nahnz):** Thin, outermost membrane enclosing the eye from the limbus back to the optic nerve, including some muscle tendons; *also called* fascia bulbi.

tenonectomy (tee-nahn-EK-tuh-mee): Surgical removal of a portion of Tenon's capsule.

tenonotomy (tee-nahn-AH-tuh-mee): Surgical procedure in which an incision is made into Tenon's capsule.

tenotomy (ten-AH-tuh-mee): Surgical procedure in which a tendon is cut (not to be confused with tenonotomy); in ophthalmic usage, referring to strabismus surgery.

tetrafoil: In optics, the higher-order aberration that distorts an image so that there are four areas in the periphery where the focus is too strong alternating with four areas where the focus is too weak; often causes blurring of vision; *also called* quadrafoil.

thermokeratoplasty (TK) (ther-moh-KAYR-uh-toh-plas-tee): Refractive surgical procedure to correct farsightedness in which heat is applied to the sclera at points around the cornea to shrink scleral tissue, thus steepening the cornea.

thimerosal (thy-MAYR-uh-sal): Mercuric preservative/ antiseptic used in some topical ophthalmic medications and contact lens care solutions; currently not much in use because of frequent allergic responses.

third cranial nerve (CN III): *Another term for* oculomotor nerve.

third nerve palsy: *Another term for* oculomotor nerve palsy.

three-mirror lens: Type of goniolens; *see also* goniolens.

three step test (3ST): *Another term for* head tilt test.

threshold: In automated visual field testing, the intensity of a target (of given size and presentation) such that there is a 50% likelihood of its being seen at that particular point.

thyroid eye disease: Set of ocular dysfunctions associated with Graves' disease.

tic: A generally brief, repetitive, involuntary, sometimes compulsive contraction of a muscle or group of muscles, usually not painful; may be exacerbated by specific stimuli (eg, stress, fatigue, medication, bright lights, etc); *see also* spasm.

tissue adhesive: *Another term for* bioadhesive.

Titmus test: Specific stereo acuity test; *see* stereo acuity.

tonic pupil: Generally *another term for* Adie's pupil.

tonography (toh-NOG-ruh-fee): A method of determining aqueous outflow by measuring changes in intraocular pressure constantly over a period of time as a weight is applied to the eye.

tonometer (toh-NOM-eh-ter): Instrument that measures intraocular pressure; **air-puff t.** type of noncontact tonometer that uses a pulse of air to measure intraocular pressure; *also called* puff t., noncontact t.; **applanation t. (A, Ap,** or **AT)** tonometer that measures intraocular pressure by quantifying the resistance of the eye to flattening; the tonometer tip flattens the cornea a specific amount and measures the pressure needed to do so; *also called* applanometer; **Goldmann t.** or

Goldmann applanation t. classic applanation tonometer design employing a split prism to create mires that indicate the endpoint of the reading; often attached to the slit lamp; **indentation t.** tonometer that measures intraocular pressure by quantifying the degree to which the eye can be indented by a given weight (eg, the Schiøtz t.); **MacKay-Marg t.** electronic pneumotonometer that measures intraocular pressure using principles of both applanation and indentation; gives a printout of every corneal contact; **noncontact t. (NCT)** *another term for* air-puff t.; **ocular blood flow pneumot. (OBF)** tonometer that measures IOP by analyzing the resistance of blood flow in the optic nerve vessels (in the globe itself versus posterior to the globe) during the systemic pulse; **Perkins t.** hand-held Goldmann tonometer; **pneumotonometer** type of tonometer that uses air pressure resistance in the instrument itself (versus that being applied to the cornea) to measure intraocular pressure; **puff t.** *another term for* air-puff t.; **rebound t.** contact tonometer that does not require topical anesthetic; **Schiøtz t.** a type of indentation tonometer; **Tono-Pen® t.** (Reichert Inc, Depew, NY) brand name of hand-held, portable pneumotonometer that gives an electronic readout of intraocular pressure when placed against the cornea.

tonometry (toh-NOM-eh-tree): The act of measuring intraocular pressure using a tonometer; **digital t.** objective method of approximating intraocular pressure by pressing against the eye with the fingers.

Tono-Pen®: *See* tonometer.

topical: General term meaning on the surface; in ophthalmic usage, generally referring to medications applied directly to the exterior adnexa or globe.

topography (toh-POG-ruh-fee): *See* corneal topography.

toric lens: Spectacle or contact lens having spherical and cylindrical components of curvature, prescribed to correct vision in an eye with astigmatism plus myopia or hyperopia; *see also* aspheric, spherocylindrical lens; *compare* spherical lens.

torsion: Rotational ocular movement along the long axis of the eye.

torticollis (tore-ti-KOL-is): Abnormal head/neck position; *see* ocular torticollis.

toxin: Substance that is poisonous/harmful to body tissues and/or systems.

toxoplasmosis (tox-soh-plaz-MOH-sis): Ocular infection caused by the protozoan *Toxoplasma gondii* and usually causing retinal lesions.

trabecular meshwork (TM) (trah-BEK-yuh-ler): In ophthalmic usage, the porous tissues at the junction of the ciliary body and sclera through which aqueous humor drains from the anterior chamber of the eye; *also called* scleral trabeculae, trabeculum.

trabeculectomy (trah-BEK-yoo-LEK-tuh-mee): General term for a surgical procedure in which tissue is removed from the trabecular meshwork, most often to treat glaucoma by allowing aqueous humor to drain more easily from the eye.

trabeculoplasty (trah-BEK-yoo-loh-plas-tee): General term for surgical procedures (most commonly describing laser surgical procedures such as argon laser trabeculoplasty [ALT]) that attempt to modify the structure of the trabecular meshwork and increase the outflow of aqueous humor in eyes with glaucoma; *see also* laser.

trabeculotomy (trah-BEK-yoo-LAH-tuh-mee): General term for a surgical procedure involving an incision into the trabecular meshwork.

trabeculum (trah-BEK-yoo-lum): *Another term for* trabecular meshwork.

trachoma (trah-KOH-muh): Inflammation of the cornea and conjunctiva caused by infection with *Chlamydia* organisms, leading to severe scarring (especially under the lids) and blindness if not treated; the leading cause of blindness worldwide, especially in third-world countries; **t. inclusion conjunctivitis (TRIC)** reference name given to the intracellular parasite that causes trachoma.

traction retinal detachment: *See* retinal detachment.

traction test: *Another term for* forced duction test.

transient ischemic attack (TIA) (is-KEE-mik): Brief interruption of blood flow to the brain, *also called* ministroke; symptoms last only minutes or up to 24 hours and can include visual disturbances as well as dizziness, numbness, slurred speech, etc.

transillumination: Evaluation of an ocular structure (often the lens and iris) by noting how light passes through it, often using a slit lamp.

transposition: Mathematical manipulation of a glasses or contact lens prescription in order to change from plus cylinder form to minus or vice versa; the procedure is as follows: algebraically add the spherical and cylindrical powers (this becomes the new spherical power), change the sign of the original cylinder (without changing its value), and rotate the axis by 90 degrees (if the original axis is 90 or less, add 90; if the original axis is over 90 degrees, subtract 90).

transpupillary thermotherapy (TTT): Use of a low-energy diode laser to treat lesions in the fundus, especially wet age-related macular degeneration.

Traquair's Island of Vision (TRAH-kwahrz): *See* Island of Traquair.

traumatic cataract: *See* cataract.

trefoil (TREE-foyl): In optics, the higher-order aberration that distorts an image so that there are three areas in the periphery where the focus is too strong alternating with three areas where the focus is too weak; often causes blurring of vision.

trephine (TREE-fyn): Surgical instrument consisting of an open cylinder with a sharp end for cutting a circular incision, typically used in ophthalmic surgery to make an incision around the edge of the cornea so it can be removed; *see also* penetrating keratoplasty.

trial frame: Specially designed, adjustable spectacle frame in which various trial lenses can be placed to measure a refractive error.

trial lens: 1. Loose spectacle lenses used in a trial frame; 2. contact lens used to check the fit before prescribing final lenses.

TRIC: Trachoma inclusion conjunctivitis; *see* trachoma.

trichiasis (tri-KY-uh-sis): Condition in which individual lashes are turned inward toward the globe and irritate ocular surface tissues.

trichomegaly (TRIK-uh-MEG-uh-lee): Abnormal increase in lash length, often associated with the use of certain ocular drugs.

trichotillomania (TRIK-uh-TIHL-oh-MAY-nee-uh): Compulsive pulling out of eyelashes due to an underlying psychiatric condition.

trichromatism (tri-KROH-muh-tiz-uhm): Condition in which all three visual pigments are present and color vision is normal; *see also* chlorolabe, cyanolabe, erythrolabe; *compare* achromatism, dichromatism, monochromatism; **anomalous t.** condition in which all three visual pigments are present but one is deficient, causing a defect in color vision; *see* specific type: deutanomaly, protanomaly, tritanomaly.

trifocal lens: Spectacle lens with three different segments that focus at near, medium, and far distances; *compare* bifocal lens; **executive t.** trifocal style where the segments run the full width of the frame; **invisible/no-line t.** *another term for* progressive addition lens.

trigeminal nerve (tri-JEM-in-ul): Cranial nerve five (CN V), the ophthalmic branch of which in part supplies sensation to the globe, eyelids, face, and forehead.

triplopia (trih-PLOH-pee-uh): Perception of three images where there is only one object; *compare* diplopia; *see also* polyopia.

tritan (TRY-tan): Color vision defect involving the blue color mechanism.

tritanomaly (try-tuh-NAHM-uh-lee): Color vision defect in which the blue pigment is partially deficient, causing blue/green and yellow/green confusion; violets are perceived normally.

tritanopia, -opsia (try-tan-OP-see-uh): Severe or total lack of the blue color mechanism; reds and greens are normal, but yellow-green through purple (including blue) appear white and gray.

trochlea (TROK-lee-uh): Ring of cartilaginous tissue attached to the frontal bone through which the tendon of the superior oblique muscle passes.

trochlear nerve (CN IV) (TROK-lee-ur): The fourth cranial nerve, a motor nerve that supplies the superior oblique muscle.

tropia (TROH-pee-uh): Constant (manifest) misalignment of the eyes in which they fail to fixate on the same object; commonly called crossed eyes; *also called* heterotropia, manifest strabismus; *see also* esotropia, exotropia, strabismus; *compare* phoria; **horizontal t.** tropia in which the eyes deviate in or out (ie, left or right); **vertical t.** tropia in which the eyes deviate up or down.

troposcope (TROH-puh-skohp): *Another term for* amblyoscope.

truncation (trun-KAY-shun): Method of stabilizing toric contact lenses by flattening one edge of the lens (usually the inferior) so that it is no longer round, thereby creating a linear edge that rests against the lid margin; truncation is employed to help prevent rotation and maintain the orientation of toric contact lenses in the proper axis; *compare* dynamic stabilization, posterior toric, prism ballast.

trypan blue (TB): Stain used as a visualization aid during anterior and posterior segment surgery.

Tscherning aberrometry (SHUR-ning ab-uh-RAHM-uh-tree): Aberrometry method in which a pattern of light spots is shone into the eye and photographed; distortions in the pattern indicate any optical aberrations that may be present in the eye.

tumbling "E": *Another term for* "E" test.

tunnel field: Nonphysiologic visual field loss in which the patient's "tunnel vision" does not expand with increased distance, as does true tunnel vision; usually associated with hysteria or malingering.

tunnel vision: True visual field defect in which only a small central portion of the visual field remains functional.

20/20: Considered to be "normal" vision, the numerator stands for the standard 20-foot test distance used in measuring distant visual acuity; the denominator represents the smallest line of test objects accurately identified by the patient from 20 feet away; 20/40 would mean that the patient could identify figures from 20 feet that the "normal" person could identify from 40 feet away (thus, the larger the denominator, the poorer the vision); corresponds to 6/6 vision (a 6-m test distance).

typoscope: Low-vision aid consisting of a rectangle of dark, nonreflective material with a narrow horizontal slit through which type can be read, thereby minimizing glare from the page and isolating the words being read.

U

UGH syndrome: Abbreviation for combination of uveitis, glaucoma, and hyphema; inflammatory condition of internal ocular structures occurring as a complication of intraocular lens implantation.

ulcer: General medical term referring to a localized, depressed lesion on the surface of a tissue; *see* corneal ulcer.

ultrasonography (uhl-truh-suh-NOG-ruh-fee): Imaging internal structures via the use of ultrasound techniques; *also called* echography.

ultrasound: Imaging technique that uses sound waves to produce an image; in ophthalmology, used to measure the axial length of the eye as well as to visualize the eye's inner structures; *see* A-scan, B-scan.

ultraviolet (UV): Portion of the electromagnetic spectrum with short wavelengths, not visible to the human eye; ultraviolet radiation causes sunburn and tanning and has been implicated in certain ocular conditions, notably corneal burns and cataract formation.

ultraviolet A (UVA) and B (UVB): The two bands of ultraviolet radiation.

ultraviolet blocker: Substance incorporated into spectacle, contact, and intraocular lenses to shield the eye from the damaging ultraviolet component of sunlight.

umbilical: In a progressive addition lens, the vertical column in which the lens power changes from distant to near; *see also* progressive addition lens.

uncorrected visual acuity (UCVA, VA$_{sc}$): Visual acuity measured without corrective lenses in place; *compare* corrected visual acuity; *see also* best corrected visual acuity.

uncrossed diplopia: *Another term for* homonymous diplopia.

undercorrection: State in which the power of corrective lenses or the effect of refractive surgery is insufficient to achieve the best visual acuity; *compare* overcorrection (definition 1).

unilateral: General anatomic term describing a structure or process appearing or occurring on only one side; in ophthalmic usage, referring to a single eye; *also called* monocular, uniocular; *compare* bilateral, contralateral, ipsilateral.

uniocular: Occurring unilaterally, only in one eye.

universal precautions: Specific rules and recommendations intended to prevent exposure to disease and/or injury (eg, hand washing, protective wear, handling of contaminated waste, etc).

upside down ptosis: *See* ptosis.

urticaria (ur-ti-KAYR-ee-uh): General medical term for an itchy rash, usually an allergic response.

uvea/uveal tract (YOO-vee-uh): The tissues of the eye that are heavily pigmented and consist primarily of blood vessels: the choroid, ciliary body, and iris (considered as a whole system);.

uveitis (yoo-vee-I-tis): Inflammation of all or part of the uvea; **anterior u.** uveitis involving only the iris (*see* iritis) and/or ciliary body (*see* iridocyclitis); **intermediate/peripheral u.** inflammation of the ciliary body and vitreous; *also called* cyclitis, pars planitis, peripheral uveitis; **phacolytic u.** uveitis resulting from degeneration and leakage of lens tissue; **posterior u.** uveitis involving some part of the posterior uveal structures: the choroid (choroiditis), retina (retinitis), retinal blood vessels (retinal vasculitis), and/or optic nerve (papillitis, optic neuritis); often referred to simply as uveitis, creating confusion as to what is meant.

V pattern: *See* esotropia, exotropia.

Van Lint block: Injection of anesthetic agents to achieve akinesia (ie, prevention of movement) of the eyelids.

vascular: Having or pertaining to blood vessels.

vasculature: The blood vessel system of a particular organ or tissue.

vasovagal reflex or response (vay-zo-VAY-guhl): Fainting or near fainting associated with the vagus nerve; in eyecare, this can occur on instillation of eye drops or contact lenses or during tonometry.

vault: *Another term for* apical clearance (definition 1).

vehicle: In pharmacology, the inert liquid or ointment in which the medication is dissolved or suspended; *see also* emulsion, solution, suspension.

venous phase: Phase of fluorescein angiography (lasts from seconds 13 to 24 after dye injection) where the dye fills the venulae and veins; *see also* fluorescein angiography, laminar flow.

vergence: 1. In optics, the gathering together or spreading apart of parallel light rays, either naturally or as a result of passing through a lens; *see also* convergence, divergence; 2. in ophthalmic usage, motion of the eyes toward or away from one another; *also called* disjunctive movements; *see also* convergence, divergence; *compare* duction.

vericella-zoster virus (VZV) (vayr-eh-SELL-uh ZOS-ter): The herpes virus that causes shingles (zoster) and chickenpox (vericella).

verification: Measuring the parameters of a contact lens, spectacle lens, or pair of spectacles to be sure that the items match what was ordered prior to dispensing to the patient.

vernal conjunctivitis: *See* conjunctivitis.

verruca vulgaris (vuh-ROO-kuh vuhl-GAYR-uhs): An epidermal wart caused by a virus.

version: Coordinated movement of both eyes in the same direction; *also called* conjugate movement.

vertex distance: Distance along the line of sight from the cornea to the back surface of a spectacle lens; *see also* effective power (of a lens).

vertex power: Focusing power of a spectacle lens measured from either of its surfaces; **back v.p.** portion of the total refractive power imparted by the posterior surface of a lens; **front v.p.** portion of the total refractive power imparted by the anterior surface of a lens.

vertical meridian: In ophthalmic use, usually referring to the vertical line dividing the visual field into right and left halves; a field defect that does come to but does not cross the vertical meridian is said to respect the vertical, and indicates a problem at or beyond the chiasm (ie, neurological); *compare* horizontal meridian.

vertigo (VUR-ti-goh): A false sense of spinning or turning.

videokeratography (VID-ee-oh-KAYR-uh-TAHG-ruh-fee): *Another term for* corneal topography.

virus: An intracellular parasite that transfers its own genetic material into the living cells of the host and causes infection (eg, herpes, adenovirus).

viscodissection: Surgical technique in which a viscoelastic substance is injected between tissues (commonly the tissues surrounding the lens nucleus) in order to separate them and facilitate subsequent manipulation; *compare* hydrodissection.

viscoelastic (viz-co-ee-LAS-tic): Any one of a number of thick gels manufactured for use in ophthalmic surgery, injected into the eye to help maintain the shape of ocular structures and as a lubricant/coating to minimize trauma from surgical instruments and implants; currently used viscoelastic materials include chondroitin sulfate, hyaluronic acid, and methylcellulose (used individually or in combination and marketed under several brand names; *see* Appendix 11).

viscous (VIS-cus): Descriptive term for the thickness of a liquid; the more viscous a fluid is, the thicker it is; in ophthalmology, generally referring to drug preparations; *see also* viscoelastic.

visible spectrum: Those electromagnetic energy waves that can be detected by the human eye, generally between 400 to 750 nanometers (red through violet).

vision: Action of the eyes, nervous system, and brain in capturing reflected light from the environment and converting it to perceived images; *see also* specific type of vision (binocular v., distance v., low v., near v., etc), visual acuity.

vision therapy or **training (VT):** Any of several systems employing ocular exercises and/or lenses to enhance development or to correct deficiencies of stereopsis, hand-eye coordination, vision, etc; *see also* orthoptics.

visual acuity (VA): Level of visual clarity; specifically, the ability to distinguish fine details, often expressed as a score on Snellen's, Jaeger's, or other vision test charts; **best corrected v.a. (BCVA)** highest level of visual acuity that can be attained with corrective lenses in place; **corrected v.a. (VA_{cc})** visual acuity measured with current corrective lenses in place; **distant v.a.** acuity for far-off tasks, especially 20 feet or more; **near v.a.** acuity at close range, especially for reading; **uncorrected v.a. (UCVA or VA_{sc})** visual acuity measured without corrective lenses in place; *see also* count finger v., hand-motion v., light perception v., light projection v., no light perception v.

visual acuity test: Method of measuring visual acuity; the test used depends upon the patient (ie, literate, responsive, etc); *see also* specific test (ie, Allen cards, "E" test, Snellen chart, etc).

visual axis: *See* axis.

visual cortex: That part of the brain responsible for vision, primarily an area in the occipital lobe known as Brodmann area 17; *also called* striate cortex.

visual efficiency: A rating based on the loss of central visual acuity and peripheral vision in the better eye of a person who is not legally blind.

visual evoked cortical potential (VECP): *Another term for* visual evoked response.

visual evoked potential (VEP): *Another term for* visual evoked response.

visual evoked response (VER): Fluctuation of brain activity in the visual cortex resulting from a visual stimulus (in a Ganzfeld bowl), measurable on electroencephalography; *also called* visual evoked cortical potential, visual evoked potential; *see also* electrophysiology; **flash VER** indicates the basic soundness of the visual system using a flashing light; **pattern VER** provides information about visual acuity using an alternating checkerboard pattern.

visual field (VF): 1. Area around the fixation point of each eye, generally circular in shape, in which objects are perceived; *also called* field of vision, peripheral vision, side vision; 2. in clinical usage, graphs representing the result of perimetry and other such tests are often simply referred to as visual fields; visual field testing is often conducted to delineate and measure areas of the retina that are damaged (eg, by glaucoma or retinal disorders), as well as to determine any portions of the optic nerve tract that might be compromised; *also called* field; *see also* perimetry.

visual field defect: Area of diminished or absent vision within the visual field; *see also* hemianopia, nerve fiber bundle defect, quadrantanopia, scotoma, tunnel field; **congruous v.f.d.** visual field defects of similar shape in both eyes; **hysterical v.f.d.** apparent area of diminished or absent vision within the visual field that cannot be correlated to ocular damage or disease and, thus, seems to have an emotional basis; the isopters have a "spiral" pattern or a tube pattern that does not expand with distance from the subject.

visual pathway: The route of nerve fibers involved in vision; order is as follows: retina (rods, cones, nerve fiber layer), optic nerve, optic chiasm, optic tract, lateral geniculate body, optic radiations, occipital cortex.

visual purple: *Another term for* rhodopsin.

vitrectomy (vih-TREK-tuh-mee): Surgical procedure involving partial or total removal of vitreous humor and any membranes, blood, or other tissue in the posterior segment; **anterior v.** vitrectomy used to remove vitreous in the anterior segment (generally present as a complication of other ocular surgery); **automated v.** vitrectomy performed using a cutting probe with irrigation and aspiration capabilities; **complete v.** removal of all vitreous from the posterior chamber; *also called* total v.; **manual v.** vitrectomy performed using scissors rather than a vitrector; *also called* scissors v.; **open-sky v.** vitrectomy performed by opening the cornea and removing the lens; **pars plana v.** vitrectomy performed by making small incisions and inserting instruments through the pars plana; **partial v.** removal of only part of the vitreous humor from the posterior chamber; **scissors v.** *another term for* manual v.; **total v.** *another term for* complete v.

vitrector (vih-TREK-ter): Surgical instrument designed for performing vitrectomy, incorporating a cutting probe with irrigation and aspiration capabilities.

vitreitis/vitritis (vih-TRY-tis): *Another term for* hyalitis.

vitreous, vitreous body/humor: Clear, fibrous, gel-like material filling the posterior segment of the eye, located behind the lens capsule and comprising about two-thirds of the total volume of the eye; typically referred to simply as the vitreous.

vitreous detachment: *Another term for* posterior vitreous detachment (PVD).

vitreous face: *Another term for* anterior hyaloid membrane.

vitreous floaters: *Another term for* floaters.

vitreous hemorrhage/bleed: Bleeding into the vitreous gel.

vitreous membrane: *Another term for* hyaloid membrane.

vitreous strands: Vitreous humor in the anterior chamber as strands of viscous, transparent tissue still attached to the hyaloid membrane.

vitreous tap: Diagnostic procedure in which a small amount of vitreous humor is removed for testing, usually to perform a culture to confirm the existence and cause of infection.

von Graefe's sign (vahn GRAY-feez): Delay in or absence of downward motion of the upper eyelid when the eye looks downward, associated with Graves' disease (which involves serious dysfunction of the thyroid gland); *compare* pseudo-von Graefe's sign.

vortex veins: Veins formed by the joining of veins draining blood from the iris, ciliary body, and choroid exiting the eye through the sclera just posterior to the equator of the globe.

wall-eyed: Lay term for exotropia; *see also* cross-eyed.

warm weather conjunctivitis: *Another term for* vernal conjunctivitis, *see entry under* conjunctivitis.

water-drinking test (WDT): Evaluation of the facility of outflow in glaucoma; the patient drinks 1 liter of water, then tonometry is performed at 15 minute intervals for 4 or more readings; a rise in IOP indicates inhibited aqueous outflow; *see also* outflow facility.

wavefront: 1. In optics, a theoretical surface composed of all points that are the same distance from an object emitting or reflecting light; 2. in refractive surgery, usually referring to the "flat" image of a distant object that may be distorted by the optical aberrations of the eye; *see also* aberration.

wavefront analysis: *Another term for* aberrometry.

wavefront analyzer: *Another term for* aberrometer.

wavefront-guided ablation: In refractive surgery, a procedure in which the optical properties of a patient's eye are measured by aberrometry, which is then used to create an excimer laser ablation pattern specifically designed to correct the myopia, hyperopia, astigmatism, or higher-order aberrations of that eye; *see also* customized ablation.

wet macular degeneration: *See* macular degeneration.

wetting angle: Angle between the surface of a drop of water and the surface of the material on which the drop lies; in ophthalmic usage, usually a description of contact lens materials, referring to the spread of moisture on the lens surface; the smaller the wetting angle, the more hydrophilic or "wettable" the material; *also called* contact angle.

white blood cell (WBC): Blood cell type that fights disease; *also called* leukocyte; types of WBCs include basophile, eosinophile, and neutrophile (*see* entries for each of these).

white of the eye: Lay term for sclera.

white-to-white measurement: Diameter of the cornea as measured from the edges of white scleral tissue.

with best correction: Notation that testing was done using lenses (trial lenses, contacts, or glasses) that allowed each eye to see to its fullest potential; *compare* with correction, without correction.

with correction (cc): Notation that testing was done with the patient wearing his or her habitual correction (glasses, contact lenses); *compare* with best correction, without correction.

"with" motion: 1. In retinoscopy, the pupillary reflex is said to be "with" when it moves in the same direction of the intercept reflex; *compare* "against" motion (definition 1), neutrality; 2. in optics, the illusion that an object viewed through a lens moves in the same direction the lens is moved; *compare* "against" motion (definition 2).

with-the-rule (WTR) astigmatism: *See* astigmatism.

without correction (sc): Notation that testing was done with the naked eye, without glasses or contact lenses; *compare* with best correction, with correction.

word blindness: *Another term for* alexia.

working distance: In retinoscopy, the distance of the retinoscope to the patient's eye; this distance must be taken into account when arriving at the refractometric measurement by reducing the amount of plus sphere measured; generally, the working distance is accepted as 66 cm, which is compensated for by reducing the measurement by 1.50 diopters (the power of the retinoscopy lens on the phoropter).

working lens: Plus-powered lens used during retinoscopy to compensate for the distance between examiner and patient; with a working distance of 66 cm, the power of the working lens is +1.50 diopters; the power of the working lens must be subtracted from the final reading in order to obtain the patient's refractive error.

Worth 4-dot or **Worth four-dot test (W4D):** Test of binocular vision or suppression; four illuminated dots (colored white, red, and green) are presented to the patient, who views them through glasses with one red and one green lens.

Wright stain: Dye used to detect and identify immune-related/inflammatory cells under the microscope.

X chromosome: The female sex chromosome; the female genome is XX; *compare* Y chromosome.

X-linked gene: A gene with a locus on the X (female) chromosome; ocular albinism and some types of color blindness are X-linked; *compare* Y-linked gene; *see also* chromosomes (sex c.), sex-linked (gene).

xanthelasma/xanthoma (zan-thuh-LAZ-muh/zan-THOH-muh): Yellowish, raised, benign growth composed of fatty tissue, generally found on the upper lids but sometimes on the lower; may be associated with elevated cholesterol.

xanthopsia (zan-THOP-see-uh): Visual disturbance in which everything appears yellow; *compare* cyanopsia, erythropsia.

xenon photocoagulator (ZEE-nahn): Device that produces intensely bright light, with ophthalmic applications similar to lasers.

xenophthalmia (zen-op-THAL-mee-uh): General term for unhealthy condition of an eye attributable to the presence of a foreign body.

xerophthalmia (zir-op-THAL-mee-uh): Dry eye condition in which the conjunctiva thickens and atrophies and the eye lacks luster.

xerosis (zihr-OH-sis): General term referring to tissue dryness.

Y chromosome: The male sex chromosome; the male genome is XY; *compare* X chromosome.

Y-linked gene: A gene with a locus on the Y (male) chromosome; *see also* chromosomes (sex c.), sex-linked (gene); *compare* X-linked gene.

Y-sutures (of crystalline lens): Tissue structure of the crystalline lens in which the ends of nuclear and cortical fibers join to form a Y shape; the anterior Y is upright and the posterior is inverted.

YAG laser: *See* Nd:YAG laser *under* laser.

yellow spot: *Another term for* the macula, referring to the macula's yellowish hue.

yoke muscles: Two extraocular muscles (one of each eye) that are neurologically paired so that they coordinate motion of both eyes in the same direction; *also called* contralateral synergists; *see also* Hering's law of simultaneous innervation.

Z

Z. terms: *Another term for* Zernike polynomials.

Zeis' glands: Oil-producing glands within the eyelids that empty into eyelash follicles; also spelled Zeiss.

Zeiss lens: *See* goniolens.

Zernike polynomials (ZER-ny-kee pah-lee-NOH-mee-uhlz): Mathematical formulas developed to describe the passage of light through a round opening such as the pupil; used to analyze the complex data gathered in aberrometry and derive measures for defocus, astigmatism, and other optical aberrations (named for Frits Zernike, Dutch mathematician who specialized in optical physics); *also called* Z. terms; *see also* aberration.

zero vergence: Quality of parallel light rays such that they do not converge or diverge.

Zinn: 1. *See* annulus of Zinn; 2. *see* zonules.

zonules or **zonules of Zinn:** Fibers that attach the edge of the lens capsule to the ciliary body; *also called* ciliary zonules.

zonulolysis or **zonulysis (zahn-yoo-loh-LY-sis):** Breakage of the zonules, occurring either naturally (from trauma) or through intentional or unintentional surgical manipulation.

zygomatic bone (zy-goh-MAT-ic): One of the bones of the orbit; commonly called the cheek bone; *also called* malar bone.

LIST OF APPENDICES

Acronyms and Abbreviations*

2°IOL: secondary IOL
2°OAG: secondary open-angle glaucoma
3ST: three step test
5-FU: 5-fluorouracil
Δ: prism, change

A: applanation tonometry
AA: accommodative amplitude
AAO: American Academy of Ophthalmology, American Academy of Optometry
ABES: American Board of Eye Surgeons
ABK: aphakic bullous keratopathy
ABO: American Board of Ophthalmology, American Board of Opticianry
abs: apostilbs
ac: before meals
AC: anterior chamber, accommodative convergence
AC/A: accommodative convergence/accommodation (ratio)
ACCC: anterior continuous curvilinear capsulorrhexis
ACES: American College of Eye Surgeons
ACD: anterior chamber depth
ACG: angle-closure glaucoma
ACIOL: anterior chamber intraocular lens implant

*Note: Not all abbreviations are accepted or approved by all offices, institutions, agencies, publications, etc. Please check your clinic's guidelines for abbreviation usage. In addition, the same abbreviation can have multiple meanings, so be cautious in using them.

ACL: anterior chamber (intraocular) lens (implant)

ACO: anterior capsular opacification

ACR: anterior curve

ACS: American College of Surgeons, Automated Corneal Shaper (Bausch & Lomb, Claremont, CA)

ADR: adverse drug reaction

AF: autofluorescence

AG: Amsler grid

AI: accommodative insufficiency

AIDS: acquired immunodeficiency syndrome

AION: anterior ischemic optic neuropathy

AK: astigmatic keratotomy, actinic keratosis, arcuate keratotomy, automated (lamellar) keratoplasty

AKC: atopic keratoconjunctivitis

ALK: automated lamellar keratoplasty

ALPI: argon laser peripheral iridoplasty

ALT: argon laser trabeculoplasty

AMA: American Medical Association

AMD: age-related macular degeneration

AMO: Allergan Medical Optics (company name)

ANSI: American National Standards Institute

AOA: American Optometric Association

AOZ: anterior optical zone

AOZD: anterior optic zone diameter

Ap: applanation tonometry

APCT: alternate prism and cover test

APD: afferent pupillary defect (Marcus Gunn pupil)

Ar: argon laser

AR: autorefraction

ARC: abnormal or anomalous retinal correspondence

ARE: acute red eye

AREDS: Age-Related Eye Disease Study

ArF: argon fluoride excimer (laser)

ArFl: argon fluoride excimer (laser)

ARM: age-related maculopathy

ARMD: age-related macular degeneration

ARP: Argyll Robertson pupil

ARVO: Association for Research in Vision and Ophthalmology

asb: apostilb

ASC: anterior subcapsular cataract

ASCRS: American Society of Cataract and Refractive Surgery

ASICO: American Surgical Instrument Company

ASR: artificial silicon retina

astig: astigmatism

AT: applanation tonometry, artificial tears

ATPO: Association of Technical Personnel in Ophthalmology

ATR: against-the-rule (astigmatism)

AUPO: Association of University Professors in Ophthalmology

a/v, A-V, A/V: arteriovenous

B9: benign

BAK: benzalkonium chloride (preservative)

BAT: Brightness Acuity Tester™ (Marco, Jacksonville, FL)

BC: base curve

BCC: basal cell carcinoma

BCVA: best corrected visual acuity

BD: base down (prism)

BDR: background diabetic retinopathy

BI: base in (prism)

bid: twice daily

BIOM: binocular indirect ophthalmic microscope

BLL: brow, lids, lashes

BM: basement membrane

BO: base out (prism)

BRA: branch retinal artery

BRAO: branch retinal artery occlusion

BRB: blood-retinal barrier

BRV: branch retinal vein

BRVO: branch retinal vein occlusion

BSCVA: best spectacle-corrected visual acuity
BSD: back surface debris
BSS: balanced salt solution
BTX: botulinum toxin
BU: base up (prism)
BUT: break-up time (tear test)
BUVA: best uncorrected visual acuity
BVP: back vertex power
BYVEP: blue-on-yellow visual evoked potential

C3F8: perfluoropropane
c: with
C/F: cell/flare
CA: carcinoma, cancer
CAB: cellulose acetate butyrate (contact lens material)
CAC: central anterior curve
CACG: chronic angle-closure glaucoma
CACT: computer-assisted corneal topography
CAI: carbonic anhydrase inhibitor
caps: capsule
CAT: computerized tomography (CT scan)
CC: corneal curvature
CCT: central corneal thickness
cd: candela
c/d: cup-to-disc ratio
CD: cylindrical dandruff
CDI: color Doppler imaging
CE: cataract extraction, complete exam
CE/IOL: cataract extraction with intraocular lens implant
c/f: cell/flare
CF: count fingers, cystic fibrosis
CI: convergence insufficiency
CIC: conjunctival impression cytology
CK: conductive keratoplasty
CL: contact lens
CLAO: Contact Lens Association of Ophthalmologists
CLE: clear lens extraction

CLEK: Collaborative Longitudinal Evaluation of Keratoconus (study)

clr: clear

cm: centimeter

CM: cutaneous melanoma

CME: cystoid macular edema

CMR: cellophane macular reflex

CMS: Centers for Medicare and Medicaid Services (U.S.)

CMV: cytomegalovirus

CN: cranial nerve

CN II: second cranial nerve (optic nerve)

CN III: third cranial nerve (oculomotor nerve)

CN IV: fourth cranial nerve (trochlear nerve)

CN V: fifth cranial nerve (trigeminal nerve)

CN VI: sixth cranial nerve (abducens nerve)

CN VII: seventh cranial nerve (facial nerve)

CNS: central nervous system

CNV: choroidal neovascularization

CO: certified orthoptist, corneal opacity

CO_2: carbon dioxide

COA®: certified ophthalmic assistant (registered trademark of the Joint Commission on Allied Health Personnel in Ophthalmology [JCAHPO])

COAG: chronic open-angle glaucoma

coll/collyr: eyewash

COMT®: certified ophthalmic medical technologist (registered trademark of JCAHPO)

conj: conjunctiva, conjunctivitis

COT®: certified ophthalmic technician (registered trademark of JCAHPO)

CPC: central posterior curve

CPO: certified paraoptometric

CPOA: certified paraoptometric assistant

CPOT: certified paraoptometric technician

CPT®: Current Procedural Terminology (registered trademark of the American Medical Association)

CRA: central retinal artery

CRAO: central retinal artery occlusion
CRNO: certified registered nurse in ophthalmology
CRP: corneal reflection pupillometer
CRT: corneal refractive therapy
CRV: central retinal vein
CRVO: central retinal vein occlusion
CSC: central serous chorioretinopathy
CSF: contrast sensitivity function
CSR: central serous retinopathy
CST: contrast sensitivity test
CT: center thickness (contact lens), computed tomography (CAT scan)
CTL: contact lens(es)
CTR: capsular tension ring
c/w: consistent with
CWS: cotton-wool spots
cyl: cylinder

d: day, disc
D: diopter(s), distance, diameter, diffusion coefficient
D&C: deep and clear
D&Q: deep and quiet
dB: decibel
DBC: distance between centers
DBL: distance between lenses
DC: dermatochalasis, discharge, discontinue, diopters (of) cylinder
DCR: dacryocystorhinostomy
dd: disc diameter
Deq: spherical equivalent
DES: dry eye syndrome, disc edges sharp
Dk: oxygen permeability
Dk/L: oxygen permeability/lens thickness (oxygen transmissibility)
DLEK: deep lamellar endothelial keratoplasty
DLK: diffuse lamellar keratitis
DLKP: deep lamellar keratoplasty

DM: diabetes mellitus
DME: diabetic macular edema, diffuse macular edema
D/N: distance and near
DNA: deoxyribonucleic acid
DO: Doctor of Osteopathy
DR: diabetic retinopathy
DS: diopter(s) sphere
DVD: dissociated vertical deviation
DW: daily wear (contact lens)

E: esophoria, eccentricity
E': esophoria at near
ECs: endothelial cells
ECCE: extracapsular cataract extraction
ECD: endothelial cell density
ECF: edematous corneal formations
ED: epithelial defect, effective diameter
EDPRG: Eye Diseases Prevalence Research Group
EDTA: ethylenediaminetetraacetate (preservative)
EEG: electroencephalography
EH: essential hypertension
EIC: epithelial iris cyst
EKC: epidemic keratoconjunctivitis
EL: eye length
ELK: endothelial lamellar keratoplasty
EOG: electro-oculogram
EOM: extraocular muscle(s)
ERG: electroretinogram
ERM: epiretinal membrane
Er:YAG: erbium:yttrium-aluminum-garnet (laser)
ET: esotropia, edge thickness (contact lenses)
ET': esotropia at near
E(T): intermittent esotropia
ETDRS: Early Treatment Diabetic Retinopathy Study
ETOH: ethanol
EUA: exam under anesthesia
EW: extended wear (contact lens)

excimer: excited dimer laser

F: focal length, focal distance
F&F: fix and follow
FA: fluorescein angiogram/angiography
FAAO: Fellow of the American Academy of Ophthalmology, Fellow of the American Academy of Optometry
FACS: Fellow of the American College of Surgeons
FAF: fundus autofluorescence (imaging)
FAP: flatter add plus (contact lens fitting)
FAZ: foveal avascular zone
FB: foreign body
FDA: Food and Drug Administration
FDP: frequency doubling perimetry
FDT: frequency-doubling technique (perimetry)
FED: Fuchs' endothelial dystrophy
FMTM: fast macular thickness map
FRCP: Fellow of the Royal College of Physicians (of England)
FRCPA: Fellow of the Royal College of Physicians (of Australia)
FRCPC: Fellow of the Royal College of Physicians (of Canada)
FRCS: Fellow of the Royal College of Surgeons (of England)
FRCSA: Fellow of the Royal College of Surgeons (of Australia)
FRCSC: Fellow of the Royal College of Surgeons (of Canada)
FTC: full to confrontation
FVP: front vertex power

GAT: Goldmann applanation tonometer
GCD: geometric center distance
GCM: good, central, maintained
GCNM: good, central, not maintained

GD: Graves' disease

GFE: gas-fluid exchange

GO: Graves' ophthalmopathy

GON: glaucomatous optic neuropathy

GP: gas permeable (contact lens)

GPC: giant papillary conjunctivitis

GPCL: gas permeable contact lens

gt: drop

gtt: drops

GVHD: graft-versus-host disease

h: hour

HE: hard exudate

HEMA: hydroxyethylmethacrylate (contact lens material)

HeNe: helium-neon (laser)

Hg: mercury

HIPAA: Health Insurance Portability and Accountability Act

HIV: human immunodeficiency virus

HM: hand motion

HOAs: higher-order aberrations

HOTV: H, O, T, and V letter test for visual acuity

HRC: high risk characteristics, harmonious retinal correspondence

HRR: Hardy-Rand-Rittler (American Optical color vision plates)

HRT: Heidelberg Retina Tomograph

hRVE: human retinal vascular endothelial (cells)

hs: at bedtime

HSK: herpes simplex keratitis

HSV: herpes simplex virus

HSV-2: herpes simplex virus-2

HTG: high-tension glaucoma

HVF: Humphrey visual field (Humphrey Instruments, San Leandro, CA)

i: one
ii: two
iii: three
I&R: insertion and removal (contact lens)
IA, I/A, I&A: irrigation and aspiration
IBI: interblink interval
ICCE: intracapsular cataract extraction
ICD: International Code of Diseases
ICE: iridocorneal endothelial syndrome
ICG: indocyanine green
ICL: implantable contact lens
ICP: intracranial pressure
ICR: intrastromal corneal ring, intermediate curve (contact lens)
IDDM: insulin-dependent diabetes mellitus
IFIS: intraoperative floppy iris syndrome
Ig: immunoglobulin
IK: interstitial keratitis
ILM: internal limiting membrane
INV: iris neovascularization
IO: inferior oblique
IOFB: intraocular foreign body
IOL: intraocular lens (implant)
ION: ischemic optic neuropathy
IOP: intraocular pressure
IPD: interpupillary distance
IR: inferior rectus, index of refraction
ISRS: International Society of Refractive Surgery
IVCM: in vivo confocal microscopy

J: Jaeger (acuity)
JCAHPO®: Joint Commission on Allied Health Personnel in Ophthalmology (registered trademark of JCAHPO)
JIA: juvenile idiopathic arthritis
JND: just noticeable difference
JRA: juvenile rheumatoid arthritis

k: oxygen solubility (contact lens)
K: cornea, keratometry, keratometric value
KC: keratoconus
KCS: keratoconjunctivitis sicca
KP: keratic precipitate
KPE: Kelman phacoemulsification
Kr: krypton (laser)

L: center thickness (contact lens)
LARP: laser reversal of presbyopia
LARS: left add/right subtract
LASEK: laser epithelial keratomileusis
Laser: light amplification by stimulated emission of radiation
LASIK: laser-assisted in-situ keratomileusis
LCVA: low-contrast visual acuity
LE: left eye
LEC: lens epithelial cells
LGV: lymphogranuloma venereum
LHT: left hypertropia
LIO: left inferior oblique, laser indirect ophthalmoscope
LK: lamellar keratoplasty
LKP: lamellar keratoplasty
LLL: left lower lid
LP: light perception
LP w/proj: LP with projection
LP w/o proj: LP without projection
LR: lateral rectus
LRP: laser reversal of presbyopia
LTG: low tension glaucoma
LTK: laser thermal keratoplasty
LUL: left upper lid
LV: low vision
LVS: low vision specialist
LXT: left exotropia

m: meter

MA: macroaneurysm, manifest astigmatism

MD: macular degeneration, medical doctor, mean defect (visual fields)

MDF: map-dot-fingerprint (corneal dystrophy)

ME: macular edema

MERG: macular electroretinogram

mfERG: multifocal electroretinogram

mfVEP: multifocal visual evoked potential

MG: Marcus Gunn pupil, myasthenia gravis

mm: millimeter

mm Hg: millimeters of mercury

Motcc: motility with correction

Motsc: motility without correction

MPT: macular photostress test

MR: manifest refraction, medial rectus

MR-DCG: magnetic resonance dacryocystography

MRI: magnetic resonance imaging

MS: multiple sclerosis

MTF: modulation transfer function

MVL: moderate visual loss

N: near

NaFl: sodium fluorescein

NAG: narrow-angle glaucoma

NCCA: noncontact corneal aesthesiometer

NCLE: National Contact Lens Examiners

NCT: noncontact tonometry/tonometer

NDA: New Drug Application

Nd:YAG: neodymium:yttrium-aluminum-garnet (laser)

NEI: National Eye Institute

NEI-VFQ: National Eye Institute Visual Function Questionnaire

neo: neovascularization

NFL: nerve fiber layer

NIDDM: noninsulin-dependent diabetes mellitus

NIH: National Institutes of Health

NLD: nasolacrimal duct
NLP: no light perception
nm: nanometer
NPA: near point of accommodation
NPC: near point of convergence
NPDR: nonproliferative diabetic retinopathy
npo: nothing by mouth
NRC: normal retinal correspondence
NS: nuclear sclerosis
NSAID: nonsteroidal anti-inflammatory drug
NSPB: National Society for the Prevention of Blindness
NTG: normal tension glaucoma
NVA: near visual acuity
NVG: neovascular glaucoma

OA: overaction (as in muscles), ophthalmic artery, optometric assistant, ophthalmic assistant
OAG: open-angle glaucoma
OBFT: ocular blood flow pneumotonometer
OC: optical center
OCP: ocular cicatricial pemphigoid
OCT: optical coherence tomographer, optical coherence tomography
OD: oculus dexter (right eye), doctor of optometry
ODM: ophthalmodynamometry
OEP: Optometric Extension Program
OHS: ocular histoplasmosis syndrome
OHT: ocular hypertension
OKN: optokinetic nystagmus
OLCR: optical low coherence reflectometer
OM: ocular melanoma
OMP: ophthalmic medical personnel
ON: optic nerve, optic neuritis, optic neuropathy
ONH: optic nerve hypoplasia, optic nerve head
OOSS: Outpatient Ophthalmic Surgery Society
OPP: ocular perfusion pressure
ORT: ocular radiotherapy

ortho-K: orthokeratology
OS: oculus sinister (left eye)
OSHA: Occupational Safety and Health Administration
OT: ophthalmic technician, optometric technician
OTC: over-the-counter (medications)
OU: oculus uterque (both eyes together)
OWS: overwear syndrome (contact lenses)
OZ: optical zone
OZD: optic zone diameter
OZR: optic zone radius

P: periphery, pupil(s)
P&I: probe and irrigate
PACT: prism and alternate cover test
PAL: progressive addition lens
PAM: Potential Acuity Meter™ (Marco, Jacksonville, FL)
PARK: photorefractive astigmatic keratectomy
PAS: peripheral anterior synechia
PBK: pseudophakic bullous keratopathy
pc: after meals
PC: posterior capsule, posterior chamber
PCCC: posterior continuous curvilinear capsulorrhexis
PCIOL: posterior chamber intraocular lens (implant)
PCL: posterior chamber (intraocular) lens (implant)
PCO: posterior capsule opacification
PCR: posterior curve
PD: prism diopters, pupillary distance
PDR: proliferative diabetic retinopathy
PDS: pigment dispersion syndrome
PDT: photodynamic therapy
PE: pigment epithelium
PEA: pre-existing astigmatism
PEE: punctate epithelial erosions
PEGS: phacoemulsification and goniosynechialysis
PERG: pattern electroretinogram
PERRLA: pupils equally round and reactive to light and
    accommodation

PFTA: preservative-free triamcinolone acetonide
PGAs: prostaglandin analogues
PGON: progressive optic neuropathy
pH: refers to the acidic or basic property of a substance
PH: pinhole
phaco: phacoemulsification
PHR: personal health record
PI: peripheral iridotomy, peripheral iridectomy
PIOL: phakic IOL
PION: posterior ischemic optic neuropathy
PK: penetrating keratoplasty
PKP: penetrating keratoplasty
pl: plano
PLT: preferred looking technique
PM: pathologic myopia
PMC: peripheral multifocal chorioretinitis
PMF: preretinal macular fibrosis
PMMA: polymethylmethacrylate
PMN: polymorphonucleocyte
PNT: pneumatic trabeculoplasty
po: by mouth
POAG: primary open-angle glaucoma
POBF: pulsatile ocular blood flow
POHS: presumed ocular histoplasmosis syndrome
POZD: posterior optic zone diameter
PPL: progressive power lens
PPV: pars plana vitrectomy
PRK: photorefractive keratectomy
PRL: preferred retinal locus
prn: as needed
PRP: panretinal photocoagulation
PRT: phenol red test
PS: posterior synechia
PSC: posterior subcapsular cataract
PSF: point spread function
PTK: phototherapeutic keratectomy
PVD: posterior vitreous detachment

PVR: proliferative vitreoretinopathy
q: every
q2h: every 2 hours
qd: every day
qh: every hour
qid: 4 times a day
QOL: quality of life
qs: as much as needed

R&R: recess and resect
RA: rheumatoid arthritis
RAP: retinal angiomatous proliferation
RAPD: relative afferent pupillary defect
RBC: red blood cell(s)
RD: retinal detachment
RE: right eye
RGC: retinal ganglion cell
RGP: rigid gas permeable (contact lens)
RHT: right hypertropia
RK: radial keratotomy
RLE: refractive lens exchange
RLF: retrolental fibroplasia (now ROP)
RLL: right lower lid
RNFL: retinal nerve fiber layer
ROP: retinopathy of prematurity (previously RLF)
RP: retinitis pigmentosa
RPE: retinal pigment epithelium
RPH: retroilluminated pinhole
rpm: revolutions per minute
RRD: rhegmatogenous retinal detachment
RTA: retinal thickness analyzer
RUL: right upper lid
Rx: prescribe

s or **sine:** without
SAC: seasonal allergic conjunctivitis
SAM: steeper add minus

SAP: standard automated perimetry
SARS: severe acute respiratory syndrome
SB: scleral buckle
SBUT: symptomatic (tear film) break-up time
SCH: subconjunctival hemorrhage
SCL: soft contact lens
SCO: spherocylindrical over-refraction
SCR: secondary curve
SE: soft exudates, side effects, spherical equivalent
SEBR: spontaneous eye blink rate
SEI: subepithelial infiltrates
SER: spherical equivalent refraction
SF6: sulfur hexafluoride
SIA: surgically induced astigmatism
sig: instructions
SIRC: surgically induced refractive change
SJS: Stevens-Johnson syndrome
SLE: slit lamp exam, systemic lupus erythematosus
SLK: superior limbic keratoconjunctivitis
SLT: selective laser trabeculoplasty
SMD: senile macular degeneration
SO: superior oblique, sympathetic ophthalmia
sol: solution
SPAC: scanning peripheral anterior chamber depth analyzer
sph: sphere/spherical
SPK: superficial punctate keratitis
SR: superior rectus
SRNV: subretinal neovascularization
SRP: surgical reversal of presbyopia
SS: Sjögren's syndrome
SSP: scleral spacing procedure
ST: straight top (bifocal/trifocal)
STCS: spatiotemporal contrast sensitivity (test)
STDR: sight-threatening diabetic retinopathy
susp: suspension
SVL: severe visual loss

SVP: spontaneous venous pulsations
SWAP: short wavelength automated perimetry

T: tonometry, tropia
tab: tablet
TASS: toxic anterior segment syndrome
TB: tuberculosis, trypan blue (dye)
TBUT: tear (film) break-up time
TCF: transciliary filtration
TCS: temporal contrast sensitivity (test)
TIA: transient ischemic attack
tid: 3 times daily
TK: thermokeratoplasty
TM: trabecular meshwork
TMH: tear meniscus height
TON: traumatic optic neuropathy
Tp: Tono-Pen® (Reichert, Inc, Depew, NY)
TRIC: trachoma inclusion conjunctivitis
TTT: transpupillary thermotherapy

UA: underaction (as in muscles)
UBM: ultrasound biomicroscopy
UCVA: uncorrected visual acuity
UFOV: useful field of vision
UGH: uveitis, glaucoma, hyphema (syndrome)
ung: ointment
ut dict: as directed
UV: ultraviolet light
UVA: ultraviolet band A
UVB: ultraviolet band B

V: vision (visual acuity), versions
VA: visual acuity
VAcc: visual acuity with correction
VAsc: visual acuity without correction
VCDR: vertical cup-to-disc ratio
VECP: visual evoked cortical potential

VEP: visual evoked potential
VER: visual evoked response
VF: visual field(s), vitreous floater
VFA: visual field abnormalities
VFD: visual field defect
VFL: visual field loss
VH: vitreous hemorrhage
VKC: vernal keratoconjunctivitis
VOD: vision right eye
VOS: vision left eye
VOU: vision both eyes
VT: vision therapy, vision training
VZV: Varicella-Zoster virus

w/u: work-up
W4D: Worth 4-Dot test
WDT: water drinking test
WHO: World Health Organization
WNL: within normal limits
WTR: with-the-rule (astigmatism)

X: exophoria
X′: exophoria at near
XFS: exfoliation syndrome
X(T): intermittent exotropia
XT: exotropia
XT′: exotropia at near

YAG: yttrium-aluminum-garnet (laser)

Medical Terminology

The good news about medical terminology is that you do not have to memorize hundreds of words. Medical terms are formed using a system… so if you know the system, you do not have to memorize a lot of words. The basis for most of these terms is Greek or Latin, but a good number of them are already in your everyday vocabulary. Many medical and anatomical terms are made up of combined words. It is just like combining English words.

All words are built around a root word, with the root word acting as the foundation (eg, ogle, yawn, destiny). Some words are made up of two root words; these are called compound words (eg, sometimes, applesauce, joystick).

We also use prefixes (ie, the word part that comes before a word [eg, pre-, un-]) and suffixes (ie, the word part that comes after a word [eg, -er, -ed, -ing]) with root words both in daily conversation and medical terminology.

A root word may be joined with a combining form to make a compound word. In medical terminology, the combining form is usually a vowel. You already know how to do this, whether you realize it or not. Take the word thermometer. Therm/o, using the combining form (o), refers to the temperature. The suffix –meter means a device used to measure.

Medical words are generally built from a root word, a combining form, and an ending of some sort. If you know the meaning of the root word and the prefix or suffix, you can pretty much figure out any medical or scientific term.

Compound words using combining forms are built. Suppose you needed a word that meant skimming over the surface of the water. Hydr/o for water, -plane for surface = hydroplane. What if you were afraid of water? Hydrophobia. Suppose you saw the word photophobia and did not know what it meant. You see –phobia and you know that it means an unnatural fear of something. What does phot/o make you think of? Maybe photograph, but this is not a fear of photographs... it is a fear of light. Now that you know that phot/o means light, you could figure out photopsia. It has something to do with light... -opsia refers to vision. So literally, it is a vision of light. Fancy name for light flashes and other such sparkles!

Let us play with this a minute. The suffix –itis means inflammation. Tonsillitis, gingivitis, cystitis. How many eye-related inflammatory words can you think of? Blepharitis, conjunctivitis, scleritis, episcleritis, uveitis, and iritis are just a few. They are inflammations of the lids, conjunctiva, sclera, episclera, uvea, and iris, respectively.

Below are some combining forms, prefixes, and suffixes useful in eye care.

Word Parts Related to Ocular Anatomy

blephar/o	lids
bulb/a	globe, eyeball
cili/o	eyelash
corne/o	cornea
cycl/o	ciliary body
dacry/o	tear
dermat/o	skin
ir/i	iris
kerat/o	cornea
lacrim/a	tear
ophthalm/o	eye
phak/o	lens

retin/o	retina
scler/o	sclera
tars/o	tarsal plate
trich	hair (lash)
uve-	uvea

WORD PARTS RELATED TO VISION, EYES, ETC

ambl/y	dim, dull
astigmat	without a point
dipl/o	double
hyper/o	above, over, excessive
ocul/o	eye
-opia	vision
-opsia	vision
-opsis	vision
opt/o, optic/o	vision
phot/o	light
presby/o	"old man" (ie, associated with age-related loss)

WORD PARTS RELATED TO SURGERY

cente-	puncture
-cise	cut
cry/o	cold
-ectomy	excise or remove a part
-orrhaphy	suturing or stitching
-ostomy	form an opening
-otomy	incise or cut into a part
-plasty	surgical repair of
therm/o	heat

OTHER USEFUL WORD PARTS

a-, an-	without
ab-	away from
ad-	toward

angi/o	blood vessel
anis/o	without equality, unequal
anti-	against
aut/o	self
carcin/o	cancer
cyst/o	bladder; any sac containing fluid
-duct	lead, conduct
dys-	bad, improper, malfunction, difficult
e-	out from
-emia	blood
end/o	within
epi-	upon, after, in addition
es/o	inside
ex/o	out, outside
extra-	outside of, beyond
gram/o	record, write
graph/o	instrument used to make a record
-graphy	actual making of a record
hemat/o	blood
hemi	half
heter/o	different
hom/o	same, common
hydr/o	pertaining to water
hyper-	over, above, beyond, up
hypo-	under, below, down
-iasis	condition, pathological state
-ism	condition with a specific cause
is/o	equal
-itis	inflammation
-lysis	disintegration
macr/o	larger than normal
mal-	bad, abnormal
megal/o	great, large
-meter	measure

micr/o	smaller than normal
mon/o	only, sole, single
morph	shape, form
mot-	move
mult/i	many
my/o	muscle
nas/o	nose
ne/o	new, young
neur/o	nerves
-oma	tumor
orth/o	straight
-osis	condition, disease
path/o, -pathy	disease
phob/o, -phobia	abnormal fear of
phor-	motion, carrying
-plegia	paralysis
pseud/o	false
ptosis	prolapse, downward displacement
punct-	pierce, prick, dot, spot
quadr-	four
schis-	split
-spasm	twitch
-scope	instrument for examining
-scopy	examining with a scope
spectr-	appearance, what is seen
sym-, syn-	with, together
therm-	heat
ton/o-	tone, pressure
tors-	twist
trop-	turn
uni-	one
vers-	turn
vert-	turn

WORD PARTS RELATED TO COLORS

alb-	white
chrom/o	color
cyan/o	blue
erythr/o	red
leuk/o	white
melan/o	black
xanth/o	yellow

PREFIXES RELATED TO LOCATION, TIME, ETC

ab-	away from
endo-	within, inner
infra-	below
pan-	entire, all
peri-	around
post-	after
pre-	before
retro-	behind
sub-	under, below
supra-	above

Atlas of Ocular Anatomy Drawings

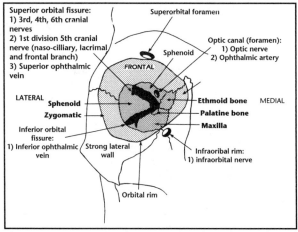

Figure A3-1. Bones and openings in the orbit. (Adapted from Nemeth SC, Shea CA. *Medical Sciences for the Ophthalmic Assistant.* Thorofare, NJ: SLACK Incorporated; 1988.)

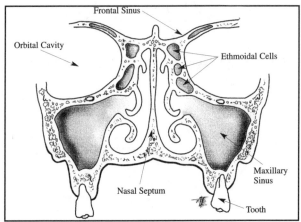

Figure A3-2. Relation of orbital cavity to sinuses. (Drawing by Ana Edwards. Reprinted with permission from Lens A, Coyne Nemeth S, Ledford JK. *Ocular Anatomy and Physiology, Second Edition.* Thorofare NJ: SLACK Incorporated; 2008.)

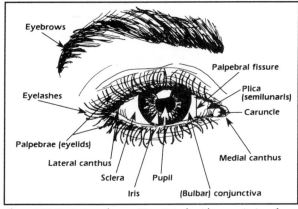

Figure A3-3. External eye. (Reprinted with permission from Nemeth SC, Shea CA. *Medical Sciences for the Ophthalmic Assistant.* Thorofare, NJ: SLACK Incorporated; 1988.)

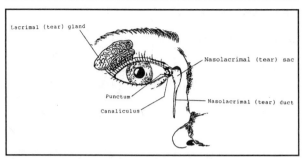

Figure A3-4. The nasolacrimal system. (Drawing by Holly Smith. Reprinted with permission from Gayton JL, Ledford, JR. *The Crystal Clear Guide to Sight for Life*. Lancaster, PA: Starburst Publishers; 1996.)

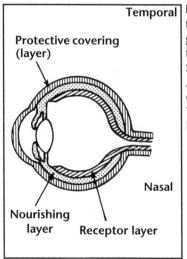

Figure A3-5. The three layers of the globe. (Adapted from Nemeth SC, Shea CA. *Medical Sciences for the Ophthalmic Assistant*. Thorofare, NJ: SLACK Incorporated; 1988.)

Figure A3-6. Segments and chambers of the globe. (Reprinted with permission from Nemeth SC, Shea CA. *Medical Sciences for the Ophthalmic Assistant*. Thorofare, NJ: SLACK Incorporated; 1988.)

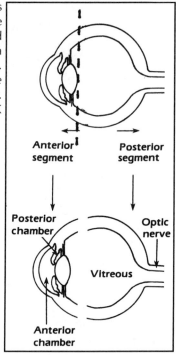

Anterior segment

Posterior segment

Posterior chamber

Optic nerve

Vitreous

Anterior chamber

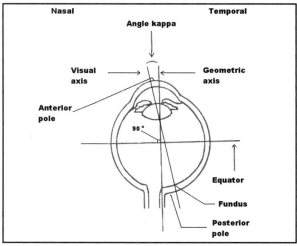

Figure A3-7. Ocular landmarks. (Reprinted with permission from Lens A, Nemeth SC, Ledford JK. *Ocular Anatomy and Physiology, Second Edition*. Thorofare, NJ: SLACK Incorporated; 2008.)

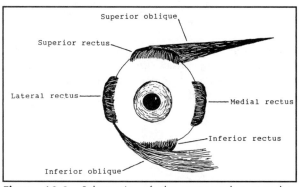

Figure A3-8. Schematic of the extraocular muscles. (Drawing by Holly Smith. Reprinted with permission from Gayton JL, Ledford JR. *The Crystal Clear Guide to Sight for Life*. Lancaster, PA: Starburst Publishers; 1996.)

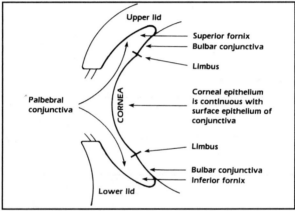

Figure A3-9. Cross-section of conjunctival topography. (Reprinted with permission from Nemeth SC, Shea CA. *Medical Sciences for the Ophthalmic Assistant.* Thorofare, NJ: SLACK Incorporated; 1988.)

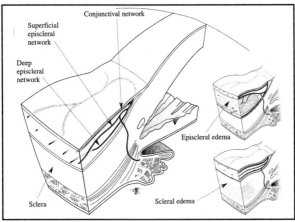

Figure A3-10. Section showing conjunctiva, episclera, and sclera. (Drawing by Ana Edwards. Reprinted with permission from Lens A, Coyne Nemeth S, Ledford JK. *Ocular Anatomy and Physiology, Second Edition.* Thorofare NJ: SLACK Incorporated; 2008.)

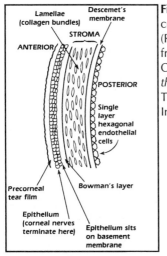

Figure A3-11. Histological cross-section of the cornea. (Reprinted with permission from Nemeth SC, Shea CA. *Medical Sciences for the Ophthalmic Assistant.* Thorofare, NJ: SLACK Incorporated; 1988.)

Figure A3-12. Optic section of the cornea as it appears under the slit lamp. (Adapted from Nemeth SC, Shea CA. *Medical Sciences for the Ophthalmic Assistant.* Thorofare, NJ: SLACK Incorporated; 1988.)

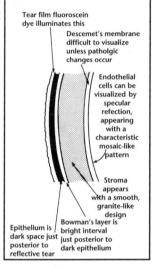

Tear film fluoroscein dye illuminates this

Descemet's membrane difficult to visualize unless patholgic changes occur

Endothelial cells can be visualized by specular refection, appearing with a characteristic mosaic-like pattern

Stroma appears with a smooth, granite-like design

Epithelium is dark space just posterior to reflective tear

Bowman's layer is bright interval just posterior to dark epithelium

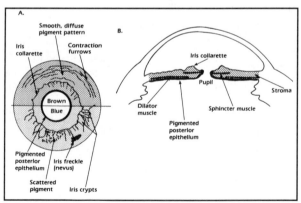

Figure A3-13. (A) External view of blue and brown irides. (B) Cross-section of iris anatomy. (Reprinted with permission from Nemeth SC, Shea CA. *Medical Sciences for the Ophthalmic Assistant.* Thorofare, NJ: SLACK Incorporated; 1988.)

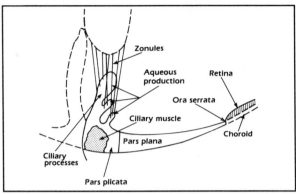

Figure A3-14. Ciliary body and related structures. (Adapted from Nemeth SC, Shea CA. *Medical Sciences for the Ophthalmic Assistant.* Thorofare, NJ: SLACK Incorporated; 1988.)

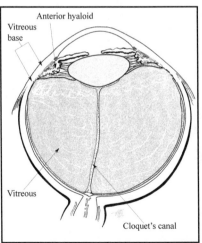

Figure A3-15. Vitreous and related structures. (Drawing by Ana Edwards. Reprinted with permission from Lens A, Langley T, Coyne Nemeth S, Shea C. *Ocular Anatomy and Physiology.* Thorofare NJ: SLACK Incorporated; 1999.)

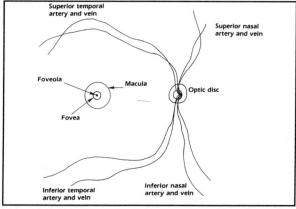

Figure A3-16. Schematic of the macula and its relationship to the posterior pole. (Adapted from Nemeth SC, Shea CA. *Medical Sciences for the Ophthalmic Assistant.* Thorofare, NJ: SLACK Incorporated; 1988.)

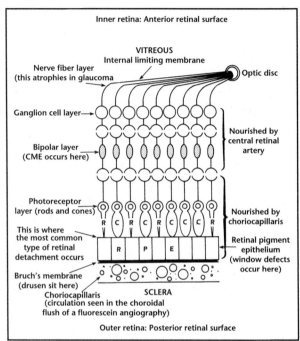

Figure A3-17. Schematic of retinal anatomy. CME = cystoid macular edema. (Adapted from Nemeth SC, Shea CA. *Medical Sciences for the Ophthalmic Assistant.* Thorofare, NJ: SLACK Incorporated; 1988.)

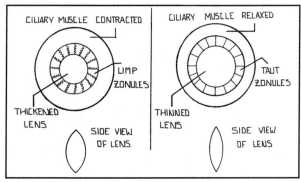

Figure A3-18. The lens and ciliary muscle in (A) accommodation and (B) relaxation. (Drawing by Holly Smith. Reprinted with permission from Ledford JK. *Exercises in Refractometry*. Thorofare, NJ: SLACK Incorporated; 1990.)

The Schematic Eye

STRUCTURE	NOTES
Cornea	IR = 1.376 Radius of central anterior surface = 7.7 mm Radius of posterior surface = 6.8 mm Refractive power of anterior surface = +48.83 D Refractive power of posterior surface = –5.88 D Total refractive power = +42.95 D Central thickness = 0.5 mm
Pupil	"Ideal" size = 2 mm to 5 mm
Aqueous	IR = 1.336
Lens	IR of cortex = 1.386 IR of nucleus = 1.406 Overall IR = 1.42 Anterior radius of curvature (unaccommodated) = 10.00 mm Anterior radius of curvature (fully accommodated) = 5.33 mm Posterior radius of curvature (unaccommodated) = 6.0 mm Posterior radius of curvature (fully accommodated) = 5.3 mm Refractive power (unaccommodated) = +19 D

IR = index of refraction; D = diopters; K = cornea

Lens (continued)	Refractive power (fully accommodated) = +33.06 D
	Thickness of nucleus = 2.419 mm
	Overall thickness = 3.6 mm

| Vitreous | IR = 1.336 |

Axial length	Overall eye length = 24.4 mm
	Distance from anterior K to anterior lens surface = 3.6 mm
	Distance from anterior K to posterior lens surface = 7.2 mm
	Distance from posterior lens surface to retina = 17.2 mm

IR = index of refraction; D = diopters; K = cornea

Reprinted with permission from Ledford J. *Certified Ophthalmic Medical Technologist Exam Review Manual*. Thorofare, NJ: SLACK Incorporated; 1997.

The Cranial Nerves

CRANIAL NERVE	NAME	MOTOR/ SENSORY	FUNCTION
I	Olfactory	Sensory	Smell
II	Optic	Sensory	Sight
III	Oculomotor	Motor	Movement of eye (MR, SR, IR, and IO), pupil constriction, accommodation, and upper lid elevation
IV	Trochlear	Motor	Movement of eye (SO)

MR = medial rectus muscle; SR = superior rectus muscle; IR = inferior rectus muscle; IO = inferior oblique muscle; SO= superior oblique muscle; LR = lateral rectus muscle

CRANIAL NERVE	NAME	MOTOR/ SENSORY	FUNCTION
V	Trigeminal	Mixed	Sensation of touch in face, nose, forehead, temple, tongue, and eye; innervation for chewing
VI	Abducens	Motor	Movement of eye (LR)
VII	Facial	Mixed	Reflex tearing, facial expression, some taste, and blinking
VIII	Vestibulocochlear (acoustic nerve)	Sensory	Hearing and equilibrium
IX	Glossopharyngeal	Mixed	Taste and swallowing

MR = medial rectus muscle; SR = superior rectus muscle; IR = inferior rectus muscle; IO = inferior oblique muscle; SO= superior oblique muscle; LR = lateral rectus muscle

CRANIAL NERVE	NAME	MOTOR/ SENSORY	FUNCTION
X	Vagus	Mixed	Taste, heart rate, breathing, digestion, and voice
XI	Spinal accessory	Motor	Innervation of neck and shoulder muscles, provides posture and rotation of head
XII	Hypoglossal	Motor	Tongue movement

Reprinted with permission from Lens A, Nemeth SC, Ledford JK. *Ocular Anatomy and Physiology, Second Edition.* Thorofare, NJ: SLACK Incorporated; 2008.

Classifications of Nystagmus

I. Normal physiologic
    A. Endpoint
    B. Induced
        1. Drugs
        2. Optokinetic
        3. Caloric
        4. Rotational
II. Congenital
    A. Motor (idiopathic)
    B. Sensory (sensory vision)
    C. Latent
III. Acquired
    A. Convergence retraction
    B. Cerebellar
        1. Opsoclonus
        2. Flutter
        3. Dysmetria
    C. Gaze—paretic
    D. Vestibular
        1. Rotary
        2. Horizontal
        3. Vertical
    E. Spasmus nutans
    F. Muscle—paretic
    G. See-saw
    H. Periodic alternating

Adapted from Cassin B, ed. *Fundamentals for Ophthalmic Technical Personnel.* Philadelphia, PA: WB Saunders; 1995.

Red Eye Differential Diagnosis

	CONJUNCTIVITIS	IRITIS	ACUTE ANGLE-CLOSURE GLAUCOMA	KERATITIS, CORNEAL FOREIGN BODY
Vision	Normal to blurring that clears with blinking	Mild blurring	Considerable blurring or haziness; halos around lights	Mild blurring
Pain	None to minor discomfort, burning, or grittiness	Moderate to aching	Severe aching	Sharp pain or foreign body sensation

	CONJUNCTIVITIS	IRITIS	ACUTE ANGLE-CLOSURE GLAUCOMA	KERATITIS, CORNEAL FOREIGN BODY
Discharge	Dependent on type: Mucopurulent—bacterial Watery—viral Watery/stringy—allergic	None	None	None to mild
Pattern of redness	Palpebral conjunctival and/or diffuse conjunctival	Conjunctival circumcorneal pattern	Diffuse conjunctival with prominent circumcorneal pattern	Conjunctival circumcorneal pattern
Pupil	Normal, reactive	Constricted—may be slightly reactive	Dilated, fixed	Normal to constricted, reactive

	CONJUNCTIVITIS	IRITIS	ACUTE ANGLE-CLOSURE GLAUCOMA	KERATITIS, CORNEAL FOREIGN BODY
Cornea	Clear	Clear to slightly hazy	Hazy	Possible visible FB, opacification, abnormal light reflex, fluorescein staining
IOP	Normal	Normal to low	High	Normal
Other		Photophobia	Possible nausea and vomiting	Possible photophobia

IOP = intraocular pressure; FB = foreign body

Reprinted with permission from Hargis-Greenshields L, Sims L. *Emergencies in Eyecare*. Thorofare, NJ: SLACK Incorporated; 1999.

The
Subjective Grading System

An important, but confusing, part of documenting abnormalities is the subjective grading system. Even the term *subjective* causes confusion because such grading occurs during the objective examination. Some clarification seems to be in order.

First, many of the patient's symptoms are subjective. These are symptoms that the patient tells us about but we cannot see, such as pain. Other findings are objective. That is, they do not involve the patient's ability to report them. We can see them ourselves when we examine the patient. Cell and flare in the anterior chamber is an objective finding; the patient did not (and cannot) tell us about it, but we can see it. Other findings fall into both realms. The patient may say, "My right eye is red," which is subjective. We can also see the injection through the slit lamp (whether the patient has reported it or not), which is objective. The slit lamp exam is an objective test.

Grading pathology and other findings, although they are discovered during the objective examination, are subjective on the part of the examiner. By subjective we mean that the assignment of a rating to a finding is dependent on the observer's opinion. You may look at the patient and grade her lid edema as 2+. Another clinician may rate the same finding (same patient, same day, and same time) as 1+ or 3+. The best we can advise you is that if you are auxiliary personnel, try to learn the grading system of your employer. As you examine more and more eyes, you will get a feel for how marked a finding is. If you are a physician, do your best to teach your grading philosophy to your staff.

With that said, we would like to offer our own opinion about how to grade your findings. Some prefer a numbered grading system. If you use this, then 0+ means that a finding is absent. 1+ would indicate that a finding is just barely perceptible. 4+ would refer to a full-blown case. Using this schematic, 2+ and 3+ would fall somewhere in between. Interjecting half steps, such as 2.5+, sometimes complicates this system. We will leave it up to you as to whether this practice is truly necessary or not.

Instead of numbers, specific terms can be used, including "none, absent, bare trace, trace, slight, moderate, marked, severe," and other such words. This is even more subjective than the numbering system. If everyone uses a scale of 0 to 4, then we have a better chance of understanding what 2+ means. Who is to say what the difference really is between "bare trace" and "trace"? (Alas, perhaps it is that nebulous 0.5 half-step!) The dilemma of subjective grading is not likely to be resolved.

GRADING INJECTION

Features	*Grade*
No injection present	0
Slight limbal (mild segmented), bulbar (mild regional), and/or palpebral injection	1
Mild limbal (mild circumcorneal), bulbar (mild diffuse), and/or palpebral injection	2
Significant limbal (marked segmented), bulbar (marked regional or diffuse), or palpebral injection	3

GRADING INJECTION (CONTINUED)

Features	Grade
Severe limbal (marked circumcorneal), bulbar (diffuse episcleral or scleral), or palpebral injection	4

Adapted from FDA document Premarket Notification Guidance Document for Daily Wear Contact Lenses. Reprinted with permission from Ledford JK, Sanders VN. *The Slit Lamp Primer, Second Edition.* Thorofare, NJ: SLACK Incorporated; 2006.

GRADING CORNEAL HAZE

Features	Grade
Clear	0
Between clear and trace; barely perceptible	0.5+
Trace; easily seen with slit lamp	1+
Mild haze	2+
Moderate haze, very pronounced, iris details still visible, anterior chamber (AC) reaction not visible	3+
Marked haze, scarring, iris details obscured	4+

Adapted from Stein HA, Cheskes AT, Stein RM. *The Excimer: Fundamentals & Clinical Use.* Thorofare, NJ: SLACK Incorporated; 1995.

GRADING CORNEAL VASCULARIZATION

Features	Grade
No vascular changes	0
Congestion and dilation of the limbal vessels; single vessel extension <1.5 mm	1
Extension of multiple vessels <1.5 mm	2
Extension of multiple limbal vessels 1.5 to 2.5 mm	3
Segmented or circumscribed extension of limbal vessels >2.5 mm or to within 3.0 mm of corneal apex	4

Adapted from FDA document Premarket Notification Guidance Document for Daily Wear Contact Lenses. Reprinted with permission from Ledford JK, Sanders VN. *The Slit Lamp Primer, Second Edition*. Thorofare, NJ: SLACK Incorporated; 2006.

GRADING CORNEAL STAINING

Features	Grade
No staining	0
Minimal superficial staining or stippling	1
Regional or diffuse punctate staining	2
Significant dense coalesced staining, corneal abrasion, or foreign body tracks	3

GRADING CORNEAL STAINING (CONTINUED)

Features	Grade
Severe abrasions >2 mm diameter, ulcerations, epithelial loss, or full-thickness abrasion	4

Adapted from FDA document Premarket Notification Guidance Document for Daily Wear Contact Lenses. Reprinted with permission from Ledford JK, Sanders VN. *The Slit Lamp Primer, Second Edition.* Thorofare, NJ: SLACK Incorporated; 2006.

GRADING ANGLES

Features	Grade
Closed angle	0
Angle extremely narrow, probable closure	1+
Angle moderately narrow, possible closure	2+
Angle moderately open, closure not possible	3+
Angle wide open, closure not possible	4+

Reprinted with permission from Ledford JK, Sanders VN. *The Slit Lamp Primer Second Edition.* Thorofare, NJ: SLACK Incorporated; 2006.

Grading Cell (1-mm Conical Beam)

Cell #	Grade
1 to 10	Trace
10 to 20	1+
20 to 30	2+
30 to 40	3+
40 up to hypopyon	4+

Reprinted with permission from Ledford JK, Sanders VN. *The Slit Lamp Primer, Second Edition.* Thorofare, NJ: SLACK Incorporated; 2006.

Grading Cortical Cataracts

Features	Grade
Gray lines, dots, and flakes aligned along the cortical fibers in periphery; visible in oblique direct illumination	1+ (early or incipient
Opaque spokes, anterior chamber may be shallower than normal for patient	2+ (immature or intumescent)
Cortex opaque up to capsule, anterior chamber may be normal depth	3+ (mature)

GRADING CORTICAL CATARACTS (CONTINUED)

Features	*Grade*
Lens is smaller, wrinkly capsule, nucleus may float in liquefied cortex	4+ (hyper-mature)

Reprinted with permission from Ledford JK, Sanders VN. *The Slit Lamp Primer, Second Edition.* Thorofare, NJ: SLACK Incorporated; 2006.

GRADING NUCLEAR SCLEROTIC CATARACTS

Lens Color	*Grade*
Gray-blue (normal)	0
Yellow overtone	1+
Light amber	2+
Reddish brown	3+
Brown or black, opaque; no fundus reflection	4+

Reprinted with permission from Ledford JK, Sanders VN. *The Slit Lamp Primer, Second Edition.* Thorofare, NJ: SLACK Incorporated; 2006.

GRADING POSTERIOR SUBCAPSULAR CATARACTS

Features	Grade
Optical irregularity on posterior capsule; visible only on retroillumination	1+
Small, white fleck	2+ (early)
Enlarged plaque; round or irregular borders	3+ (moderate)
Opaque plaque	4+ (advanced)

Reprinted with permission from Ledford JK, Sanders VN. *The Slit Lamp Primer, Second Edition.* Thorofare, NJ: SLACK Incorporated; 2006.

Slit Lamp Findings for Systemic Diseases and Conditions

Some of these findings are admittedly rare.

Conjunctivitis *can include conjunctival redness, conjunctival edema, excessive tearing, and matter/discharge.*

See also notes on medications used to treat ocular conditions (Appendix 13).

For other complications of systemic disorders, see Appendix 10.

abuse (physical): Lid bruises and swelling, lid burns, subconjunctival hemorrhage (may be numerous and tiny), corneal abrasion, hyphema, traumatic cataract, lens subluxation.

acne: *See* rosacea.

acquired immunodeficiency syndrome (AIDS): Exophthalmos; conjunctivitis (recurrent infections); dry eye; Kaposi's sarcoma (reddish-blue vascular nodules) of lids, palpebral conjunctiva, or orbit.

albinism: Nystagmus, white brows and lashes, reddish iris.

alcoholism: Ptosis, nystagmus, iris paralysis.

allergies: Conjunctivitis, congestion of conjunctival blood vessels, dry eye (secondary to medication), iritis (seasonal).

anemia: Subconjunctival hemorrhage.

ankylosing spondylitis: Iritis.

arteriosclerosis: Arcus senilis.

asthma: Conjunctivitis, cataract (secondary to corticosteroid treatment).

Bell's palsy: Incomplete or absent lid closure, exposure keratitis.

breast cancer: Metastatic lesion to angle, metastatic lesion to iris, other metastatic lesions (visible mass, redness), symptoms of metastatic lesions (exophthalmos, hyphema).

cancer: *See* breast cancer, colon cancer, leukemia, lung cancer, and melanoma.

Candida albicans **(yeast):** Swelling of lacrimal gland, lid "thrush," conjunctivitis, stringy mucus, keratitis, pseudomembranes.

carotid artery disease: Dilation of conjunctival blood vessels, iritis.

chickenpox (varicella): Vesicles on lid, conjunctivitis, abnormal pupil, superficial punctate keratitis, iritis.

chlamydia: Lid swelling, conjunctival injection, conjunctivitis, conjunctival pseudomembranes, keratitis, corneal vascularization.

colon cancer: Metastatic lesions (visible mass, redness), symptoms of metastatic lesions (exophthalmos, hyphema).

craniofacial syndromes: Exophthalmos, nystagmus, exposure keratitis, coloboma.

diabetes: Xanthelasma, corneal wrinkles, rubeosis of iris, loss of iris pigment, cataract, asteroid hyalosis.

Down syndrome: Nystagmus, epicanthal folds, keratoconus, iris spots, Brushfield's spots (gray or white spots around the edge of the iris), cataract.

eczema: Lid crusting, scaling, and oozing (blepharitis); conjunctivitis; conjunctival thickening; congestion of conjunctival blood vessels; dry eyes; keratoconus; cataract.

emphysema: Cataract (secondary to corticosteroid treatment).

endocarditis: Nystagmus, tiny red dots on conjunctiva, anisocoria, iritis.

facial deformity syndromes: Microphthalmos, downsloping lid slant, nystagmus, lower lid coloboma, dermoid cysts of the globe, cataract.

German measles (rubella; congenital defects following maternal infection): Microphthalmos, nystagmus, corneal edema, corneal clouding, iris atrophy, aniridia, cataract.

German measles (acute postnatal cases): Follicular conjunctivitis.

gonorrhea (neonatorum): Edema of orbit, lid edema, congestion of conjunctival blood vessels, conjunctival chemosis, purulent conjunctivitis, conjunctival pseudomembranes, keratitis, corneal perforation, iritis.

gout: Episcleritis, scleritis, corneal crystals, iritis.

hay fever: Conjunctivitis, congestion of conjunctival blood vessels, dry eye (secondary to medication), iritis (seasonal).

Herpes simplex (congenital defects following maternal infection): Cataract.

Herpes simplex (acute postnatal cases): Lid lesions, follicular conjunctivitis, limbal dendrites, corneal dendrites, corneal edema.

Herpes zoster: *See* shingles.

histoplasmosis: Conjunctivitis.

hypercholesterolemia: Arcus senilis, xanthelasma.

hypervitaminosis: Exophthalmos, calcium deposits in conjunctiva, band keratopathy, cataract.

influenza: Keratitis.

leprosy: Lash loss (brows and lids), paralysis of lid, thickened corneal nerves, corneal pannus, corneal scarring, corneal perforation, keratitis, iritis, iris nodules, cataract.

leukemia: Exophthalmos, metastatic lesions (visible mass, redness), symptoms of metastatic lesions (exophthalmos, hyphema).

lung cancer: Metastatic lesion to angle, metastatic lesion to iris, other metastatic lesions (visible mass, redness), symptoms of metastatic lesions (exophthalmos, hyphema).

lupus: Roundish lesions on lids, congestion of conjunctival blood vessels, episcleritis, keratitis, iridocyclitis.

malaria: Conjunctivitis, keratitis, iritis.

malnutrition: Lid edema, conjunctival chemosis, dry eye, keratopathy.

Marfan syndrome: Nystagmus, blue sclera, off-center pupil, multiple pupils, pupillary membrane, subluxed lens.

measles (rubeola): Koplik's spots (tiny white grain surrounded by a red round area) on caruncle or conjunctiva, catarrhal conjunctivitis (inflammation with discharge), keratitis, iritis.

melanoma: Metastatic lesions (visible mass, redness), symptoms of metastatic lesions (exophthalmos, hyphema).

menopause: Increased wrinkling of skin, ectropion, entropion, ptosis, dermatochalasis, dry eye.

mononucleosis: Swelling (indicating infection of the lacrimal gland), lid edema, conjunctivitis.

multiple sclerosis: Nystagmus, ptosis, anisocoria.

mumps: Swelling (indicating infection of the lacrimal gland), conjunctivitis, episcleritis, scleritis, unilateral keratitis, stromal keratitis and vascularization (interstitial keratitis), iritis.

muscular dystrophy disorders: Ptosis, dry eye, cataract.

myasthenia gravis: Ptosis, abnormal pupil.

neurofibromatosis (von Recklinghausen's disease): Exophthalmos, thickened lid margins, lid neurofibroma, cafe-au-lait marks on lids, ptosis, limbal neurofibroma, prominent corneal nerves, iris nodules.

occlusive vascular disorder (progressive): Dilation of conjunctival vessels, iritis.

parathyroid (overactive): Calcification of conjunctiva, corneal opacities (calcium deposits), band keratopathy.

parathyroid (underactive): Blepharospasm, conjunctivitis, keratitis, cataract.

Parkinson's disease: Eyelid tremors, diminished blinking.

peptic ulcer disease: Iritis.

psoriasis: Scaling lid skin, blepharitis, exfoliated scales in conjunctival sac, conjunctivitis, corneal infiltrates, corneal erosion, corneal vascularization.

rheumatoid arthritis: Conjunctivitis, dry eye, episcleritis, scleritis, scleral thinning, keratitis sicca, band keratopathy, corneal melting, iritis, cataract.

rosacea: Blepharitis, conjunctivitis, multiple chalazia, keratitis, corneal ulcers, corneal infiltrates, corneal pannus, iritis.

rubeola: *See* measles.

rubella: *See* German measles.

sarcoidosis: Swelling of lacrimal gland, sarcoid lid nodule, episcleral nodule, keratic precipitates, corneal edema, iritis.

scleroderma: Scarring of lid margin, keratitis, corneal ulceration, cataract.

shingles (Herpes zoster): Vesicles on lid, ptosis, lid edema, lid redness, incomplete lid closure, scleritis, keratitis, exposure keratitis, corneal edema, infiltrates, iritis.

sickle cell disease: Comma-shaped conjunctival vessels.

sinus problems: Conjunctivitis, congestion of conjunctival blood vessels, dry eye (secondary to medication), iritis (seasonal).

smallpox (variola): Lid lesions, trichiasis, symblepharon (lid adheres to the globe), conjunctivitis, severe keratitis, leukoma (white corneal opacity), iritis, patchy iris atrophy, vitreous opacity.

smoking: Dry eye, cataract.

temporal (cranial) arteritis: Iritis.

temporal (giant cell) arteritis: Ptosis, iritis.

third nerve palsy (oculomotor nerve palsy): Ptosis, anisocoria.

thyroid (overactive): Exophthalmos, orbital puffiness, lid retraction, lid lag, incomplete lid closure, exposure keratitis, keratoconjunctivitis of superior limbus.

thyroid (underactive): Periorbital edema, loss of outer third of brows, lid edema, mild cortical lens opacities.

toxoplasmosis (congenital and acquired): Conjunctivitis, leukocoria ("white pupil"), vitreous haze.

tuberculosis: Scleritis, phlyctenular keratoconjunctivitis (tiny red pustules on conjunctiva and/or cornea).

vaccinia: Lid infection, cellulitis, lid vesicles, blepharitis, conjunctivitis, keratitis, corneal perforation, vitreous opacity.

varicella: *See* chickenpox.

variola: *See* smallpox.

vitamin A deficiency: Foamy patches on bulbar conjunctiva, conjunctival dryness, corneal dryness, corneal haze, corneal perforation.

vitamin B deficiency: Conjunctival dryness, corneal dryness.

vitamin C deficiency: Subconjunctival hemorrhage.

Systemic Disorders and Their Effects on the Eye*

DISORDER	OCULAR COMPLICATIONS
I. Cardiovascular	
A. Atherosclerosis/ carotid artery disease	Retinal artery obstruction
B. Endocarditis	Conjunctival and retinal hemorrhage (Roth's spot) Infection Artery occlusion
C. Hypertension	Narrowing, twisting, and fibrosis of retinal blood vessels Retinal hemorrhage Papilledema Cotton-wool spots
D. Mitral valve prolapse	Retinal vessel occlusion
II. Endocrine	
A. Diabetes	Leaking and rupturing of retinal blood vessels Neovascularization of retinal vessels Iris rubeosis Retinal detachment

* See also Appendix 9

DISORDER	OCULAR COMPLICATIONS
A. Diabetes (cont)	Macular edema
	Increased incidence of glaucoma and cataract
B. Graves' disease	Inflammation of extraocular muscles (EOMs)
	Corneal exposure
	Compression of optic nerve
C. Hypothyroid	Partial loss of eyebrows and eyelashes
	Keratoconus
	Cataracts
	Optic atrophy
D. Pituitary tumor	Visual field loss
	Optic atrophy
	Nerve palsy

III. Infections

A. AIDS	Swelling of retinal vessels
	Cotton-wool patches
	Kaposi's sarcoma of lids, conjunctiva, or orbit
B. Chlamydia	Trachoma (redness; corneal neovascularization; trichiasis; scarring of lids, conjunctiva, and cornea)
C. Herpes simplex	Corneal opacity
D. Influenza	Conjunctivitis
	Dacryoadenitis

DISORDER	**OCULAR COMPLICATIONS**
E. Lyme disease	Conjunctivitis Periorbital edema Corneal infiltrates Uveitis Endophthalmitis
F. Measles (rubeola)	Conjunctivitis Subconjunctival hemorrhage Superficial keratitis
G. Shingles (Herpes zoster)	Corneal and lid lesions Inflammation of conjunctiva, sclera, and uvea
H. Syphilis	Eyelid chancre Argyll Robertson pupil Swelling of optic disc Optic atrophy EOM weakness
I. Toxoplasmosis	Chorioretinitis
J. Tuberculosis	Ocular tubercles

IV. Connective tissue disease

A. Lupus	Scleritis Damage to lacrimal gland Optic neuritis Cotton-wool spots
B. Multiple sclerosis	Optic neuritis Paralysis of EOMs Nystagmus

DISORDER	**OCULAR COMPLICATIONS**
C. Rheumatoid arthritis	Keratoconjunctivitis sicca Scleritis Episcleritis Uveitis (in juveniles)
D. Temporal arteritis	Ischemic optic neuritis Weakness of EOMs

V. Muscle disorders

A. Muscular dystrophy	Weakness of EOMs (causing diplopia) Weakness of levator muscle (causing ptosis)
B. Myasthenia gravis	Weakness of EOMs Ptosis

VI. Blood dyscrasias

A. Anemia	Pale conjunctiva Retinal hemorrhage Cotton-wool spots and hard exudates
B. Leukemia	Optic nerve compression Elevated intraocular pressure (IOP)
C. Sickle cell disease	Neovascularization Vitreous hemorrhage Retinal detachment Elevated IOP

VII. Age-related disorders

A. Elderly	Cataract Macular degeneration

DISORDER	**OCULAR COMPLICATIONS**
A. Elderly (cont)	Dry eye Increased incidence of glaucoma Increased incidence of infection Presbyopia (first noticed around age 40) Loss of skin and muscle tone (entropion, ectropion, dermatochalasis, EOM dysfunction, ptosis)
B. Prematurity	O_2 damage to retina Impeded development of retinal blood vessels Retinal detachment Retinal scarring

VIII. Environmental disorders

A. Alcoholism	Visual field defects Nerve palsies Optic atrophy Alcohol amblyopia Decreased color vision Cataracts
B. Child abuse	Retinal and vitreal hemorrhage Periorbital bruising and swelling Subconjunctival hemorrhage Orbital fractures Hyphema Dislocated lens Retinal detachment

Disorder	**Ocular Complications**
C. Malnutrition	Night blindness Retinopathy Corneal ulceration/necrosis
D. Smoking	Chronic conjunctivitis Increased risk of nuclear sclerosis Increased risk of macular degeneration Increased optic nerve damage in glaucoma Nystagmus Optic neuropathy
IX. Genetic disorders	
A. Albinism	Blue-gray to pink iris Nystagmus Decreased visual acuity Strabismus Photophobia
B. Down syndrome	Short, slanted palpebral fissures Epicanthal folds Strabismus Nystagmus Myopia Cataracts Keratoconus Brushfield's spots
X. Neoplastic disorders	
A. Cancer	Ocular metastasis (iris most common)

DISORDER	**OCULAR COMPLICATIONS**
B. Non-Hodgkin's lymphoma	Proptosis Conjunctival growths Diplopia Lacrimal gland infiltration

XI. Other disorders/conditions

A. Chronic obstructive pulmonary disease	Dilation of retinal vessels Retinal hemorrhage Darkening of blood vessels (conjunctiva and retina)
B. Gout	Conjunctivitis Episcleritis Scleritis Elevated IOP Uric acid crystals (cornea or sclera)
C. Pregnancy	Minor refractive shifts Difficulty with accommodation Drop in IOP Mild ptosis Hyperpigmentation of lids
D. Sarcoidosis	Bilateral anterior uveitis Granulomas Optic neuritis Optic atrophy

Ophthalmic Drugs

Note: See numbered lists starting on p. 361 for further information. The following is a list of brand name drugs available in the United States. (Note: A few are offered as generic only; these are labeled.) Please consult each drug's literature for further information. Mention of specific products is not intended as an endorsement by the author or publisher. A few medications are listed twice; this is because the ingredients vary from the drop to the ointment form. While it is impossible to list every ophthalmic medication on the market and medications may be discontinued or recalled, we have done our best to ensure that these tables are accurate. Viscoelastics and irrigating solutions are not listed in a separate table.

BRAND NAME	USE(S)	LIST NUMBER
5-FU	Glaucoma surgery (inhibits scarring)	1
Acular	Nonsteroidal anti-inflammatory	3
Acular LS	Nonsteroidal anti-inflammatory	3
Acular PF	Nonpreserved nonsteroidal anti-inflammatory	3
Adrucil	Glaucoma surgery (inhibits scarring)	1

Brand Name	Use(s)	List Number
Advanced Eye Relief All Clear AR	Decongestant	7
Advanced Eye Relief	Nonpreserved artificial lubricant	2
Advanced Eye Relief Environmental	Preserved artificial lubricant	2
Advanced Eye Relief PF	Nonpreserved artificial lubricant	2
Advanced Eye Relief Night Time	Nonpreserved artificial lubricant	2
Advanced Eye Relief Rejuvenation	Preserved artificial lubricant	2
Advanced Eye Wash	Irrigating solution (extraocular)	
Akarpine	Glaucoma	4
AK-Beta	Glaucoma	4
AK-Cide	Steroidal anti-inflammatory/antibacterial	6
AK-Con	Decongestant	7
AK-Con-A	Decongestant/antihistamine	7, 8
AK-Dex	Steroidal anti-inflammatory	3
AK-Dilate	Mydriasis	1
AK-Fluor	Dye study of fundus/iris	1
AK-NACL	Corneal edema	1
AK-Pentolate	Cycloplegia	1
AK-Poly-Bac	Antibiotic	5
AK-Pred	Steroidal anti-inflammatory	3

Brand Name	Use(s)	List Number
AK-Pro	Glaucoma	4
AK-Rinse	Irrigating solution (extraocular)	
AK-Spore	Antibiotic	5
AK-Spore HC	Steroidal anti-inflammatory/antibiotic	6
AK-T-Caine	Anesthetic	1
AK-Taine	Anesthetic	1
AK-Tob	Antibiotic	5
AK-Trol	Steroidal anti-inflammatory/antibiotic	6
AKWA Tears	Preserved artificial lubricant (drop)	2
AKWA Tears	Nonpreserved artificial lubricant (ointment)	2
Alamast	Mast cell stabilizer	8
Alaway	Antihistamine	8
Albalon	Decongestant	7
Alcaine	Anesthetic	1
All Clear Redness Reliever	Decongestant/lubricant	7
Allersol	Decongestant	7
Alocril	Mast cell stabilizer	8
Alomide	Mast cell stabilizer	8
Alphagan-P	Glaucoma	4

Brand Name	Use(s)	List Number
Alrex	Steroidal anti-inflammatory	3
Amvisc	Viscoelastic	
Amvisc Plus	Viscoelastic	
AquaSite	Preserved artificial lubricant	2
Aquify	Preserved artificial lubricant	2
Atropine Care	Cycloplegia	1
Atrosulf	Cycloplegia	1
Avastin	Wet ARMD	1
Azopt	Glaucoma	4
Betagan	Glaucoma	4
Betimol	Glaucoma	4
Betoptic	Glaucoma	4
Betoptic-S	Glaucoma	4
BioGlo	Corneal dye	1
BioLon	Viscoelastic	
Bion Tears	Nonpreserved artificial lubricant	2
Bleph-10	Antibacterial	5

ARMD = age-related macular degeneration

Brand Name	Use(s)	List Number
Bleph-30	Antibacterial	5
Blephamide	Steroidal anti-inflammatory/antibacterial	6
Blephamide SOP	Steroidal anti-inflammatory/antibacterial	6
Blinx	Irrigating solution (extraocular)	1
Blueron	Surgical aid/stain	1
Botox	Inhibits muscle response	1
Botox Cosmetic	Inhibits muscle response	1
Carbastat	Glaucoma	4
Carboptic	Glaucoma	4
Cardio-green	Angiographic study	1
Cetamide	Antibacterial	5
Ciloxin	Antibiotic	5
Clarif-Eye	Decongestant	7
Clarine	Decongestant	7
Clear Eyes	Preserved artificial lubricant	2
Clear Eyes ACR	Decongestant/astringent	7
Clear Eyes Redness Relief	Decongestant/lubricant	7
Clear Eyes Seasonal Relief	Decongestant/astringent	7
Clear View	Decongestant	7

Brand Name	Use(s)	List Number
Collyrium Fresh Eyes	Irrigating solution (extraocular)	6
Cortisporin	Steroidal anti-inflammatory/antibiotic	4
Cosopt	Glaucoma	8
Crolom	Mast cell stabilizer	1
Cyclogyl	Cycloplegia	1
Cyclomydril	Cycloplegia/mydriasis	1
Cylate	Cycloplegia	1
Dendrid	Antiviral	5
Dexacine	Steroidal anti-inflammatory/antibiotic	6
Dexasporin	Steroidal anti-inflammatory/antibiotic	6
Diamox	Glaucoma	4
DisCoVisc	Viscoelastic	
Duovisc	Viscoelastic	
Econopred Plus	Steroidal anti-inflammatory	3
Eflone	Steroidal anti-inflammatory	3
Elestat	Antihistamine	8
Emadine	Antihistamine	8
Endogel	Viscoelastic	
Enlon	Diagnosis of myasthenia gravis	1
Epifrin	Glaucoma	4

Brand Name	Use(s)	List Number
E-Pilo	Glaucoma	4
Epinal	Glaucoma	4
Eye-Sine	Decongestant	7
Eye Stream	Irrigating solution (extraocular)	
Eyevisc	Viscoelastic	
Eyevisc Plus	Viscoelastic	
Eye Wash Solution	Irrigating solution (extraocular)	
Flarex	Steroidal anti-inflammatory	3
Fluor-I-Strips	Corneal dye	1
Fluor-op	Steroidal anti-inflammatory	3
Fluoracaine	Anesthetic/stain	1
Fluorescite	Dye study of fundus/iris	1
FluoreStrips	Corneal dye	1
Fluorets	Corneal dye	1
Fluress	Anesthetic/stain	1
FML	Steroidal anti-inflammatory	3
FML Forte	Steroidal anti-inflammatory	3
FML-S	Steroidal anti-inflammatory/antibacterial	6
FML SOP	Steroidal anti-inflammatory	3

Brand Name	Use(s)	List Number
Ful-Glo	Corneal dye	1
Gelbag	Viscoelastic	
Gelbag Plus	Viscoelastic	
Geneyes	Decongestant	7
Genoptic	Antibiotic	5
Gentak	Antibiotic	5
GenTeal	Preserved artificial lubricant	2
GenTeal Gel	Preserved artificial lubricant	2
GenTeal Mild	Preserved artificial lubricant	2
GenTeal Moderate	Preserved artificial lubricant	2
GenTeal PF	Nonpreserved artificial lubricant	2
GenTeal Severe	Preserved artificial lubricant	2
Glaucon	Glaucoma	4
Glycerin (generic)	Reducing corneal edema	1
Gonak	Coupling agent applied to diagnostic lens	1
Goniosoft	Coupling agent applied to diagnostic lens	1
Goniosol	Coupling agent applied to diagnostic lens	1
Healon	Viscoelastic	
Healon GV	Viscoelastic	

Brand Name	Use(s)	List Number
Healon 5	Viscoelastic	5
Herplex	Antiviral	3
HMS	Steroidal anti-inflammatory	1
Homatropine (generic)	Cycloplegia	2
Hypotears	Preserved artificial lubricant	2
Hypotears PF	Nonpreserved artificial lubricant	1
IC-Green	Angiographic study	3
Inflamase Forte	Steroidal anti-inflammatory	3
Inflamase Mild	Steroidal anti-inflammatory	4
Iopidine	Glaucoma	4
Ismotic	Glaucoma	1
Isopto Atropine	Cycloplegia	4
Isopto Carbachol	Glaucoma	4
Isopto Carpine	Glaucoma	5
Isopto Cetamide	Antibacterial	1
Isopto Homatropine	Cycloplegia	1
IsoptoHyoscine	Cycloplegia	2
Isopto Tears	Preserved artificial lubricant	2
Iquix	Antibiotic	5

Brand Name	Use(s)	List Number
Lacrilube NP	Nonpreserved artificial lubricant	2
Lacrilube SOP	Preserved artificial lubricant	2
Lacrisert	Artificial lubricant	2
Liquifilm	Steroidal anti-inflammatory	3
Liquifilm Tears	Preserved artificial lubricant	2
Lotemax	Steroidal anti-inflammatory	3
Lucentis	Wet ARMD	1
Lumigan	Glaucoma	4
Macugen	Wet ARMD	1
Maxidex	Steroidal anti-inflammatory	3
Maxitrol	Steroidal anti-inflammatory/antibiotic	6
MiniDrops	Nonpreserved artificial lubricant	2
Miochol-E	Rapid miosis during surgery	1
Miostat	Rapid miosis during surgery	1
Mitomycin C (generic)	Wet ARMD	1
Moisture Eyes	Preserved artificial lubricant	2
Mucomyst	Mucolytic	1

ARMD = age-related macular degeneration

Brand Name	Use(s)	List Number
Murine Plus	Decongestant	7
Murine Tears	Preserved artificial lubricant	2
Murine Tears Plus	Decongestant/lubricant	7
Muro-128	Hyperosmolar for corneal edema	1
Murocel	Preserved artificial lubricant	2
Murocoll 2	Cycloplegia/mydriasis	1
Mydfrin	Mydriasis	1
Mydral	Mydriasis	1
Mydriacyl	Cycloplegia	1
Napha-Forte	Decongestant	7
Naphcon	Decongestant	7
Naphcon-A	Decongestant/antihistamine	7
Natacyn	Antifungal	5
Nature's Tears	Nonpreserved lubricant	2
Neocidin	Antibiotic	5
Neocin	Antibiotic	5
Neo-Decadron	Steroidal anti-inflammatory/antibiotic	6
Neo-Deca-Gen	Steroidal anti-inflammatory/antibiotic	6
Neo-Dexide	Steroidal anti-inflammatory/antibiotic	6

Brand Name	Use(s)	List Number
Neofrin	Mydriasis	1
Neopolydex	Steroidal anti-inflammatory/antibiotic	6
Neopolytracin	Antibiotic	5
Neosporin	Antibiotic	5
Neotricin HCL	Steroidal anti-inflammatory/antibiotic	6
Nevanac	Nonsteroidal anti-inflammatory	3
Nutra-Tears	Preserved artificial lubricant	2
Ocuclear	Decongestant	7
Ocucoat	Preserved artificial lubricant	2
Ocucoat (injectable)	Viscoelastic	
Ocucoat PF	Nonpreserved artificial lubricant	2
Ocufen	Nonsteroidal anti-inflammatory	3
Ocuflox	Antibiotic	5
Oculinum	Muscle relaxant	1
OcuNefrin	Decongestant/lubricant	7
Ocu-Pred	Steroidal anti-inflammatory	3
Ocupress	Glaucoma	4
OCuSOFT	Irrigating solution (external)	
Ocusulf-10	Antibacterial	5

Brand Name	Use(s)	List Number
Ocutracin	Steroidal anti-inflammatory/antibiotic	6
Opcon-A	Antihistamine/decongestant	7, 8
Ophthaine	Anesthetic	1
Ophthetic	Anesthetic	1
Opti-Clear	Decongestant	7
Opticrom	Mast cell stabilizer	8
Opticyl	Cycloplegia	1
Optigene 3	Decongestant	7
OptiPranolol	Glaucoma	4
Optivar	Antihistamine/mast cell stabilizer	8
Optive	Preserved artificial lubricant	2
Osmitrol	Glaucoma	4
Osmoglyn	Glaucoma	4
P#E1	Glaucoma	4
Paracaine	Anesthetic	1
Paremyd	Mydriasis	1
Pataday	Antihistamine	8
Patanol	Antihistamine	8
Pentolair	Cycloplegia	1
Phenoptic	Mydriasis	1

Brand Name	Use(s)	List Number
Phospholine iodide	Glaucoma	4
Pilocar	Glaucoma	4
Pilopine HS	Glaucoma	4
Piloptic	Glaucoma	4
Polycin-B	Antibiotic	5
Poly-Dex	Steroidal anti-inflammatory/antibiotic	6
Poly-Pred	Steroidal anti-inflammatory/antibiotic	6
Polysporin	Antibiotic	5
Polytracin	Antibiotic	5
Polytrim	Antibiotic	5
Pontocaine	Anesthetic	1
Pred Forte	Steroidal anti-inflammatory	3
Pred G	Steroidal anti-inflammatory/antibiotic	6
Pred Mild	Steroidal anti-inflammatory	3
Propine	Glaucoma	4
ProVisc	Viscoelastic	
Quixin	Antibiotic	5
Rayflo	Viscoelastic	
Redness Relief	Decongestant	7

Brand Name	Use(s)	List Number
Redness Reliever	Decongestant	7
Refresh	Nonpreserved artificial lubricant	2
Refresh Celluvisc	Nonpreserved artificial lubricant	2
Refresh Dry Eye Therapy	Nonpreserved artificial lubricant	2
Refresh Endura	Nonpreserved artificial lubricant	2
Refresh Liquigel	Preserved artificial lubricant	2
Refresh Plus	Nonpreserved artificial lubricant	2
Refresh PM	Nonpreserved artificial lubricant	2
Refresh Tears	Preserved artificial lubricant	2
Restasis	Immunomodulator for k. sicca	1
Retisert	Steroidal anti-inflammatory (retinal implant)	3
Rev-Eyes	Reverse mydriasis	1
Rohto V. Cool	Decongestant	7
Rohto V. Ice	Decongestant/astringent	7
Rohto Zi	Preserved artificial lubricant	2
Romycin	Antibiotic	5
Sandimmune	Immunosuppressant	1
Sochlor	Hyperosmotic	1
SoftGlo	Corneal dye	1

BRAND NAME	USE(S)	LIST NUMBER
Soothe	Nonpreserved artificial lubricant	2
Stye	Nonpreserved artificial lubricant	2
Sulf-10	Antibacterial	5
Sulfacel-15	Antibiotic	5
Sulfamide	Steroidal anti-inflammatory/antibacterial	6
Systane	Preserved artificial lubricant	2
Tearisol	Preserved artificial lubricant	2
Tears Again Liquid Gel	Preserved artificial lubricant	2
Tears Again MC	Preserved artificial lubricant	2
Tears Again Night & Day Gel	Nonpreserved artificial lubricant	2
Tears Again Nighttime Relief	Nonpreserved artificial lubricant	2
Tears Again Ointment	Nonpreserved artificial lubricant	2
Tears Again Solution	Preserved artificial lubricant	2
Tears Naturale	Preserved artificial lubricant	2
Tears Naturale Forte	Preserved artificial lubricant	2
Tears Naturale Free	Nonpreserved artificial lubricant	2
Tears Naturale PM	Nonpreserved artificial lubricant	2
Tears Naturale II	Preserved artificial lubricant	2
Tears Renewed	Preserved artificial lubricant	2
Tensilon	Diagnosis of myasthenia gravis	1

Brand Name	Use(s)	List Number
TheraTears	Nonpreserved artificial lubricant	2
Timoptic	Glaucoma	4
Timoptic XE	Glaucoma	4
Tobradex	Steroidal anti-inflammatory/antibiotic	6
Tobrex	Antibiotic	5
Travatan	Glaucoma	4
Travatan Z	Glaucoma	4
Tropicacyl	Cycloplegia	1
Trusopt	Glaucoma	4
Tysine	Decongestant	7
Ultratears	Preserved artificial lubricant	2
Vasocidin	Steroidal anti-inflammatory/antibacterial	6
Vasocine	Steroidal anti-inflammatory/antibacterial	6
Vasoclear	Decongestant	7
Vasoclear-A	Decongestant/astringent	7
Vasocon	Decongestant	7
Vasocon-A	Decongestant/antihistamine	7, 8
Vexol	Steroidal anti-inflammatory	3
Vigamox	Antibiotic	5
Viroptic	Antiviral	5

Brand Name	Use(s)	List Number
Viscoat	Viscoelastic	7, 8
Visine-A	Decongestant/antihistamine	7
Visine AC	Decongestant/astringent	7
Visine Advanced Relief	Decongestant/lubricant	2
Visine Long Lasting	Preserved artificial lubricant	7
Visine LR	Decongestant	7
Visine Original	Decongestant	7
Visine Pure Tears	Nonpreserved artificial lubricant	2
Visine Tears	Preserved artificial lubricant	2
VisionBlue	Surgical aid/stain	1
Visudyne	Photodynamic therapy (ARMD)	1
Vitrasert	Antiviral	5
Vitrax	Viscoelastic	2
Viva-Drops	Nonpreserved artificial lubricant	2
Voltaren	Nonsteroidal anti-inflammatory	3
Xalatan	Glaucoma	4
Zaditor	Mast cell stabilizer/antihistamine	8
Zincfrin	Decongestant/astringent	7
Zylet	Steroidal anti-inflammatory/antibiotic	6
Zymar	Antibiotic	5

ARMD = age-related macular degeneration

List 1

Diagnostics/Miscellaneous

Note: All drugs are in topical drop form unless otherwise noted

Brand Name	Generic Name	Use
5-FU	Fluorouracil (injection)	Glaucoma surgery (OLU)
Adrucil	Fluorouracil (injection)	Glaucoma surgery (OLU)
AK-Dilate	Phenylephrine	Mydriasis
AK-Fluor	Fluorescein (injection)	Dye study of fundus/iris
AK-NACL	Sodium chloride (gtt/ung)	Corneal edema
AK-Pentolate	Cyclopentolate	Cycloplegia
AK-T-Caine	Tetracaine	Anesthetic
AK-Taine	Proparacaine	Anesthetic
Alcaine	Proparacaine	Anesthetic
Atropine Care	Atropine	Cycloplegia
Atrosulf	Atropine	Cycloplegia

gtt = drop; ung = ointment; OLU = off-label use

Brand Name	Generic Name	Use
Avastin	Bevacizumab	Inhibits neovascularization (OLU)
BioGlo	Fluorescein (strip)	Corneal stain
Blueron	Patent blue	Surgical aid/stain
BOTOX	Botulinum toxin type A (injection)	Inhibits muscle response
BOTOX Cosmetic	Botulinum toxin type A (injection)	Inhibits muscle response
Cardio-green	Indocyanine green (injection)	Angiographic study
Cyclogyl	Cyclopentolate	Cycloplegia
Cyclomydril	Cyclopentolate/phenylephrine	Cycloplegia/mydriasis
Cylate	Cyclopentolate	Cycloplegia
Enlon	Edrophonium	Diagnosis of myasthenia gravis
Fluor-I-Strips	Fluorescein (strip)	Corneal stain
Fluoracaine	Proparacaine/fluorescein	Anesthetic/stain
Fluorescite	Fluorescein (injection)	Dye study of fundus/iris
FluoreStrips	Fluorescein (strip)	Corneal stain
Fluorets	Fluorescein (strip)	Corneal stain
Fluress	Benoxinate/fluorescein	Anesthetic/stain
Ful-Glo	Fluorescein (strip)	Corneal stain

gtt = drop; ung = ointment; OLU = off-label use

Brand Name	Generic Name	Use
Glycerin (generic)	Glycerin	Topical osmotic
Gonak	Methylcellulose	Coupling agent applied to diagnostic lens
Goniosoft	Methylcellulose	Coupling agent applied to diagnostic lens
Goniosol	Methylcellulose	Coupling agent applied to diagnostic lens
Homatropine (generic)	Homatropine	Cycloplegia
IC-Green	Indocyanine green (injection)	Angiographic study
Isopto Atropine	Atropine	Cycloplegia
Isopto Homatropine	Homatropine	Cycloplegia
Isopto-Hyoscine	Scopolamine	Cycloplegia
Lucentis	Ranibizumab	Inhibits neovascularization
Macugen	Pegaptanib	Inhibits neovascularization
Miochol-E	Acetylcholine (intraocular)	Rapid miosis during surgery
Miostat	Carbachol (intraocular)	Rapid miosis during surgery
Mitomycin C (generic)	Mitomycin C	Inhibits neovascularization (OLU)

gtt = drop; ung = ointment; OLU = off-label use

Brand Name	Generic Name	Use
Mucomyst	Acetylcystine	Reduces mucus (OLU)
Muro-128	Sodium chloride (gtt/ung)	Corneal edema
Murocoll 2	Scopolamine/phenylephrine	Cycloplegia/mydriasis
Mydfrin	Phenylephrine	Mydriasis
Mydral	Tropicamide	Cycloplegia
Mydriacyl	Tropicamide	Cycloplegia
Neofrin	Phenylephrine	Mydriasis
Oculinum	Botulinum toxin type A (injection)	Muscle relaxant
Ophthaine	Proparacaine	Anesthetic
Ophthetic	Proparacaine	Anesthetic
Opticyl	Cyclopentolate	Cycloplegia
Paracaine	Proparacaine	Anesthetic
Paremyd	Hydroxyamphetamine	Mydriasis
Pentolair	Cyclopentolate	Cycloplegia
Phenoptic	Phenylephrine	Mydriasis
Pontocaine	Tetracaine	Anesthetic
Restasis	Cyclosporine	Immunomodulator for k. sicca

gtt = drop; ung = ointment; OLU = off-label use

Brand Name	Generic Name	Use
Rev-Eyes	Dapiprazole	Reverse mydriasis
Sandimmune	Cyclosporine	Immunosuppressant used in PK
Sochlor	5% NaCl	Corneal edema
SoftGlo	Fluorescein (strip)	Corneal stain
Tensilon	Edrophonium	Diagnosis of myasthenia gravis
Tropicacyl	Tropicamide	Cycloplegia
VisionBlue	Trypan blue	Surgical aid/stain
Visudyne	Verteporfin	Photodynamic therapy

gtt = drop; ung = ointment; OLU = off-label use; PK = penetrating keratoplasty

LIST 2

Artificial Ocular Lubricants

BRAND NAME	TYPE OF LUBRICANT	FORM
Advanced Eye Relief	Nonpreserved	Drops
Advanced Eye Relief Environmental	Preserved	Drops
Advanced Eye Relief PF	Nonpreserved	Drops
Advanced Eye Relief Night Time	Nonpreserved	Ointment
Advanced Eye Relief Rejuvenation	Preserved	Drops
AKWA Tears	Preserved	Drops
AKWA Tears	Nonpreserved	Ointment
AquaSite	Preserved	Drops
Aquify	Preserved	Drops
Bion Tears	Nonpreserved	Drops
Clear Eyes	Preserved	Drops
GenTeal	Preserved	Drops
GenTeal Gel	Preserved	Gel

Brand Name	Type of Lubricant	Form
GenTeal Mild	Preserved	Drops
GenTeal Moderate	Preserved	Drops
GenTeal PF	Nonpreserved	Drops
GenTeal Severe	Preserved	Drops
Hypotears	Preserved	Drops
Hypotears	Nonpreserved	Ointment
Hypotears PF	Nonpreserved	Drops
Isopto Tears	Preserved	Drops
Lacrilube NP	Nonpreserved	Ointment
Lacrilube SOP	Preserved	Ointment
Lacrisert	N/A	Pellet
Liquifilm Tears	Preserved	Drops
MiniDrops	Nonpreserved	Drops
Moisture Eyes	Preserved	Ointment
Murine Tears	Preserved	Drops
Murocel	Preserved	Drops
Nature's Tears	Nonpreserved	Mist
Nutra-Tears	Preserved	Drops
Ocucoat	Preserved	Drops

BRAND NAME	TYPE OF LUBRICANT	FORM
Ocucoat PF	Nonpreserved	Drops
Optive	Preserved	Drops
Refresh	Nonpreserved	Drops
Refresh Celluvisc	Nonpreserved	Drops
Refresh Dry Eye Therapy	Nonpreserved	Drops
Refresh Endura	Nonpreserved	Drops
Refresh Liquigel	Preserved	Gel
Refresh Plus	Nonpreserved	Drops
Refresh PM	Nonpreserved	Ointment
Refresh Tears	Preserved	Drops
Rohto Zi	Preserved	Drops
Soothe	Nonpreserved	Drops
Stye	Nonpreserved	Ointment
Systane	Preserved	Drops
Tearisol	Preserved	Drops
Tears Again Liquid Gel	Preserved	Gel
Tears Again MC	Preserved	Drop
Tears Again Night & Day Gel	Nonpreserved	Gel
Tears Again Nighttime Relief	Nonpreserved	Ointment

BRAND NAME	TYPE OF LUBRICANT	FORM
Tears Again Ointment	Nonpreserved	Ointment
Tears Again Solution	Preserved	Drops
Tears Naturale	Preserved	Drops
Tears Naturale Forte	Preserved	Drops
Tears Naturale Free	Nonpreserved	Drops
Tears Naturale PM	Nonpreserved	Ointment
Tears Naturale II	Preserved	Drops
Tears Renewed	Preserved	Drops
TheraTears	Nonpreserved	Drops
Ultratears	Preserved	Drops
Visine Long Lasting	Preserved	Drops
Visine Pure Tears	Nonpreserved	Drops
Visine Tears	Preserved	Drops
Viva-Drops	Nonpreserved	Drops

L**IST** 3

Anti-Inflammatories

B**RAND** N**AME**	G**ENERIC** N**AME**	T**YPE**
Acular	Ketorolac	NSAID
Acular LS	Ketorolac	NSAID
Acular PF	Ketorolac	Nonpreserved NSAID
AK-Dex	Dexamethasone	Steroid/anti-inflammatory
AK-Pred	Prednisolone	Steroid/anti-inflammatory
Alrex	Loteprednol	Steroid/anti-inflammatory
Econopred Plus	Prednisolone	Steroid/anti-inflammatory
Eflone	Fluorometholone	Steroid/anti-inflammatory
Flarex	Fluorometholone	Steroid/anti-inflammatory
Fluor-op	Fluorometholone	Steroid/anti-inflammatory
FML	Fluorometholone	Steroid/anti-inflammatory

NSAID = nonsteroidal anti-inflammatory

BRAND NAME	GENERIC NAME	TYPE
FML Forte	Fluorometholone	Steroid/anti-inflammatory
FML SOP	Fluorometholone	Steroid/anti-inflammatory
HMS	Medrysone	Steroid/anti-inflammatory
Inflamase Forte	Prednisolone	Steroid/anti-inflammatory
Inflamase Mild	Prednisolone	Steroid/anti-inflammatory
Liquifilm	Fluorometholone	Steroid/anti-inflammatory
Lotemax	Loteprednol	Steroid/anti-inflammatory
Maxidex	Dexamethasone	Steroid/anti-inflammatory
Nevanac	Nepafenac	NSAID
Ocufen	Flurbiprofen	NSAID
Ocu-Pred	Prednisolone	Steroid/anti-inflammatory
Pred Forte	Prednisolone	Steroid/anti-inflammatory
Pred Mild	Prednisolone	Steroid/anti-inflammatory
Retisert	Fluocinolone	Steroid/anti-inflammatory
Vexol	Rimexolone	Steroid/anti-inflammatory
Voltaren	Diclofenac	NSAID

NSAID = nonsteroidal anti-inflammatory drug

List 4

Glaucoma Medications

Brand Name	Generic	Class
Akarpine	Pilocarpine	Miotic
AK-Beta	Levobunolol	Nonselective β blocker
AK-Pro	Dipivefrin	α, β adrenergic agonist
Alphagan-P	Brimonidine	Pure α-2 adrenergic agonist
Azopt	Brinzolamide	CAI
Betagan	Levobunolol	Nonselective β blocker
Betimol	Timolol	Nonselective β blocker
Betoptic	Betaxolol	Selective β-1 blocker
Betoptic-S	Betaxolol	Selective β-1 blocker
Carbastat	Carbachol	Miotic (intraocular)
Carboptic	Carbachol	Miotic

α = alpha; β = beta; CAI = carbonic anhydrase inhibitor

BRAND NAME	GENERIC	CLASS
Cosopt	Timolol/dorzolamide	Nonselective β blocker/CAI
Diamox	Acetazolamide oral	CAI
Epifrin	Epinephrine	α,β adrenergic agonist
E-Pilo	Pilocarpine/epinephrine	Miotic/α,β adrenergic agonist
Epinal	Epinephrine	α,β adrenergic agonist
Glaucon	Epinephrine	α,β adrenergic agonist
Iopidine	Apraclonidine	Pure α-2 adrenergic agonist
Ismotic	Isosorbide oral	Hyperosmotic
Isopto Carbachol	Carbachol	Miotic
Isopto Carpine	Pilocarpine	Miotic
Lumigan	Bimatoprost	Prostaglandin
Ocupress	Carteolol	Nonselective β blocker
OptiPranolol	Metipranolol	Nonselective β blocker
Osmitrol	Mannitol intravenous	Hyperosmotic
Osmoglyn	Glycerin oral	Hyperosmotic
P#E1	Pilocarpine/epinephrine	Miotic/α,β adrenergic agonist
Phospholine iodide	Echothiophate	Miotic

α = alpha; β = beta; CAI = carbonic anhydrase inhibitor

Brand Name	Generic	Class
Pilocar	Pilocarpine	Miotic
Pilopine HS	Pilocarpine gel	Miotic
Piloptic	Pilocarpine	Miotic
Propine	Dipivefrin	α,β adrenergic agonist
Timoptic	Timolol	Nonselective β blocker
Timoptic XE	Timolol gel	Nonselective β blocker
Travatan	Travoprost	Prostaglandin
Travatan Z	Travoprost	Prostaglandin
Trusopt	Dorzolamide	CAI
Xalatan	Latanoprost	Prostaglandin

α = alpha; β = beta; CAI = carbonic anhydrase inhibitor

List 5

Anti-Infectives

Brand Name	Ingredient(s)	Use	Form(s)
AK-Poly-Bac	Polymyxin/bacitracin	Antibiotic	ung
AK-Spore	Polymyxin B/neomycin/gramicidin	Antibiotic	gtt
AK-Spore	Polymyxin B/neomycin/bacitracin	Antibiotic	ung
AK-Tob	Tobramycin	Antibiotic	gtt
Bleph-10	Sulfacetamide	Antibacterial	gtt/ung
Bleph-30	Sulfacetamide	Antibacterial	gtt
Cetamide	Sulfacetamide	Antibacterial	ung
Ciloxin	Ciprofloxacin	Antibiotic	gtt/ung
Dendrid	Idoxuridine	Antiviral	gtt
Genoptic	Gentamicin	Antibiotic	gtt/ung
Gentak	Gentamicin	Antibiotic	gtt/ung

gtt = drop; ung = ointment; inj = injection

Brand Name	Ingredient(s)	Use	Form(s)
Herplex	Idoxuridine	Antiviral	gtt
Isopto Cetamide	Sulfacetamide	Antibacterial	gtt
Iquix	Levofloxacin	Antibiotic	gtt
Natacyn	Natamycin	Antifungal	gtt
Neocidin	Polymyxin B/neomycin/bacitracin	Antibiotic	ung
Neocin	Polymyxin B/neomycin/gramicidin	Antibiotic	gtt/ung
Neopolytracin	Polymyxin B/neomycin/bacitracin	Antibiotic	ung
Neosporin	Polymyxin B/neomycin/bacitracin	Antibiotic	ung
Neosporin	Polymyxin B/neomycin/gramicidin	Antibiotic	gtt
Ocuflox	Ofloxacin	Antibiotic	gtt
Ocusulf-10	Sulfacetamide	Antibiotic	gtt
Polycin-B	Polymyxin B/bacitracin	Antibiotic	ung
Polysporin	Polymyxin/bacitracin	Antibiotic	ung
Polytracin	Polymyxin/bacitracin	Antibiotic	ung
Polytrim	Polymyxin B/trimethoprim	Antibiotic	gtt
Quixin	Levofloxacin	Antibacterial	gtt
Romycin	Erythromycin	Antibiotic	ung

gtt = drop; ung = ointment; inj = injection

Brand Name	Ingredient(s)	Use	Form(s)
Sulf-10	Sulfacetamide	Antibacterial	gtt
Sulfacel-15	Sulfacetamide	Antibacterial	gtt
Tobrex	Tobramycin	Antibiotic	ung
Vigamox	Moxifloxacin	Antibiotic	gtt
Viroptic	Trifluridine	Antiviral	gtt
Vitrasert	Ganciclovir	Antiviral	implant
Zymar	Gatifloxacin	Antibiotic	gtt

gtt = drop; ung = ointment; inj = injection

LIST 6

Anti-Infective/Anti-Inflammatory Combinations

BRAND NAME	INGREDIENTS	USE	FORM(S)
AK-Cide	Sulfacetamide/prednisolone	ster/slf	gtt/ung
AK-Spore HC	Bacitracin/neomycin/polymyxin B/hydro-cortisone	ster/antib	ung
AK-Spore HC	Neomycin/polymyxin B/hydrocortisone	ster/antib	gtt
AK-Trol	Neomycin/polymyxin B/dexamethasone	ster/antib	gtt/ung
Blephamide	Sulfacetamide/prednisolone	ster/slf	gtt/ung
Blephamide SOP	Sulfacetamide/prednisolone	ster/slf	ung
Cortisporin	Bacitracin/neomycin/polymyxin B/hydrocortisone	ster/antib	ung
Cortisporin	Neomycin/polymyxin B/hydrocortisone	ster/antib	gtt
Dexacine	Neomycin/polymyxin B/dexamethasone	ster/antib	ung

ster = steroid; slf = sulfonamide; antib = antibiotic; gtt = drop; ung = ointment

Brand Name	Ingredients	Use	Form(s)
Dexasporin	Neomycin/polymyxin B/dexamethasone	ster/antib	gtt
FML-S	Sulfacetamide/fluorometholone	ster/slf	gtt
Maxitrol	Neomycin/polymyxin B/dexamethasone	ster/antib	gtt/ung
NeoDecadron	Neomycin/dexamethasone	ster/antib	gtt/ung
Neo-Deca-Gen	Neomycin/dexamethasone/gentamicin	ster/antib	gtt
Neo-Dexide	Neomycin/decamethasone	ster/antib	gtt
Neopolydex	Neomycin/polymyxin B/dexamethasone	ster/antib	gtt/ung
Neotricin HCL	Neomycin/bacitracin//polymyxin B/ hydrocortisone	ster/antib	ung
Ocutracin	Neomycin/bacitracin/polymyxin B/ hydrocortisone	ster/antib	gtt
Poly-Dex	Neomycin/polymyxin B/dexamethasone	ster/antib	gtt/ung
Poly-Pred	Neomycin/polymyxin B/prednisolone	ster/antib	gtt
Pred G	Gentamicin/prednisolone	ster/antib	gtt
Sulfamide	Sulfacetamide/prednisolone	ster/slf	gtt/ung
Tobradex	Tobramycin/dexamethasone	ster/antib	gtt/ung
Vasocidin	Sulfacetamide/prednisolone	ster/slf	gtt/ung
Vasocine	Sulfacetamide/prednisolone	ster/slf	ung
Zylet	Tobramycin/loteprednol	ster/antib	gtt

ster = steroid; slf = sulfonamide; antib = antibiotic; gtt = drop; ung = ointment

LIST 7

Decongestants/Combinations

BRAND NAME	GENERIC NAME/ ACTIVE INGREDIENT(S)	USE(S)
Advanced Eye Relief All Clear AR	Naphazoline	Decongestant
AK-Con	Naphazoline	Decongestant
AK-Con-A	Naphazoline/pheniramine	Decongestant/antihistamine
Albalon	Naphazoline	Decongestant
All Clear Redness Reliever	Naphazoline/polyethylene glycol	Decongestant/lubricant
Allersol	Naphazoline	Decongestant
Clarif-Eye	Tetrahydrozoline	Decongestant
Clarine	Tetrahydrozoline	Decongestant
Clear Eyes ACR	Naphazoline/zinc/glycerin	Decongestant/astringent
Clear Eyes Redness Relief	Naphazoline/glycerin	Decongestant/lubricant
Clear Eyes Seasonal Relief	Naphazoline/zinc	Decongestant/astringent
Clear View	Tetrahydrozoline	Decongestant

Brand Name	Generic Name/ Active Ingredient(s)	Use(s)
EyeSine	Tetrahydrozoline	Decongestant
Geneyes	Tetrahydrozoline	Decongestant
Murine Plus	Tetrahydrozoline	Decongestant
Murine Tears Plus	Tetrahydrozoline/polyvinyl alcohol/povidone	Decongestant/lubricant
Napha-Forte	Naphazoline	Decongestant
Naphcon	Naphazoline	Decongestant
Naphcon-A	Naphazoline/pheniramine maleate	Decongestant/antihistamine
Ocuclear	Oxymetazoline	Decongestant
OcuNefrin	Phenylephrine	Decongestant/lubricant
Opcon-A	Naphazoline/pheniramine maleate	Decongestant/antihistamine
Opti-Clear	Tetrahydrozoline	Decongestant
Optigene 3	Tetrahydrozoline	Decongestant
Redness Relief	Naphazoline	Decongestant
Redness Reliever	Tetrahydrozoline	Decongestant
Rohto V. Cool	Naphazoline	Decongestant

Brand Name	Generic Name/ Active Ingredient(s)	Use(s)
Rohto V. Ice	Tetrahydrozoline/zinc	Decongestant/astringent
Tysine	Tetrahydrozoline	Decongestant
Vasoclear	Naphazoline	Decongestant
Vasoclear-A	Naphazoline/zinc	Decongestant/astringent
Vasocon	Naphazoline	Decongestant
Vasocon-A	Naphazoline/antazoline	Decongestant/antihistamine
Visine-A	Naphazoline/pheniramine maleate	Decongestant/antihistamine
Visine AC	Tetrahydrozoline/zinc sulfate	Decongestant/astringent
Visine Advanced Relief	Tetrahydrozoline	Decongestant/lubricant
Visine LR	Oxymetazoline	Decongestant
Visine Original	Tetrahydrozoline	Decongestant
Zincfrin	Phenylephrine/zinc	Decongestant/astringent

List 8

Anti-Allergenics

BRAND NAME	INGREDIENTS	TYPE
AK-Con-A	Pheniramine/naphazoline	Decongestant/antihistamine
Alamast	Pemirolast	MCS
Alaway	Ketotifen	Antihis
Alocril	Nedocromil	MCS
Alomide	Lodoxamide	MCS
Crolom	Cromolyn	MCS
Elestat	Epinastine	Antihis
Emadine	Emedastine	Antihis
Opcon-A	Pheniramine/naphazoline	Antihis/decon
Opticrom	Cromolyn	MCS
Optivar	Azelastine	MCS/antihis

MCS = mast cell stabilizer; antihis = antihistamine; decon = decongestant

Brand Name	Ingredients	Type
Pataday	Olopatadine	Antihis
Patanol	Olopatadine	Antihis
Vasocon-A	Antazoline/naphazoline	Antihis/decon
Visine-A	Pheniramine/naphazoline	Antihis/decon
Zaditor	Ketotifen	MCS/antihis

MCS = mast cell stabilizer; antihis = antihistamine; decon = decongestant

Lasers in Ophthalmology

LASER	WAVELENGTH	ACTION	USES
I. Thermal Argon	Blue-green (488 to 515 nm) Low energy Continuous wave	Photocoagulation Absorbed by hemoglobin, melanin, and xanthophyll	Retinal vascular disease Choroidal neovascularization Trabeculoplasty Iridotomy Suture lysis
Krypton	Red (647 nm) Continuous wave	Photocoagulation Absorbed by melanin, to a lesser degree by hemoglobin (not absorbed by retinal vessels and xanthophyll)	Same as argon but deeper choroid

LASER	WAVELENGTH	ACTION	USES
Krypton (cont)		Passes more readily through lens opacities and vitreous hemorrhages	
CO_2	Infrared Long wavelength Low penetration	Photovaporization (photo-evaporation) Absorbed by water	Skin lesions Fine, bloodless skin incisions Cautery
Tunable dye	Adjustable (green to red)	Photocoagulation Variably absorbed by melanin, hemoglobin, and xanthophyll	Same as argon and krypton
Diode laser	Infrared (805 nm)	Photocoagulation Sometimes used in conjunction with ICG dye	Retinal vascular disease Choroidal neovascularization

LASER	WAVELENGTH	ACTION	USES
Frequency-doubled YAG	Green (532 nm) Continuous wave	Photocoagulation	Same as krypton
II. Ionizing Q-switched YAG	Infrared (1064 nm) Pulsed laser	Photodisruption (cold, cutting) Very tiny spot sizes	Incisions/cutting Synechotomy Capsulotomy Vitreous adhesions Iridotomy
III. Photochemical Excimer	UV light (photo-evaporation)	Photoablation Breaks chemical bonds of tissues	Corneal opacities Refractive surgery
Photodynamic therapy	Red-infrared (665 to 732 nm)	Causes chemical changes that result in vascular occlusion and cellular disruption	Malignant tumors Choroidal neovascularization

Laser	Wavelength	Action	Uses
Photodynamic therapy (cont)		Used in conjunction with photosensitive agents	

Reprinted with permission from Ledford J. *Certified Ophthalmic Medical Technologist Exam Review Manual*. Thorofare, NJ: SLACK Incorporated; 2000.

Ocular and Systemic Effects of Topical Ocular Drugs

DRUG TYPE	OCULAR EFFECTS	SYSTEMIC EFFECTS
Decongestant	Increased redness Dryness Pupil dilation Transient stinging	Nervousness Decreased heart rate Headache, nervousness
Corticosteroids	PSC cataract Elevated IOP (no symptoms)	Stomach ulcers Psychoses Muscle weakness Bone weakness
NSAIDs	Transient stinging Follicular conjunctivitis	Stomach upset Stomach ulcers

Drug Type	Ocular Effects	Systemic Effects
NSAIDs (continued)		Vomiting Promote asthma
Antibiotics	Transient stinging Allergic reaction Redness Photophobia Depigmentation of eyelids	Dermatitis Digestive upset
Antivirals	Transient stinging Corneal toxicity	Contact dermatitis
Direct-acting adrenergics	Transient stinging Redness	Arousal of sympathetic nervous system
Beta blockers	Transient stinging	Decreased heart rate Slowed breathing Depression Confusion

DRUG TYPE	OCULAR EFFECTS	SYSTEMIC EFFECTS
Beta blockers (continued)		Dizziness
		Digestive upset
		Headache
		Rash
		Insomnia
		Impotence
		Decreased appetite
Miotics	Transient stinging	Brow headache
	Blurred vision	Sweating
	Miosis	Salivation
	Accommodative spasm	Digestive upset
	Posterior synechiae	Decreased heart rate
		Flushing
		Tremors
		Difficulty breathing
		Lethargy

Drug Type	Ocular Effects	Systemic Effects
Carbonic anhydrase inhibitors	Conjunctival irritation	Bitter taste
Prostaglandins	Transient stinging Redness Irritation Browning of iris Trichomegaly Blood pressure variation	Headache Cold/flu/sinus symptoms Digestive upset Anxiety/depression Angina/chest pain

Reprinted with permission from Ledford J. *The Complete Guide to Ocular History Taking.* Thorofare, NJ: SLACK Incorporated; 1999.

Troubleshooting Glasses Problems

PROBLEM	POSSIBLE CAUSE	CORRESPONDING ACTION
Inadequate distant vision	Lenses are not what was prescribed	Repeat refractometry.
	Inadequate refractometry DBC off (induced prism)	Lensometry Mark centers, measure DBC, compare to DBC of old glasses and patient's PD; check location of centers with glasses on patient.
	Vertex distance off	Check vertex distance of old and new glasses; use over-refractometry and VD of trial frames, or use Halberg clips.
	New hyperope or new fully corrected hyperope	Educate; doctor may use cycloplegia to ease patient into correction; doctor may back off on amount to ease patient into full correction.

Problem	Possible Cause	Corresponding Action
Inadequate distance vision (cont)	Previously overcorrected myope	Educate; doctor may add a bit of minus to ease patient into correct Rx.
	Lenses warped/scratched	Visual inspection.
Inadequate near vision		
1. Has to hold reading too close	Over-plused (see below)	Reassess patient needs; over-refractometry; try Rx in trial frame; have patient measure working distances to desk, music stand, etc.
2. Has to hold reading too far back	Over-minused (see below)	
	Either of these may be caused by failure to reckon with addition or subtraction of power in distance portion of lenses; failure of prescriber to analyze patient's needs (may be aggravated by poorly done history)	

Problem	Possible Cause	Corresponding Action
Inadequate near vision (continued)		
3. Unclear	Single-vision reading glasses made using distance PD	Mark centers, measure DBC, compare to distant and near PDs.
	DBC off (not looking through optical centers)	Mark centers, measure DBC, compare to PD; check location of centers with glasses on patient.
	Patient not holding material at proper distance	Educate; reassess patient's needs; over-refractometry; try Rx in trial frame; have patient measure working distance to desk, computer, etc.
Eyes feel tired, drawn, pull	DBC is off (induced prism)	Mark centers, measure DBC of old and new glasses, compare with patient's PD; check location of centers with glasses on patient.
	DBC matches PD, but patient is used to the incorrect PD of old glasses	As above; prescriber may decide to ease patient into correct DBC by changing it gradually.

PROBLEM	POSSIBLE CAUSE	CORRESPONDING ACTION
Eyes feel tired, drawn, pull (continued)	Change in base curve	Measure base curve of old and new lenses.
	Accommodative imbalance	Repeat refractometry, being careful to balance.
	Image-size disparities	Check base curve of old and new lenses.
	Astigmatic change	Re-check refractometry; have patient turn axis dial on phoropter/trial frame to clear position.
Swimmy-headed/ nausea	Base curve change	Measure base curve of old and new lenses.
	DBC is off (induced prism)	Mark centers, measure DBC of old and new lenses, compare to patient's PD; check location of centers with glasses on patient.
	Image size disparities	Check base curve of old and new lenses.

PROBLEM	POSSIBLE CAUSE	CORRESPONDING ACTION
Swimmy-headed / nausea (cont)	Accommodative imbalance	Repeat refractometry, being careful to balance.
Can't walk in bifocals	Patient failing to tuck chin	Educate.
	Executive-style segs	Prescriber may choose to try different seg type.
	Segs too high	Visualize
Loss of midrange	Bifocal power was increased to improve near acuity.	Educate; consider trifocals.
	Failure to analyze patient needs (may be aggravated by poorly done history)	Reassess patient's needs; over-refractometry; try Rx in trial frame; have patient measure working distances to desk, typewriter, etc.
Distortion/slant, "stepping down"	Base curve change	Check base curve of old and new lenses.
	Increase in magnification from addition of plus power	Compare lensometry of old and new lenses, consult optician.

PROBLEM	POSSIBLE CAUSE	CORRESPONDING ACTION
Distortion/slant, "stepping down" (continued)	Increase in magnification from change in lens shape	Educate, compare new and old lens size and shape, consult optician.
	Increased pantoscopic tilt ("face form")	Compare tilt of old and new frames on patient, consult optician.
	Progressive change in the power of the lens from the optical center to the periphery	Educate—give time to adjust; doctor may consider a change in lens curvature.
	DBC is off (induced prism)	Mark centers, measure DBC of old and new lenses, compare with patient's PD; check location of centers with glasses on patient.
Straight lines are bowed	Yoked prism (induced prism in which the base is in the same direction in both lenses)	Mark centers, check location of centers with glasses on patient.
	Changing from glass to plastic lenses (barrel-shaped distortion in minus and pincushion-shaped in plus lenses).	Verify material of old and new lenses; educate; doctor may consider returning to original material.

PROBLEM	POSSIBLE CAUSE	CORRESPONDING ACTION
Straight lines are bowed (continued)	Intolerant to addition of or change in astigmatic correction	Recheck refractometry; have patient turn axis dial on phoropter/trial frame to clearest position; doctor may back off the amount of cylinder to ease patient into correction.
"Standing in a hole"	Yoked prism (base down in both lenses)	Mark centers, check location of centers with glasses on patient.
"Standing on a hill"	Yoked prism (base up in both lenses	Mark centers, check location of centers with glasses on patient.
Double vision	DBC off (induced prism) when reading	Mark centers, measure DBC of old and new lenses, compare with patient's PD; check location of centers with glasses on patient.
	Single-vision reading glasses made with distance PD	Mark centers, measure DBC, compare with distance and near PD.

PROBLEM	POSSIBLE CAUSE	CORRESPONDING ACTION
Double vision (cont)	Segs asymmetrically placed with regard to pupils	Visual inspection
	Anisometropia (difference in refractive error between two eyes causing image-size disparity)	Reassess patient needs; prescriber may suggest a slab-off.
Magnification	Increase in plus power	Educate; prescriber may choose to add plus more slowly (ie, back off a little) to ease patient into full correction.
	Increase in size of lens	Educate.
	Base curve change	Read base curve of old and new lenses.
Minification	Over-minused	Recheck refractometry, preferably with cycloplegia; try fogging and duochrome.
	Base curve change	Read base curve of old and new lenses.

PROBLEM	POSSIBLE CAUSE	CORRESPONDING ACTION
Headaches (new)	DBC is off (induced prism)	Mark centers, measure DBC of old and new lenses, compare to patient's PD; check location of centers with glasses on patient.
	Accommodative imbalance	Recheck refractometry, being careful to balance.
	Base curve change	Measure base curve of old and new lenses.
	Image-size disparities	Check base curve of old and new lenses.
	Base curve change	Check base curve of old and new lenses.
Vague discomfort ("just not right")	Change in astigmatic correction/ sensitive to small changes in astigmatic correction	Recheck refractometry; have patient turn axis dial on phoropter/trial frame to clearest position.
	DBC is off (induced prism)	Mark centers, measure DBC of old and new lenses, compare to patient's PD; check location of centers with glasses on patient.

PROBLEM	POSSIBLE CAUSE	CORRESPONDING ACTION
Vague discomfort (cont)	Incorrect pantoscopic tilt	Compare tilt of old and new frames on patient; consult optician.
Glasses do not relieve migraines, redness, conjunctivitis, etc.	These symptoms do not have refractive origin. Patient has failed to understand the purpose and capabilities of correction.	Educate; treat pathology.

Normal Values of Common Blood Tests

1. Complete blood count (CBC)—Checks the number of red blood cells, white blood cells, and platelets present in a blood sample. Normal values are:
   > White blood cell count: 4500 to 10,000/cu mm
   > Platelet count: 150,000 to 400,000/cu mm
   > Red cell count:
   >> Male: 4.7 to 6.1 million/cu mm
   >> Female: 4.2 to 5.4 million/cu mm
   > Hemoglobin:
   >> Male: 13.8 to 17.2 g/dL
   >> Female: 12.1 to 15.1 g/dL
   > Hematocrit:
   >> Male: 40.7% to 50.3%
   >> Female: 36.1% to 44.3%

2. Prothrombin time—Evaluates the ability of the blood to clot. A normal value is between 11 and 13.5 seconds.

3. Blood glucose level—Used to detect the presence of diabetes and to monitor its treatment. Normal fasting blood glucose level is up to 100 mg/dL.

4. Rheumatoid factor—A test for rheumatoid arthritis. Normal value depends on the method used.

5. Erythrocyte sedimentation rate (sed rate)—Indicates the presence and intensity of an inflammatory process such as arthritis or cancer. It is not specific for any one disease.

Normal values (Westergren) are:
>   Male, <50: 0 to 15 mm/hr
>   Male, >50: 0 to 20 mm/hr
>   Female, <50: 0 to 20 mm/hr
>   Female, >50: 0 to 30 mm/hr

6. Creatinine and blood urea nitrogen (BUN)—Both creatinine and BUN are tests of kidney function. Normal values are:
>   Creatinine: 0.8 to 1.4 mg/dL
>   BUN: 7 to 20 mg/dL

7. Potassium—3.7 to 5.2 mmol/L

8. Sodium—135 to 145 mmol/L

9. Calcium—8.5 to 10.2 mg/dL

Note: Some normals vary slightly according to the patient's age, the laboratory, and the test manufacturer.

Adapted from Bittinger M. *General Medical Knowledge for Eyecare Paraprofessionals.* Thorofare, NJ: SLACK Incorporated; 1999. Values updated on MedLine Plus Medical Encyclopedia. http://medlineplus.gov. Accessed August 5, 2007.

The Metric System

The metric system is a system for measuring length, weight, and volume. It is used in most English-speaking countries, although its acceptance in the United States has been slow.

The beauty of the metric system lies in the fact that it is based on multiples of 10. In addition, the same prefixes indicating fractions of units can be applied to all three types of measurements.

The base metric unit for length is the meter. The gram is the base for weight, and the liter for volume. Metric Fraction Prefixes (p. 406) shows the prefixes that are most useful in the eyecare field. These prefixes can be combined to any of the base units. For example, the terms *kilometer*, *kilogram*, and *kiloliter* all refer to 10^3 of their respective units (ie, 1000 m, gm, or l).

The metric system is widely used in the scientific community. Because of this, most of the formulas used in optics are written to use metric units. If your measurements are taken in nonmetric units (eg, inches, pounds, or fluid ounces), you will need to be able to convert them to metric units in order to work the formula. Common conversions are shown in Appendix 17.

It is also important to note that while measurements may be given in the metric system, the formula may call for a different fraction unit. For example, the formula for focal length is $D = 1 \div F$ where D is the power of the lens in diopters and F is the focal length in meters. However, you may be given the focal length in centimeters. It is important to know the formula and to read the question carefully in order to be sure that you are working with the correct units. If not, it is easy to go from one unit to the other by moving the decimal point accordingly.

At times, it may also be necessary to be able to convert visual acuity measurements from those based on 20 feet to those based on the metric system (6 m is standard). Visual Acuity Equivalents (p. 405) gives these conversions.

METRIC FRACTION PREFIXES

Prefix	*Part of Base Unit*
Kilo	10^3 or base unit x 1000
Hecto	10^2 or base unit x 100
Deci	10^{-1} or base unit x 0.1
Centi	10^{-2} or base unit x 0.01
Milli	10^{-3} or base unit x 0.001
Micro	10^{-6} or base unit x 0.000001

Base units: meter (length), liter (liquid measurement), square meters (square measurement), gram (weight), and cubic meters (cubic measure).

VISUAL ACUITY EQUIVALENTS

Based on 20 Feet	*Based on 6 Meters*
20/40	6/120
20/300	6/90
20/200	6/60
20/100	6/30
20/80	6/24
20/70	6/21
20/60	6/18
20/50	6/15
20/40	6/12
20/30	6/9
20/25	6/7.5
20/20	6/6
20/15	6/4.5
20/10	6/3

Reprinted with permission from Lens A. *Optics, Retinoscopy, and Refractometry, Second Edition.* Thorofare, NJ: SLACK Incorporated; 2006.

English and Metric Conversion

LINEAR MEASURE

1 centimeter = 0.3937 inch (centimeters x 0.3937 = inches)
1 inch = 2.54 centimeters (inches x 2.54 = centimeters)
1 foot = 0.3048 meter (feet x 0.3048 = meters)
1 meter = 39.37 inches/1.0936 yards (meters x 39.37 = inches)
1 yard = 0.9144 meter (yards x 0.9144 = meters)
1 kilometer = 0.621 mile
1 mile = 1.609 kilometers

SQUARE MEASURE

1 square centimeter = 0.1550 square inch
1 square inch = 6.452 square centimeters
1 square foot = 0.0929 square meter
1 square meter = 1.196 square yards
1 square yard = 0.8361 square meter
1 hectare = 2.47 acres
1 acre = 0.4047 hectare
1 square kilometer = 0.386 square mile
1 square mile = 2.59 square kilometers

WEIGHT MEASURE

1 gram = 0.035 ounce (grams x 0.035 = ounces)
1 ounce = 28.35 grams (ounces x 28.35 = grams)
1 kilogram = 2.2 pounds (kilograms x 2.2 = pounds)
1 pound = 0.4536 kilogram (pounds x 0.4536 = kilograms)

WEIGHT MEASURE (CONTINUED)

1 metric ton = 0.98421 English ton
1 English ton = 1.016 metric tons

VOLUME MEASURE

1 cubic centimeter (cc) = 0.061 cubic inch (cc x 0.061 = inches^3)
1 cubic inch = 16.39 cubic centimeters (inches^3 x 16.39 = cc)
1 cubic foot = 0.0283 cubic meter
1 cubic meter = 1.308 cubic yards
1 cubic yard = 0.7646 cubic meter
1 liter = 1.0567 quarts
1 quart dry = 1.101 liters
1 quart liquid = 0.9463 liter
1 gallon = 3.78541 liters
1 peck = 8.810 liters
1 hectoliter = 2.8375 bushels

Adapted with permission from Jacobs K, Jacobs L. *Quick Reference Dictionary for Occupational Therapy*. 3rd ed. Thorofare, NJ: SLACK Incorporated; 2001.

Weights and Measures

LINEAR MEASURE

12 inches = 1 foot
3 feet = 1 yard (0.9144 meter)
5.5 yards = 1 rod
40 rods = 1 furlong/220 yards
8 furlongs = 1 statute mile/1760 yards
5280 feet = 1 statute or land mile
3 miles = 1 league
6076.11549 feet = 1 international nautical mile (1852 meters)

DRY MEASURE

2 pints = 1 quart
8 quarts = 1 peck
4 pecks = 1 bushel/2150.42 cubic inches

ANGULAR AND CIRCULAR MEASURE

60 seconds = 1 minute
60 minutes = 1 degree
90 degrees = 1 right angle
180 degrees = 1 straight angle
360 degrees = 1 circle

SQUARE MEASURE

144 square inches = 1 square foot
9 square feet = 1 square yard
30.25 square yards = 1 square rod

SQUARE MEASURE (CONTINUED)

160 square rods = 1 acre
640 acres = 1 square mile

TROY WEIGHT

24 grains = 1 pennyweight
20 pennyweights = 1 ounce
12 ounces = 1 pound, Troy

CUBIC MEASURE

1728 cubic inches = 1 cubic foot
27 cubic feet = 1 cubic yard

LIQUID MEASURE

4 gills = 1 pint
2 pints = 1 quart
4 quarts = 1 gallon/231.0 cubic inches

AVOIRDUPOIS WEIGHT

27.34375 grains = 1 dram
16 drams = 1 ounce
16 ounces = 1 pound/0.45359237 kilogram
100 pounds = 1 short hundredweight
20 short hundredweights = 1 short ton

Reprinted with permission from Jacobs K, Jacobs L. *Quick Reference Dictionary for Occupational Therapy.* 3rd ed. Thorofare, NJ: SLACK Incorporated; 2001.

Optical Formulas

It is always vital to use the correct units of measurement when using any formula. See Appendix 17 for English and metric conversions.

FOCAL DISTANCE/LENGTH

Distance from a lens to the point at which rays of light converge to a focal point.

$F = 1 \div D$
where
F = focal length in meters
D = lens power in diopters

DIOPTRIC POWER OF A LENS

$D = 1 \div F$
where
D = lens power in diopters
F = focal length in meters

TOTAL NOMINAL POWER OF A LENS

$P1 + P2 = PT$
where
P1 = front surface power of the lens in diopters
P2 = back surface power of the lens in diopters
PT = total dioptric power of the lens

OBJECT/IMAGE RELATIONSHIP

$U + D = V$

where

U = vergence of the object rays at the lens in diopters

D = power of the lens in diopters

V = vergence of the image rays at the lens in diopters

SNELL'S LAW (THE BASIC LAW OF REFRACTION)

Optical formula defining the refraction of light as it passes from one medium to another.

$n \sin i = n' \sin i'$

where

n = IR of the first medium

n' = IR of the second medium

i = angle of incidence

i' = angle of refraction

INDEX OF REFRACTION (REFRACTIVE INDEX)

$IR = S \div M$

where

S = the speed of light (186,282 miles per second)

M = speed of light in the medium

DIOPTRIC POWER OF A PRISM (Δ)

$P = C \div D$

where

P = prism power in diopters

C = displacement of image in centimeters

D = distance from the prism in meters

PRENTICE'S LAW/RULE OF INDUCED PRISM

Optical formula defining the amount that a ray of light deviates (measured in prism diopters, Δ) from its original straight path when passing through a point at a given distance (measured in centimeters, cm).

$\Delta = D \times OC$
where
Δ = induced prism in prism diopters
D = dioptric power of lens
OC = decentration of optical center in centimeters

Note: If the induced prism is oriented up or down, any cylinder must be added to the sphere power if its axis is horizontal (or nearly so). If induced prism is oriented in or out, cylinder must be added to sphere power if its axis is vertical (or nearly so). If cylinder is oblique, add half of the cylinder to the sphere power.

SPHERICAL EQUIVALENT

$SE = A + (B \div 2)$
where
A = spherical component of prescription
B = cylindrical component of prescription

TRANSPOSITION

Optical formula for changing plus cylinder refractions to minus cylinder and vice versa.

1. Add sphere and cylinder algebraically, being careful of + and –
2. Change sign of cylinder
3. Rotate axis by 90°

POWER OF A MIRROR

$P = 2 \div r$
where
P = power in diopters
r = radius of curvature (in meters) of the mirror

POWER OF MAGNIFIERS

Important note: A working distance of 40 cm (16 in) is the standard basis for the manufacturing of low vision magnifiers, hence the 4.0 found in the formula below. Some manufacturers base their lens power on a standard of 25 cm (10 inches) rather than 40, and the "X" value should instead be multiplied by 2.5. This is also referred to as "X." Yes, it is confusing. And yes, it can lead to incorrect powers when ordering low vision aids. You should read the dioptric power of any magnifier you order to be sure it is what the patient needs.

$D = X \times 4.0$
where
D = lens power in diopters
X = the "X" power of the magnifier

MINIMUM (NEEDED) LENS BLANK SIZE

$ED + [(A + DBL) - PD] + 2$ mm
where
ED = effective diameter of the frame in mm
A = A measurement of the frame in mm
DBL = distance between lenses in mm
PD = patient's pupillary distance in mm

VOGEL'S FORMULA FOR BASE CURVE SELECTION

Plus lens (glass):
BC = SE + 6
where
BC = base curve
SE = spherical equivalent of lens

Minus lens (glass):
BC = (SE ÷ 2) + 6
where
BC = base curve
SE = spherical equivalent of lens

Manual Alphabet
for Communicating
With the Hearing Impaired*

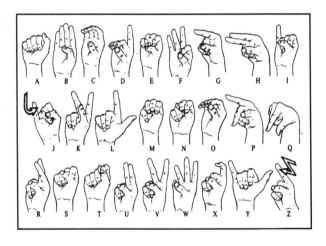

*This table is intended for use in reading alphabetic visual acuity charts.

Reprinted with permission from the National Technical Institute for the Deaf, Rochester, NY.

The Braille Alphabet

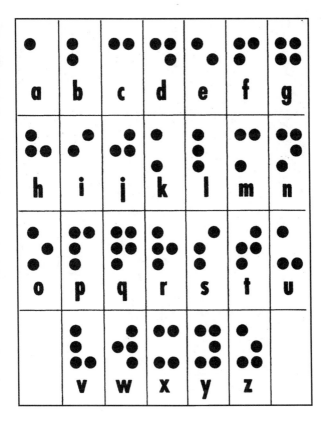

Reprinted with permission from the American Printing House for the Blind, Louisville, Ky.

English-to-Spanish
Ocular History Flowchart

To use this flowchart, the examiner and the patient
look at the text together. The examiner points to specific questions needed for the history, and the patient
points to the appropriate answer for that question.

To the patient/Al paciente:
When the examiner points to a question, please point to
the appropriate answer.
Cuando el examinador señala a una pregunta, señala por
favor a la respuesta apropiada.

A. Chief Complaint
(*Note*: See also Table A22-1 on p. 437)

Are you having a problem with your eyes?
¿Tiene usted un problema con sus ojos?

    no   yes
    no   sí

        What type of problem? (To the examiner: Each of
        the numbered items below has a detailed list of
        questions farther in this outline.

        ¿Qué tipo del problema?

            1. change in vision
                cambio en la visión

            2. pain
                dolor

3. "specks" or "cobwebs" in vision
   las "motas" o las "telarañas" en la visión

4. redness
   rojez

5. double vision
   diplopía

6. vision blacks out
   los negros de la visión fuera

(*Note*: If the patient is a child, see also Table A22-2 on pp. 438-439)

Have you ever had surgery to either eye?
¿Ha tenido jamás usted la cirugía a cualquier ojo?

    no   yes
    no   sí

cataract	glaucoma	laser	other
de la catarata	del glaucoma	el láser	otro

Which eye?
¿Cuál ojo?

right	left	both
el derecho	dejó	ambos

How long ago?
¿Hace mucho tiempo?

days	weeks	months	years
de días	de semanas	de meses	años

1. Change in Vision/Cambio en la Visión

Is the decrease in vision:
Es la disminución en la visión:

up close?	far away?	both?
¿Arriba el fin?	¿Muy lejos?	¿Ambos?

Which eye?
¿Cuál ojo?

right	left	both
derecho	izquierdo	ambos

Has the change been sudden or gradual? Or does it come and go?
¿Ha sido el cambio repentino o gradual? ¿O viene y va?

sudden	gradual	comes and goes
repentino	gradual	viene y va

2. Pain/Dolor

Which eye?
¿Cuál ojo?

right	left	both
derecho	izquierdo	ambos

How long has this been going on?
¿Cuán tiempo ha estado pasando esto?

days	weeks	months
días	semanas	meses

Describe the pain:
Describa el dolor:

dull	stabbing	throbbing	ache
embotado	punzante	dolor pulsando	achaques

Does it come and go? Or is it constant?
¿Viene y va? ¿O es constante?

constant	comes and goes
la constante	viene y va

How long does the pain last?
¿Cuanto tiempo dura el dolor?

seconds	several minutes	half hour
segundos	varios minutos	media hora

several hours
varias horas

Is the eye red?
¿Es el ojo rojo?

no	yes
no	sí

3. Floaters/Las "motas" o las "telerañas" en la visión

Which eye?
¿Cuál ojo?

right	left	both
derecho	izquierdo	ambos

How long has this been going on?
¿Cuanto tiempo ha estado pasando esto?

days	weeks	months	years
días	semanas	meses	años

Have you also seen flashes of light in that eye? (Maybe in the dark, when you move your eye?)
¿Ha visto también los destellos de la luz en ese ojo? ¿(Quizá en la oscuridad, cuando usted mueve su ojo)?

no	yes
no	sí

4. Redness/Rojo

Which eye?
¿Cuál ojo?

right	left	both
el derecho	izquierdo	ambos

How long has this been going on?
¿Cuanto tiempo ha estado pasando esto?

days	weeks	months	years
días	semanas	meses	años

Has there been a discharge from the eye(s)?
¿Ha habido una descarga del ojo (ojos)?

no	yes
no	sí

clear, watery tears
lágrimas claras y aguadas

stringy
fibroso

lids stuck together in mornings
las tapas atascaron juntos en mañanas

white
blanco

green
verde

bloody
manche de sangre

Is there also pain?
¿Hay también dolor?

no   yes
no   sí

Has your vision changed as well?
¿Ha cambiado su visión también?

no   yes
no   sí

5. Double vision/Diplopía

How long has this been going on?
¿Cuanto tiempo ha estado pasando esto?

days	weeks	months	years
días	semanas	meses	años

Is your vision double all the time? Or does it come and
   go?
¿Es su visión doble todo el tiempo? ¿O viene y va?

constant   comes and goes
constante   viene y va

Is your vision only double with or without your glasses on?
¿Es su visión sólo doble con o sin sus gafas?

only happens with glasses off
sólo suceda con gafas lejos

only happens with glasses on
sólo sucede con gafas puesta

Is the double vision up close or at a distance?
¿Está la diplopía es cercao a distancia?

up close	at a distance	both
cerca	a distancia	ambos

What happens if you cover one eye?
¿Qué sucede si usted cubre un ojo?

double vision goes away   vision is still double
la diplopía se va   la visión es todavía doble

Double when you cover the right eye?
¿Duplica cuando usted cubre el ojo correcto?

no	yes
no	sí

Double when you cover the left eye?
¿Duplica cuando usted cubre el ojo izquierdo?

no	yes
no	sí

What are the doubled images like?
¿Como son las imágenes duplicadas?

side by side
el lado a el lado

up and down from each other
arriba o abajo de uno al otro

diagonal
diagonal

like a "ghost image" (as when the TV is not tuned in quite right)
como una "imagen fantasma" (como cuando la televisión no es sintonizada bastante correcto)

6. Vision Blacks Out

Which eye?
¿Cuál ojo?

right	left	both
derecho	izquierdo	ambos

Has the change been sudden or gradual? Or does it come and go?
¿Ha sido el cambio repentino o gradual? ¿O viene y va?

sudden	gradual	comes and goes
repentino	gradual	viene y va

How long does an episode last?
¿Cuanto tiempo dura un episodio?

several seconds
varios segundos

several minutes
de minutos

half an hour
varias media hora

several hours
varias media hora
Do you have a headache afterwards?
¿Tiene usted un dolor de cabeza después?

no	yes
no	sí

How long has this been going on?
¿Cuán largo ha estado pasando esto?

days	weeks	months	years
de días	de semanas	de meses	años

Is there pain in the eye?
¿Hay el dolor en el ojo?

no	yes
no	sí

Does the vision black out totally, or is it "smoky"?
¿Fuera totalmente, o hace la visión negra es "llena de humo"?

blacks out totally	smoky
los negros fuera totalmente	lleno de humo

Is it like a "curtain" comes over your vision?
¿Está como una "cortina" viene sobre su visión?

no	yes
no	sí

Have you seen any flashes of light?
¿Ha visto usted cualquier destello de la luz?

no   yes
no   sí

B. Ocular History/Historia Ocular

Do you wear glasses?
Usa usted gafas?

no   yes
no   sí

Are they for distance, close up, or both?
¿Son ellos para la distancia, cierran, o ambos?

distance	close up	both
el fin de la distancia	cerca	ambos

How old are your glasses? (Please hold up a finger for each year.)
¿Qué edad son sus gafas? (Por favor asidero arriba un dedo para cada años).

Do you wear contact lenses?
¿Usa usted lentillas?

no   yes
no   sí

Have you ever had injury to either eye?
¿Ha tenido jamás usted una herida a cualquier ojo?

no   yes
no   sí

Type of injury:
El tipo de la herida:

    laceration
    cuerpo extraño

    foreign body
    cuerpo extraño

    chemical splash
    salpicadura químico

    scratched cornea
    rasguñó a cornea

    burn
    queme

    "black eye"
    "ojo amoratado"

Which eye?
¿Cuál ojo?

right	left	both
derecho	izquierdo	ambos

Have you ever had surgery to either eye?
¿Ha tenido jamás usted la cirugía a cualquier ojo?

no	yes
no	sí

cataract	glaucoma	laser	other
catarata	glaucoma	láser	otro

Which eye?
¿Cuál ojo?

right   left   both
derecho   izquierdo   ambos

C. General Medical History/Historia Médico

Do you have diabetes?
¿Tiene usted la diabetes?

no   yes
no   sí

Do you use shots? Or pills?
¿Utiliza usted los disparos? ¿O las píldoras?

Is your blood sugar under control?
¿Está su nivel de azúcar en la sangre bajo control?

no   yes
no   sí

How many years have you known that you are diabetic?
¿Cuántos años ha sabido usted que usted es diabético?

1 to 5   5 to 10   10 to 20

Do you have high blood pressure?
¿Tiene ud la hipertensión?

no   yes
no   sí

Are you allergic to any medications?
¿Es usted alérgico a alguna medicina?

> no   yes
> no   sí
>> penicillin   codeine   sulfa
>> penicilina   codeine   sulfa
>>
>> topical anesthetic (numbing drops)
>> anestésico tópico (entumeciendo gotas)
>>
>> other
>> otro

Women: Are you, or could you be, pregnant?
Las mujeres: ¿Es usted, o podría ser usted, embarazada?

> no   yes
> no   sí
>> How many months?
>> ¿Cuántos meses?
>>
>>> 1 to 3   4 to 6   7 to 9

D. Family History/Historia Familiar

Has anyone in your family had cataracts?
¿Tiene cualquiera en su familia tuvo las cataratas?

> no   yes
> no   sí
>
>> parent   sibling   grandparent
>> padres   abuelos   hermanos

Has anyone in your family had glaucoma?
¿Tiene cualquiera en su familia tuvo glaucoma?

    no   yes
    no   sí

parent	sibling	grandparent
padres	abuelos	hermanos

Has anyone in your family had macular degeneration?
¿Tiene cualquiera en su familia tuvo degeneración macu-
    lara?

    no   yes
    no   sí

parent	sibling	grandparent
padres	abuelos	hermanos

Are there any diabetics in your family?
¿Hay cualquier diabético en su familia?

    no   yes
    no   sí

parent	sibling	grandparent
padres	abuelos	hermanos

TABLE A22-1

Common History Modifiers

Which eye?
¿Cuál ojo?

right	left	both
derecho	izquierdo	ambos

How long ago did it start?
¿Hace quanto mucho tiempo que empezó?

hours	days	weeks
de horas	de días	de semanas

months	years
meses	años

Did the problem start suddenly? Or gradually? Or does it come and go?
¿Empezó el problema de repente? ¿O gradualmente? ¿O viene y va?

suddenly	gradually	comes and goes
repentino	gradual	viene y va

On a scale of one to five, how severe is the problem?
¿En una escala de uno a cinco, que severo es el problema?

0   1 2 3   4 5

no problem	very severe
no problema	muy severo

TABLE A22-2

Additional Questions for Pediatric Exam

Does the child seem to have trouble seeing?
¿Tiene problemas con la visión el niño?

    no   yes
    no   sí

       school sent home note
       la escuela mandó un nota a la casa

       sits close to the TV
       se sienta cerca a la televisión

       holds things close to see
       tiene las cosas cerca para ver

       squints
       estrabismos

Do you notice that an eye drifts in or out?
¿Advierte usted que un ojo lleva en o fuera?

    no   yes
    no   sí

       drifts in
       los deriva en

       drifts out
       los deriva fuera

       All the time, or just sometimes?
       ¿Todo el tiempo, o apenas a veces?

all the time	sometimes
todo el tiempo	a veces

Which eye?
¿Cuál ojo?

right	left	can't tell
derecho	izquierdo	no puede decir

both
ambos

Has anyone else in the family had this problem?
¿Tiene cualquiera más en la familia que tuvo este problema?

no	yes
no	sí

parent	sibling	grandparent	aunt/uncle
padres	de abuelos	hermanos	tía/tío

Certification as Paraoptometric and Ancillary Ophthalmic Personnel

The eyecare field is vast. It provides many opportunities for motivated persons to advance themselves. Information given here is taken from the most recent data available prior to publication; contact your certifying body for the most current information.

PARAOPTOMETRY

The American Optometric Association, Paraoptometric Section, offers three levels of certification: certified paraoptometric (CPO), certified paraoptometric assistant (CPOA), and certified paraoptometric technician (CPOT). One must qualify to take the written exam at each level, and there are several options. First, for job-trained candidates, qualification is earned by working in the field; in addition, CPOA candidates must first earn the CPO rank, and CPOT candidates must hold current CPOA status. Alternately, candidates may qualify for the exams during their last semester in an optometric assistant or accredited technician program. Those passing the CPOT written exam must additionally pass a skills examination before the title is awarded.

Topics covered in the CPO exam are basic sciences (anatomy, disorders, terminology, surgery, basic pharmacology), clinical principles and procedures (eye examination, refractive status, contact lenses), ophthalmic optics and dispensing (prescription, lenses, dispensing), and professional issues (eyecare specialists and ancillary personnel, practice management).

Exam criteria for the CPOA includes practice management (office procedures, patient handling, office finances, professional issues), ophthalmic optics and dispensing (prescriptions, lenses, frame selection, adjustment, and dispensing), basic procedures (purpose and preliminary testing procedures, recording, pupillary responses, case history, visual acuity, color vision, stereo acuity, examination instrumentation), special procedures (contact lenses, tonometry, visual fields, sphygmomanometry, first aid, low vision surgery), refractive status of the eye and binocularity (refractive errors, refractive conditions, eye movements, binocular vision), and basic ocular anatomy and physiology (general anatomy and physiology, basic functions of anatomical structures, common pathological and functional disorders, basic ocular pharmacology).

The written exam for CPOT covers pretesting procedures (case history, visual acuity, vision screening and preliminary testing techniques, color vision, stereo acuity), clinical procedures (keratometry, tonometry, visual fields, sphygmomanometry, contact lenses, vision therapy, triage/first aid, low vision, special ocular procedures), ophthalmic optics and dispensing (optical principles of light, prescriptions, lenses, frame selection, adjustment), refractive status of the eye and binocularity (refractive errors, refractive conditions, eye movements, binocular vision), anatomy and physiology (general anatomy and physiology, the eye), and practice management (office management, professional issues, government rules and regulations).

The CPOT practical exam utilizes three stations. Station 1 is case history and pretesting. Station 2 is contact lens, dilation, and blood pressure procedures. Station 3 is neutralization and ophthalmic dispensing.

For information on the home study course and to obtain more details for the examinations, contact:

American Optometric Association, Paraoptometric Section
243 N. Lindbergh Blvd.
St. Louis, MO 63141
Phone: 1-800-365-2219
Fax: 1-314-991-4101
Web site: www.aoa.org
E-mail: ps@theaoa.org

The American Optometric Association has put together a self-study course that is especially recommended (but not required) for those seeking certification. Ordering information can be obtained at the address above. In addition to the home study course, there are other study materials available for those who wish to prepare for examinations. *The Basic Bookshelf for Eyecare Professionals* (a 24-book set published by SLACK Incorporated) was written to include all the exam content areas one needs to review for the tests. Information needed by each certification level is pointed out in the margin of the series books, although the older designations of OptA and OptT are used in original editions. Series titles *Certified Ophthalmic Assistant Exam Review, Second Edition* and *Certified Ophthalmic Technician Exam Review, Second Edition* each contain an appendix to refer CPO, CPOA, and CPOT candidates to questions that pertain to their exams as well.

OPHTHALMIC MEDICAL PERSONNEL

Note: JCAHPO, COA, COT, COMT, OCT, and CCOA are all registered trademarks of the Joint Commission on Allied Health Personnel in Ophthalmology.

JCAHPO Certifications

COA, COT, AND COMT

Those assisting in ophthalmology, generically known as ophthalmic medical personnel (OMP), can be certified at three levels: certified ophthalmic assistant (COA), certified ophthalmic technician (COT), and certified ophthalmic medical technologist (COMT). There are also subspecialty certifications in ophthalmic surgery, coding specialist, and corporate ophthalmic assistant. The certifying body is the Joint Commission on Allied Health Personnel in Ophthalmology (JCAHPO).

Those who wish to take the computer-based examinations in ophthalmology must first qualify. One option is to enroll in a formal training program leading to the desired credential.

Most OMPs, however, are job trained. In this case, you must qualify by working in the field for a specified length of time. Your physician-sponsor must sign a form indicating that you are proficient at certain tasks. Job-trained COT candidates must hold the COA title, and COMT applicants must already have their COT. At the COA level, one must first take and pass either the American Academy of Ophthalmology (AAO) Independent Study Course or the Canadian Home Study Course. At the COT and COMT levels, increasing amounts of approved continuing education credits are required. In addition, once the candidate has passed the written exam for the COT or COMT, a practical exam must be taken as well. At the COT level, this practical is in the form of a computer simulation. (Contact JCAHPO for up-to-date details.) Those who have certified since 1997 may also be awarded college credits from the American Council on Education for their credentials.

The exam at the COA level includes questions covering history taking (presenting complaint/history of presenting illness, past ocular history, family history, systemic illness [past and present], medications, allergies and drug reactions, partially sighted patient), basic skills and lensometry (methods of measuring/recording acuity, color vision testing, lensometry, A-scan biometry, exophthalmometry, Amsler grid, Schirmer tests, evaluation of pupils, estimation of anterior chamber depth), patient services (ocular dressings and shields, drug delivery, spectacle principles, assisting patients, minor surgery), basic tonometry (applanation, noncontact, complications/contraindications, scleral rigidity, factors altering intraocular pressure), instrument maintenance (15 different classes of instruments), and general medical knowledge (CPR, anatomy, physiology, systemic diseases, ocular diseases, ocular emergencies, metric conversions, microbial control).

The prospective COT exam covers COA level material as well as clinical optics (optics, retinoscopy, refractometry, advanced spectacle principles, low vision aids), basic ocular motility (EOM actions, strabismus, amblyopia detection, evaluation assessment methods), visual fields (visual pathways, visual fields, methods of measuring the visual field, techniques, errors in testing, defects from disease), contact lenses (basic principles, fitting procedures, patient instruction, trouble-shooting problems, verification of lenses), intermediate tonometry (aqueous humor dynamics, glaucoma, indentation), ocular pharmacology (types, strengths, actions, and complications of 13 drug classes), and photography (basics, fundus photography, defects/artifacts). The skills evaluation is computer simulated and covers lensometry (nonautomated, including bifocal or trifocal add), retinoscopy/refinement, detection and identification of phoria or tropia using appropriate cover tests, automated visual field testing, keratometry, and applanation tonometry.

Candidates for the COMT level are tested on the COA and COT content areas in addition to microbiology (inflammatory response, microscopy, staining, culture media, specimen collection and processing), advanced tonometry (pathophysiology of glaucoma, tonometry theory, managing tonometry problems), advanced visual fields (advanced principles of testing, etiology, and description of less common defects), advanced color vision (physiology/theory, defects, advanced testing techniques), advanced clinical optics (advanced refractometry, advanced optics), advanced ocular motility (amblyopia, anatomy/physiology of EOMs, binocular function, advanced strabismus), advanced photography (fluorescein angiography, slit lamp, external, specular micrography, film processing), advanced pharmacology (basic concepts of topical medications, mechanism of action and desired effects), special instruments and techniques (13 techniques, including lasers), and advanced general medical knowledge (ocular manifestation of systemic diseases, low vision/blindness, ocular disease, trauma).

During the practical exam, the COMT candidate must calibrate, adjust, and perform applanation tonometry; retinoscopy (plus or minus cylinder), cross cylinder, refinement of refractive error; keratometry; lensometry (read power and mark centers of spectacle lenses), frame measurements, lens clock (base curve and approximate lens power), PD, near point of accommodation (NPA), amplitude of accommodation, vertex distance, measure contact lenses (power, thickness, and base curve); cover test, prism measurement, Maddox rod measurement, and range of motion; near point of convergence (NPC), duction limitations, convergence and divergence, stereo acuity; demonstrate ability to take fundus photos, identify errors in technique of photos (slit lamp, fundus, and fluorescein angiogram), identify phases of fluorescein angiography from photographs, perform axial length measurement, assess pupil function, perform tangent screen, calibrate and perform bowl perimetry, and perform Amsler grid test.

In order to keep one's credentials (whether obtained through a formal program or independently), proof of continuing education must be submitted periodically. Continuing education credits are given for JCAHPO-approved classes and self-study.

THE OPHTHALMIC SURGERY SUBSPECIALTY

Those working in the field of ophthalmic surgery have a JCAHPO category of their own. To qualify to take the exam, the candidate must either have graduated from an OMP program that included classroom and supervised experience in ophthalmic surgical assisting or have 18 months of work experience.

The test categories include preoperative preparation of patient, instruments, aseptic technique, ophthalmic anesthesia, surgical procedures (covering 10+ categories), surgical complications, ophthalmic surgical pharmacology, and minor surgery.

THE OPHTHALMIC CODING SPECIALIST

JCAHPO and the American Academy of Ophthalmic Executives (AAOE) have developed this certification to test the coding knowledge of those in eye care. The exam covers 18 areas: ICD-9, CPT©, E&M, eye codes, modifiers, special testing services, major surgery, minor surgery, retina, pediatrics, oculoplastics, dispensing, vision rehabilitation, anterior segment, cornea, glaucoma, compliance, and neuro-ophthalmology.

CORPORATE CERTIFIED OPHTHALMIC ASSISTANT (CCOA)

There are many industry people who have studied ophthalmology and would like to earn a credential to demonstrate that commitment. To qualify for the exam, one must complete an independent study course, obtain 12 Group A JCAHPO CE credits, and give evidence of being employed by an ophthalmic company.

The exam criteria are the same as that for COA (see pp. 444-445).

REGISTERED OPHTHALMIC ULTRASOUND BIOMETRIST (ROUB)

To be eligible for the registered ophthalmic ultrasound biometrist (ROUB) exam, the candidate may be an OMP certified by JCAHPO (with 2000+ hours of work experience), a graduate of an ophthalmic assisting program, or an ultrasound biometrist with 4000+ hours of work experience plus continuing education credits. The exam covers keratometry, physics, instrumentation, instrument settings, examination techniques, sources of error, and intraocular lens power calculations.

For current criteria for any of the JCAHPO exams, contact:

JCAHPO
2025 Woodland Dr.
St. Paul, MN 55125-2998
Phone: 1-800-284-3737
Fax: 1-651-731-0410
E-mail: jcahapo@jcahpo.org
Web site: www.jcahpo.org

For the ophthalmic assisting home study courses, contact:

AAO
Clinical Education Division
P.O. Box 7424
San Francisco, CA 94120
Phone: 1-415-561-8540
Fax: 1-415-561-8557
or

Southern Alberta Institute of Technology
1301 16th Ave, NW
Calgary, Alberta, Canada T2M OL4
Phone: 1-403-284-7248

There is a rich source of printed material to assist a willing learner in achieving higher levels of education. *The Basic Bookshelf for Eyecare Professionals* (a set of 24 books by SLACK Incorporated) offers *Certified Ophthalmic Assistant Exam Review, Second Edition; Certified Ophthalmic Technician Exam Review, Second Edition;* and *Certified Ophthalmic Medical Technologist Review*, which provide hundreds of exam-type questions in every content area. These books are useful for exam candidates as well as for general review. JCAHPO has developed a study guide for COA and COT applicants, each including 20 sample questions, available at the address or Web site listed above.

CERTIFIED RETINAL ANGIOGRAPHER (CRA)

The Ophthalmic Photographers' Society (OPS) provides credentials for Certified Retinal Angiographer (CRA) for those who perform fluorescein angiography exams and other photography of the eye. Candidates must submit a portfolio of their work (see OPS Web site for criteria; includes 19 slides and three angiograms) and an endorsement by a sponsoring employer (including verification of a minimum of 2 years of retinal angiography experience). The written exam covers ocular anatomy and physiology as they apply to retinal photography (including identification of pathology), patient management, film and digital photography, data and image management, safety, fundus photography, fluorescein angiography, indocyanine green angiography, optical coherence tomography, and pharmacology. The practical exam includes film photography, retinal photography, and simulated fluorescein angiography. (CRA is a registered trademark of OPS.)

The Ophthalmic Photographers' Society, Inc
1869 West Ranch Road
Nixa, MO 65714-8262
Phone: 1-800-403-1677
Fax: 1-417-724-8450
Web site: www.opsweb.org

CERTIFIED OPTICAL COHERENCE TOMOGRAPHER (OCT)

OPS now offers certification for those with proficiency in performing optical coherence tomography. As part of the application process, candidates must submit a portfolio of their work (see OPS Web site for criteria; includes about 18 images) and an endorsement by a sponsoring employer (including verification of a minimum 1 year of tomography experience). The written exam covers ocular anatomy and its application to OCT imaging, concepts of pathology as related to OCT imaging, patient management, OCT equipment and properties, OCT interpretation, and safety. Use OPS contact information for more details.

CERTIFIED ORTHOPTIST

The American Orthoptic Council offers national certification as a Certified Orthoptist (CO). Candidates must attend a 24-month accredited program; admission generally includes an interview. Before sitting for the exam, the candidate must have a baccalaureate degree. There is a written exam as well as an oral/practical exam.

American Orthoptic Council
3914 Nakoma Rd
Madison, WI 53711
Phone: 1-608-233-5383
Fax: 1-608-263-4247
Web site: www.orthoptics.org
email: lwfranceco@att.net

National Contact Lens Certified, National Contact Lens Certified, Advanced

The National Contact Lens Examiners (NCLE) offers a basic and advanced certification as a contact lens fitter.

Eligible candidates for the basic exam (National Contact Lens Certified [NCLC]) are at least 18 years old and have a GED or high school diploma. The basic exam covers prefit and assessment, diagnostic fit and evaluation, lens dispensing and patient education, follow up visits, and administrative procedures.

The advanced level is National Contact Lens Certified, Advanced Certification (NCLC-AC). To sit for this exam, the candidate must have work experience and complete selected education modules. Alternately, a COT, COMT, or NCLE (of at least 1 year's duration) may take the exam. Content areas include prefit, preparation, and evaluation; determine lens type and design contact lens parameters; instruction and delivery; follow-up visits; professional, personnel, and customer relations; sales and marketing; business; physical management; and professional development.

NCLE
6506 Loisdale Rd, Suite 209
Springfield, VA 22150
Phone: 1-703-719-5800
Fax: 1-703-719-9144
Web site: www.abo-ncle.org

Certified Ophthalmic Executive (COE)

The American Society of Ophthalmic Administrators (ASOA) offers Certified Ophthalmic Executive (COE) certification to those with at least 3 years' experience in medical practice management, one of which must be in ophthalmology. The exam criteria includes basic ophthalmic knowledge, finance and accounting, marketing, operations, management, information systems, human resources, and risk management and regulatory compliance.

> ASOA
> 4000 Legato Rd, Suite 700
> Fairfax, VA 22033
> Phone: 1-800-451-1339
> Fax: 1-703-591-0614
> Web site: www.asoa.org

Much of the material in this appendix is reprinted and updated with permission from Borover B, Langley T. *Office and Career Management for the Eyecare Paraprofessional.* Thorofare, NJ: SLACK Incorporated; 1997.

Web Sites Related to Eyecare

Note: The number of Web sites pertaining to eyecare is tremendous; it was impossible to list them all, so this is just a select few (especially in the Manufacturers/Suppliers section). In addition, sites periodically change their URLs or cease altogether. (Be warned: sometimes abandoned sites are taken over by other, surprising folks!) We have done our best to ensure that this listing is accurate as of publication time. There are many good sites that are not listed because of space and time constraints; however, most of those given here also have links to other such sites. It is also important to note that while we have separated sites into categories, some sites offer multiple services (eg, have membership information as well as patient education articles).

PROFESSIONAL ORGANIZATIONS

MedMark
www.medmark.org/oph/oph.html
The ultimate link site for organizations (both professional and public) on all things eye related; also institutes, clinics, colleges, education/training, consumer sites, general information sources, journals, projects, and much more.

American Academy of Ophthalmology (AAO)
www.aao.org
Includes news, official journals, meeting announcements, member search, links, member services, and patient information.

American Academy of Optometry (AAO)
www.aaopt.org
Includes news from AAO, meeting announcements, links, optometry bulletin board, member services, and patient information.

American Association of Certified Orthoptists (AACO) and The American Orthoptics Council
www.orthoptics.org
Includes training, continuing education, membership info, journal, and links.

American Board of Ophthalmology (ABO)
www.abop.org
Includes history and mission statement; examination application, requirements, dates, and deadlines; requirements for recertification; links; and patient information.

American Medical Association (AMA)
www.ama-assn.org
Includes news, publications, patient information, and member services.

American Optometric Association (AOA)
www.aoa.org
Primarily for the general public (patient information, media information, links to state optometry associations) but also includes member services, news, meeting information, and policy statements.

American Society of Cataract and Refractive Surgery (ASCRS)
www.ascrs.org
Includes news from ASCRS, official journals, member search, meeting announcements, links, member services, and patient information.

American Society of Ocularists (ASO)
www.ocularist.org
Includes member search, information on publication and meetings, and patient information.

American Society of Ophthalmic Registered Nurses (ASORN)
http://webeye.ophth.uiowa.edu/ASORN
Includes information on educational programs and certification, publications, member services, and job listings.

American Society of Retina Specialists
www.asrs.org
Online journal, news, annual meeting information, member referrals, and more.

Association for Education and Rehabilitation of the Blind and Visually Impaired
www.aerbvi.org
Membership organization for professionals involved in education and rehabilitation. Conferences, continuing education, events, resources, forums, membership application, and more.

Association of Regulatory Boards of Optometry
www.arbo.org
General information, directory of optometry boards, meetings, publications, and links.

Association of Technical Personnel in Ophthalmology (ATPO)
www.atpo.org
About ATPO; salary report, newsletter, professional development, job listings, membership, links (including formal OMP programs), and online continuing education credits.

Contact Lens Association of Ophthalmologists (CLAO)

www.clao.org

Includes information on membership, publications, courses, and meetings; member referrals.

International Perimetric Society (IPS)

http://webeye.ophth.uiowa.edu/ips

About perimetry, the IPS, meeting information, IPS news, membership list, IPS proceedings and abstracts, and perimetry standards.

Joint Commission on Allied Health Personnel in Ophthalmology

www.jcahpo.org/newsite/index.htm

About JCAHPO, ophthalmic medical assisting, certification, education and research foundation, continuing education program listing, news, and events.

Ophthalmic Photographers' Society

www.opsweb.org

Membership, photo gallery, publications, educational programs, certification, educational information about photography, and informative self-test with explanatory answers.

Opticians Association of America

www.oaa.org

General information, membership information, job opportunities, speaker database, and membership directory.

Optical Society of America

www.osa.org

Optics and photonics research, applications, and industry news.

The American Society of Ophthalmic Plastic and Reconstructive Surgery (ASOPRS)

www.asoprs.org

Includes member directory, fellowships, official journals, meeting announcements, links, member services, information on activities of ASOPRS Foundation, and patient information.

OTHER ORGANIZATIONS

American Diabetes Association (ADA)

www.diabetes.org

Primarily for patients but also has information for health care professionals. Includes news of interest to diabetics; association news, publications, and services; diabetes research information; and links.

American Foundation for the Blind

www.afb.org

"Expands possibilities for people with vision loss" via information, education, links (including employment), and more. Resources for the visually impaired, caregiver/advocate, employer, and professional.

Association for Macular Diseases, the Macula Foundation, Inc, and the LuEsther T. Mertz Retinal Research Center

www.macula.org

Site for both patients and professionals. Includes detailed information about the eye and macular degeneration (extensive, excellent graphics), activities of association and foundation, research grants, meetings, and links.

Eye Bank Association of America (EBAA)
www.restoresight.org
Includes news, information for patients, member services, and links.

Foundation Fighting Blindness (FFB)
www.blindness.org
Official site of organization supporting research and treatment of retinal degenerative diseases; information, chat, news.

The Glaucoma Foundation
www.glaucoma-foundation.org
Includes information on research programs, donations, patient information, news, and publications.

Lighthouse International
www.lighthouse.org
Low vision resources: publications, courses, advocacy, eye conditions, eyecare, low vision, newsletters, volunteers, and links.

The Low Vision Gateway
www.lowvision.org
Provides internet links to resources (information, professionals, rehab), organizations, disorders, support groups, and much more.

Macular Degeneration Network
www.macular-degeneration.org
Patient education on macular degeneration, conference news for providers, and virtual book store.

Macular Degeneration Foundation
www.eyesight.org
Patient education and support on macular degeneration and related conditions of low vision; articles, newsletter.

National Association for Visually Handicapped
www.navh.org
For patients, family, and friends who need anything from large print books to the latest on their particular condition. Health care professionals are welcome here as well.

National Eye Institute
www.nei.nih.gov
News items, funding availability, and links to several full-text pamphlets and booklets for the general public. Topics include age-related macular degeneration, cataract, diabetic retinopathy, and glaucoma.

National Federation of the Blind
www.nfb.org
"Voice of the Nation's Blind." Advocacy, information, resources, products and technology, and publications for the blind.

The National Organization for Albinism and Hypopigmentation
www.albinism.org
Online community; information for professionals, parents, and teachers; and events, projects, and links.

Retinopathy of Prematurity and Related Diseases
www.ropard.org
Information for adult patients and parents of patients (including suggestions for toys and play), online newsletter, and sells 2 videos on ROP for parents and health practitioners.

Reference and Education (Professional)

Academy for Certification of Vision Rehabilitation & Education Professionals
www.acvrep.org
Certification information for those working with the visually impaired. Disciplines include orientation and mobility, vision rehabilitation therapy, and low vision therapy.

Atlas of Ophthalmic Images
www.eyeatlas.com
Color photos of the eye and ocular conditions, includes an invitation to contribute your own photos.

eMedicine Journal
www.emedicine.com/oph/index.shtml
Medical references and patient info about most any ocular condition.

The Eye Exam
www.medicine.ucsd.edu/clinicalmed/eyes.htm
Takes you through a virtual eye exam, including photos of normal and disorders; how to's: external exam, visual acuity, extraocular muscles, visual field, pupil evaluation, and direct ophthalmoscopy.

The Joy of Visual Perception
www.yorku.ca/eye/toc.htm
Site explores the eye and vision in an easy-to-understand format, some of which is interactive. Topics include optics, anatomy, visual acuity, color vision, neurology, etc.

eyetec.net
www.eyetec.net
Hints on passing JCAHPO certification exams (including practice tests for sale) and online continuing education credits.

Eyeweb.org
www.eyeweb.org
Case presentations, photographic atlas, ophthalmology lectures, and online quizzes (click on Medical Students).

Handbook of Ocular Disease Management
www.revoptom.com/handbook
Information on how to manage dozens of commonly encountered ocular diseases: signs and symptoms, pathophysiology, recommendations on management and treatment, and "clinical pearls."

Medscape
www.medscape.com/ophthalmology
Information on ophthalmology news, resources, CME, conferences, journals and references, discussion, and patient education. Free registration.

Merck Manual of Diagnosis and Therapy Eye Disorders
www.merck.com/mmpe/sec09.html
Eleven chapters on the eye from Merck Manual's online medical library.

National Library of Medicine
www.nlm.nih.gov
Health information, library services, research programs, and clinical trials. Health information offers Medlineplus (drug information, current health news, patient education) and Medline/Pub Med (searches 4600 biomedical journals). Also information on AIDS/HIV, cancer, health services, toxicology, and more.

Ophthalmic Hyperguide
www.ophthalmic.hyperguides.com
Tutorials, lectures, and online tests for a variety of ocular disorders; requires password (free).

OphthalWorld
www.ophthalworld.com
"For anything and everything in ophthalmology"; newsletters, products, conferences, articles (posts unsolicited), case discussion, job opportunities, free sign-up, some areas of site restricted to members only.

Paraoptometric Center of the American Optometric Association
www.aoa.org/x4859.xml
Certification information, downloads, news, education services, and training programs.

VisionCareCE
www.visioncarece.com
CE articles for opticians, optometrists, and other eye-care professionals (prices vary).

Journals

American Journal of Ophthalmology (AJO)
www.ajo.com
Table of contents, information for contributors, links, and some other information available for free. Full content requires paid subscription.

American Orthoptic Journal (AOJ)
www.aoj.org
Site of the official journal of the American Association of Certified Orthoptists (AACO). Includes table of contents, searchable abstracts, continuing medical education quiz, subscription and contributor information, and some information on AACO.

Contact Lens Spectrum
www.clspectrum.com
Includes table of contents, back issues, news, patient information, subscriptions, and contact lenses and solutions summary.

Digital Journal of Ophthalmology (DJO)
www.djo.harvard.edu
Includes online articles, grand rounds, multimedia reviews, links, and information for patients and contributors.

MDLinx (ophthalmology)
www.mdlinx.com/OphthoLinx
Gives highlights of articles in various ophthalmic journals. One may then access the abstract and article on the journal's Web site for a fee. Provides free email newsletters on a variety of ophthalmic topics/specialties as well as resources, ophthalmology news, information on conferences, and more.

Ocular Surgery News
www.osnsupersite.com
A news magazine designed for ocular professionals. Full-text news items, information about conferences and meetings, and full-color discussions of current surgical techniques. OSN is just one link on this "super" site.

Ophthalmic Journals on the World Wide Web
www.medbioworld.com
This site has links to ophthalmic journals, news, organizations, reference tools, and resources. At the home window, select Topic Links. In the next window, type "ophthalmology" into the links search box.

Primary Care Optometry News
www.pconsupersite.com
News and articles, practice management, legislation, and technology.

Review of Ophthalmology
www.revophth.com
Articles, archive, events, ideas, email newsletter, and CME.

20/20 Magazine
www.2020mag.com
Information on lenses and frames. Features include fashion, technology, marketing, and conference info.

SUPPLIERS/MANUFACTURERS

Akorn Inc
www.akorn.com
Pharmaceutical/medical products; ophthalmic products: surgical instruments and products, pharmaceuticals, and medical office products.

Alcon
www.alconlabs.com
Consumer/professional information; products (over-the-counter: contact lens care, lubricants; prescription: glaucoma, allergy, infection, etc; IOLs, LASIK), conditions, and studies.

Allergan
www.allergan.com
Product information for eyecare professionals and consumers. Products: neurotoxin, lubricants, therapeutics (glaucoma, infection, allergy, etc).

Bausch & Lomb
www.bausch.com
Contact lenses and supplies, patient education on conditions/treatments, pharmaceutical products (glaucoma, vitamins, allergy, etc), and microsurgical instruments.

Carl Zeiss, Inc
www.zeiss.com
Patient education on vision and eyeglasses; professional information for labs, retail, and offices; technical articles on lens design, etc. (Note: Not to be confused with Carl Zeiss Meditech Inc.)

CIBA Vision
www.cibavision.com
Contact lenses and supplies, surgical and IOLs; also patient education on many vision/eye topics.

Commercial Web Sites (this is the site's title)
www.oftal.it/commerci.htm
Links to commercial sites in eyecare.

Humphrey (Carl Zeiss Meditec)
www.humphrey.com
Sales and service for automated perimeters, lasers, slit lamps, OTC; news and events.

Innovative Imaging Inc
www.eye-imaging.com
Diagnostic ophthalmic ultrasound instrumentation (A-scan/B-scan), course list, echography accessories, and case studies.

Johnson & Johnson
www.jnjvision.com
Patient education on contacts; professionals need a company-supplied code to log onto the professional area.

Marco Ophthalmics
www.marcooph.com
Ophthalmic products (refractors, slit lamps, stands, trial sets, projectors, etc), distributors, and conventions.

MedOp Inc
www.medicalophthalmics.com
Vitamins; online and printable brochures on various topics, mostly nutritional.

Novartis Ophthalmics
www.novartisophthalmics.com
Parent company of CIBA; professional and consumer sites; product listing, eye condition information, articles, and media.

OptiSearch

www.optisearch.com

Frames online: search by manufacturer, collection, specifications, or product. Also offers manufacturer directory.

Precision Optical Co

www.precision-optical-co.com

Products (lenses, frames, sunglasses, etc), services (full lab services), and specials.

APPENDIX 25

Suggested Reading

American Academy of Ophthalmology. *Clinical Optics: Section Three*. San Francisco, CA: Author; 2005.

American Academy of Ophthalmology. *Introducing Ophthalmology: A Primer for Office Staff*. San Francisco, CA: Author; 2002.

American Academy of Ophthalmology. *Pediatric Ophthalmology and Strabismus: Section Six*. San Francisco, CA: Author; 2006.

American Optometric Association, Jameson M. *Self-Study Course for Paraoptometric Assisting*. 2nd ed. Burlington, MA: Butterworth-Heinemann; 2000.

Bartlett JD, Jaanus SD. *Clinical Ocular Pharmacology*. 4th ed. Burlington, MA: Butterworth-Heinemann; 2001.

Bittinger M. *General Medical Knowledge for Eyecare Paraprofessionals*. Thorofare, NJ: SLACK Incorporated; 1999.

Borover B, Langley T. *Office and Career Management for the Eyecare Paraprofessional*. Thorofare, NJ: SLACK Incorporated; 1997.

Boess-Lott R, Stecik S. *The Ophthalmic Surgical Assistant*. Thorofare, NJ: SLACK Incorporated; 1999.

Brady FB. *A Singular View: The Art of Seeing With One Eye*. 6th ed. Vienna, VA: Author; 2004.

Brown B. *The Low Vision Handbook for Eyecare Professionals*. 2nd ed. Thorofare, NJ: SLACK Incorporated; 2007.

Carlson NB, Kurtz D. *Clinical Procedures for Ocular Examination*. 3rd ed. New York, NY: McGraw-Hill Professional Publishing; 2004.

Carlton J. *Frames and Lenses*. Thorofare, NJ: SLACK Incorporated; 2000.

Casser L, Fingeret M. *Atlas of Primary Eyecare Procedures*. 2nd ed. New York, NY: McGraw-Hill; 1997.

Cassin B. *Fundamentals for Ophthalmic Technical Personnel*. Philadelphia, PA: WB Saunders; 1995.

Chern KC, Foley E, Reddy A, Koo J. *Ophthalmic Office Procedures*. New York, NY: McGraw-Hill; 2004.

Choplin N, Edwards R. *Visual Fields*. Thorofare, NJ: SLACK Incorporated; 1998.

Contact Lens Association of Ophthalmologists. *Contact Lenses: The CLAO Guide to Basic Science and Clinical Practice*. 3nd ed. Dubuque, IA: Kendall/Hunt Pub. Co; 1995.

Contact Lens Association of Ophthalmologists. *CLAO Home Study Course for Contact Lens Technicians, 3rd ed*.

Corboy JM. *The Retinoscopy Book: An Introductory Manual for Eye Care Professionals*. 5th ed. Thorofare, NJ: SLACK Incorporated; 2003.

Cubbidge RP. *Eye Essentials: Visual Fields*. Burlington, MA: Butterworth-Heinemann; 2005.

Cunningham D. *Clinical Ocular Photography*. Thorofare, NJ: SLACK Incorporated; 1998.

Daniels K. *Contact Lenses*. Thorofare, NJ: SLACK Incorporated; 1999.

Dornic D. *Ophthalmic Pocket Companion*. 6th ed. Burlington, MA: Butterworth-Heinemann; 2002.

DuBois L. *Clinical Skills for the Ophthalmic Examination: Basic Procedures*. 2nd ed. Thorofare, NJ: SLACK Incorporated; 2006.

Duvall B, Kershner RM. *Ophthalmic Medications and Pharmacology*. 2nd ed. Thorofare, NJ: SLACK Incorporated; 2006.

Duvall BS, Lens A, Werner EB. *Cataract and Glaucoma for Eyecare Paraprofessionals*. Thorofare, NJ: SLACK Incorporated; 1999.

Fannin TE, Grosvenor T. *Clinical Optics*. 2nd ed. Burlington, MA: Butterworth-Heinemann; 1996.

Freeman M, Hull C. *Optics*. 11th ed. Burlington, MA: Butterworth-Heinemann; 2004.

Friedman NJ, Kaiser PK. *Essentials of Ophthalmology*. Philadelphia, PA: Saunders; 2007.

Gayton JL, Kershner RM. *Refractive Surgery for Eyecare Paraprofessionals*. Thorofare, NJ: SLACK Incorporated; 1997.

Gayton JL, Ledford JR. *The Crystal Clear Guide to Sight for Life*. Lancaster, PA: Starburst Publishers; 1996.

Gimbel HV, Penno AEA. *LASIK Complications: Trends and Techniques*. 3rd ed. Thorofare, NJ: SLACK Incorporated; 2004.

Goldberg S, Trattler W. *Ophthalmology Made Ridiculously Simple*. 3rd ed. Miami, FL: Medmaster; 2005.

Gwin N. *Overview of Ocular Disorders*. Thorofare, NJ: SLACK Incorporated; 1999.

Hansen VC. *A Systematic Approach to Strabismus*. Thorofare, NJ: SLACK Incorporated; 1998.

Hargis-Greenshields L, Sims L. *Emergencies in Eyecare*. Thorofare, NJ: SLACK Incorporated; 1999.

Harvey W, Franklin A. *Eye Essentials: Routine Eye Examination*. Burlington, MA: Butterworth-Heinemann; 2005.

Henson DB. *Visual Fields*. Oxford, UK: Oxford University Press; 1996.

Herrin MP. *Instrumentation for Eyecare Paraprofessionals.* Thorofare, NJ: SLACK Incorporated; 1999.

Hunter DG, West CE. *Last Minute Optics: A Concise Review of Optics, Refraction, and Contact Lenses.* Thorofare, NJ: SLACK Incorporated; 1996.

James CB, Benjamin L. *Ophthalmology: Investigation and Examination Techniques.* Burlington, MA: Butterworth-Heinemann; 2006.

Jose RT, ed. *Understanding Low Vision.* New York, NY: American Foundation for the Blind; 1983.

Kaiser PK, Friedman N, Pineda R. *The Massachusetts Eye and Ear Infirmary Illustrated Manual of Ophthalmology.* 2nd ed. Philadelphia, PA: Saunders; 2004.

Kanski JJ. *Clinical Ophthalmology: A Synopsis.* Burlington, MA: Butterworth-Heinemann; 2004.

Kanski JJ. *Clinical Ophthalmology: A Systematic Approach.* 6th ed. Burlington, MA: Butterworth-Heinemann; 2007.

Kline LB, Bajandas FJ. *Neuro-Ophthalmology Review Manual, Revised Fifth Edition.* Thorofare, NJ: SLACK Incorporated; 2004.

Kline LB, ed. *Neuro-Ophthalmology: Section 5.* San Francisco, CA: American Academy of Ophthalmology; 2005.

Krueger R, Applegate R, MacRae S. *Wavefront Customized Visual Correction: The Quest for Super Vision II.* Thorofare, NJ: SLACK Incorporated; 2004.

Ledford JK. *Certified Ophthalmic Assistant Exam Review Manual.* 2nd ed. Thorofare, NJ: SLACK Incorporated; 2003.

Ledford JK. *Certified Ophthalmic Technician Exam Review Manual.* 2nd ed. Thorofare, NJ: SLACK Incorporated; 2004.

Ledford JK. *Certified Ophthalmic Medical Technologist Exam Review Manual*. Thorofare, NJ: SLACK Incorporated; 2000.

Ledford JK. *The Complete Guide to Ocular History Taking*. Thorofare, NJ: SLACK Incorporated; 1999.

Ledford JK, ed. *Handbook of Clinical Ophthalmology for Eyecare Professionals*. Thorofare, NJ: SLACK Incorporated; 2001.

Ledford JK, Pineda R. *The Little Eye Book: A Pupil's Guide to Understanding Ophthalmology*. Thorofare, NJ: SLACK Incorporated; 2002.

Ledford JK, Sanders VN. *The Slit Lamp Primer*. 2nd ed. Thorofare, NJ: SLACK Incorporated; 2006.

Lens A. *Optics, Retinoscopy, and Refractometry*. 2nd ed. Thorofare, NJ: SLACK Incorporated; 2006.

Lens A. *LASIK for Technicians*. Thorofare, NJ: SLACK Incorporated; 2002.

Lens A, Nemeth SC, Ledford JK. *Ocular Anatomy and Physiology*. 2nd ed. Thorofare, NJ: SLACK Incorporated; 2008.

Macnaughton J. *Eye Essentials: Low Vision Assessment*. Burlington, MA: Butterworth-Heinemann; 2005.

Milder B, Rubin ML, Weinstein GW. *The Fine Art of Prescribing Glasses Without Making a Spectacle of Yourself*. 3rd ed. Gainesville, FL: Triad Publishing Company; 2004.

Hom MM. *Mosby's Ocular Drug Consult*. St. Louis, MO: Mosby; 2006.

Newmark E, ed. *Ophthalmic Medical Assisting: An Independent Study Course*. 4th ed. San Francisco, CA: American Academy of Ophthalmology; 2006.

Pavan-Langston D, ed. *Manual of Ocular Diagnosis and Therapy*. 5th ed. Philadelphia, PA: Lippincott Williams & Wilkins; 2002.

Physicians' Desk Reference for Ophthalmic Medicines 2007. 35th ed. Ft. Worth, TX: Thomson Healthcare; 2006.

Pickett K. *Overview of Ocular Surgery and Surgical Counseling.* Thorofare, NJ: SLACK Incorporated; 1999.

Riordan-Eva P, Asbury T, Whitcher JP, eds. *Vaughan & Asbury's General Ophthalmology.* 16th ed. New York, NY: Lange Medical Books/McGraw-Hill; 2004.

Rubin ML. *Optics for Clinicians.* Gainesville, FL: Triad Publishing Company; 1993.

Saine PJ, Tyler ME. *Ophthalmic Photography: Retinal Photography, Angiography, and Electronic Imaging.* 2nd ed. Burlington, MA: Butterworth-Heinemann; 2001.

Scheiman M. *Understanding and Managing Vision Deficits: A Guide for Occupational Therapists.* 2nd ed. Thorofare, NJ: SLACK Incorporated; 2002.

Schwartz GS. *The Eye Exam: A Complete Guide.* Thorofare, NJ: SLACK Incorporated; 2006.

Schuman JS, Puliafito CA, Fujimoto JG. *Everyday OCT: A Handbook for Clinicians and Technicians.* Thorofare, NJ: SLACK Incorporated; 2007.

Simon JW, Calhoun JH. *A Child's Eyes: A Guide to Pediatric Primary Care.* Gainesville, FL: Triad Publishing Co; 1998.

Spalton DJ, Hitchings RA, Hunter P. *Atlas of Clinical Ophthalmology With CD-ROM.* 3rd ed. St. Louis, MO: Mosby Ltd; 2005.

Stein HA, Slatt BJ, Stein RM, Freeman MI. *Fitting Guide for Rigid and Soft Contact Lenses: A Practical Approach.* 4th ed. St. Louis, MO: Mosby-Year Book; 2002.

Stein HA, Stein RM, Freeman MI. *The Ophthalmic Assistant: A Guide for Ophthalmic Medical Personnel.* 8th ed. St. Louis, MO: Mosby; 2006.

Taylor D, Hoyt CS. *Pediatric Ophthalmology and Strabismus*. 3rd ed. Philadelphia, PA: Saunders Ltd; 2005.

Van Boemel GB. *Special Skills and Techniques*. Thorofare, NJ: SLACK Incorporated; 1999.

Note: Just because a book is out of print does not mean it is not obtainable. Try an online search!

WE'D LIKE YOUR FEEDBACK!

If there are terms that you feel should be included, definitions that you think should be changed or added to, or any other ideas you have to improve the *Quick Reference Dictionary of Eyecare Terminology*, please let us know. E-mail your suggestions to bookspublishing@slackinc. com

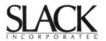